Lecture Notes in Computational Vision and Biomechanics

Volume 21

This book is the twenty-first volume to be published under the Book Series "Lecture Notes in Computational Vision and Biomechanics (LNCV&B)".

The research related to the analysis of living structures (Biomechanics) has been a source of recent research in several distinct areas of science, for example, Mathematics, Mechanical Engineering, Physics, Informatics, Medicine and Sport. However, for its successful achievement, numerous research topics should be considered, such as image processing and analysis, geometric and numerical modelling, biomechanics, experimental analysis, mechanobiology and enhanced visualization, and their application to real cases must be developed and more investigation is needed. Additionally, enhanced hardware solutions and less invasive devices are demanded.

On the other hand, Image Analysis (Computational Vision) is used for the extraction of high-level information from static images or dynamic image sequences. Examples of applications involving image analysis can be the study of motion of structures from image sequences, shape reconstruction from images and medical diagnosis. As a multidisciplinary area, Computational Vision considers techniques and methods from other disciplines, such as Artificial Intelligence, Signal Processing, Mathematics, Physics and Informatics. Despite the many research projects in this area, more robust and efficient methods of Computational Imaging are still demanded in many application domains in Medicine, and their validation in real scenarios is matter of urgency.

These two important and predominant branches of Science are increasingly considered to be strongly connected and related. Hence, the main goal of the LNCV&B book series consists of the provision of a comprehensive forum for discussion on the current state of the art in these fields by emphasizing their connection. The book series covers (but is not limited to):

- Applications of Computational Vision and Biomechanics
- Biometrics and Biomedical Pattern Analysis
- Cellular Imaging and Cellular Mechanics
- Clinical Biomechanics
- Computational Bioimaging and Visualization
- Computational Biology in Biomedical Imaging
- Development of Biomechanical Devices
- Device and Technique Development for Bio-medical Imaging
- Experimental Biomechanics
- Gait & Posture Mechanics
- Grid and High Performance Computing for Computational Vision and Biomechanics
- Image Processing and Analysis
- Image Processing and Visualization in Biofluids
- Image Understanding
- Material Models

- Mechanobiology
- Medical Image Analysis
- Molecular Mechanics
- Multi-Modal Image Systems
- Multiscale Biosensors in Biomedical Imaging
- Multiscale Devices and Biomems for Biomedical Imaging
- Musculoskeletal Biomechanics
- Multiscale Analysis in Biomechanics
- Neuromuscular Biomechanics
- Numerical Methods for Living Tissues
- Numerical Simulation
- Software Development on Computational Vision and Biomechanics
- Sport Biomechanics
- Virtual Reality in Biomechanics
- Vision Systems

In order to match the scope of the LNCV&B book series, each book must include contents relating to or combining both Image Analysis and Biomechanics. Proposals for new books are welcome and should be submitted to the editors of the book series.

The Editors would like to take this opportunity to thank once again to all members of the Advisory Board for their support and help in the scientific managing tasks of this book series, and also to Nathalie Jacobs and Anneke Pot to offer their assistance.

More information about this series at http://www.springer.com/series/8910

João Manuel R.S. Tavares
R.M. Natal Jorge
Editors

Computational and Experimental Biomedical Sciences: Methods and Applications

ICCEBS 2013–International Conference on Computational and Experimental Biomedical Sciences

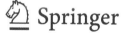 Springer

Editors
João Manuel R.S. Tavares
Universidade do Porto
Porto
Portugal

R.M. Natal Jorge
Universidade do Porto
Porto
Portugal

ISSN 2212-9391   ISSN 2212-9413   (electronic)
Lecture Notes in Computational Vision and Biomechanics
ISBN 978-3-319-36844-3   ISBN 978-3-319-15799-3   (eBook)
DOI 10.1007/978-3-319-15799-3

Printed on acid-free paper

Springer International Publishing AG Switzerland is part of Springer Science+Business Media (www.springer.com)

Preface

The main aim of the *International Conference on Computational and Experimental Biomedical Sciences (ICCEBS)* is to solidify knowledge in the fields of bioengineering and biomedical engineering. The use of more robust, affordable and efficient techniques and technologies with application in biomedical sciences is presently a subject of huge interest and demand, and this conference is intended to be a privileged discussion forum to define their key stakeholders. The aim of *ICCEBS* is to bring together researchers from around the world representing several scientific fields related to biomedical sciences, including engineering, medicine, biomechanics, bioengineering, biomaterials, experimental mechanics, computer sciences, computational mathematics, hardware developers and manufactures, electronic and instrumentation and materials science.

This book contains the full papers presented at *ICCEBS 2013–1st International Conference on Computational and Experimental Biomedical Sciences*, which was organized in Azores, in October 2013. *ICCEBS 2013* brought together researchers representing several fields, such as biomaterials, biomechanics, engineering, medicine, mathematics, medical imaging, orthopaedics, rehabilitation and statistic. The included works present and discuss new trends in those fields, using several methods and techniques, including active shape models, constitutive models, isogeometric elements, genetic algorithms, level sets, material models, neural networks, optimization and the finite element method, in order to address more efficiently different and timely applications involving biofluids, computer simulation, computational biomechanics, image-based diagnosis, image processing and analysis, image segmentation, image registration, scaffolds, simulation and surgical planning.

The editors would like to take this opportunity to thank the members of the *ICCEBS 2013* Program Committee, and to all the authors for sharing their works, experiences and knowledge, making possible its dissemination through this book.

João Manuel R.S. Tavares
R.M. Natal Jorge

Organising Committee

Conference Co-chairs

João Manuel R.S. Tavares
Faculdade de Engenharia da Universidade do Porto
Porto, Portugal
Email: tavares@fe.up.pt
URL: www.fe.up.pt/~tavares

R.M. Natal Jorge
Faculdade de Engenharia da Universidade do Porto
Porto, Portugal
Email: rnatal@fe.up.pt

Conference Program Committee

Adelia Sequeira–Universidade de Lisboa, Portugal
Alexandre X. Falcão–Universidade Estadual de Campinas, Brazil
Ana Mafalda Reis–Universidade do Porto, Portugal
André Marçal–Universidade do Porto, Portugal
André Vital Saúde–Universidade Federal de Lavras, Brazil
Ansgar Koene–University of Birmingham, UK
Cathy Holt–Cardiff University, UK
Christos Constantinou–Stanford University, USA
Christos Grecos–University of West of Scotland, UK
Constantine Kotropoulos–Aristotle University of Thessaloniki, Greece
Daniela Iacoviello–Università degli Studi di Roma "La Sapienza", Italy
Eduardo Borges Pires–Universidade de Lisboa, Portugal
Eduardo Soudah–International Center for Numerical Methods in Engineering, Spain
Elsa Azevedo–Universidade do Porto, Portugal

Emmanuel Audenaert–Ghent University Hospital, Belgium
Eugenio Oñate–Universitat Politècnica de Catalunya, Spain
Fatima L.S. Nunes–Universidade de São Paulo, Brazil
Filipa Sousa–Universidade do Porto, Portugal
Fiorella Sgallari–University of Bologna, Italy
Francisco P.M. Oliveira–Universidade do Porto, Portugal
Gerhard A. Holzapfel–Graz University of Technology, Austria
Hemerson Pistori–Dom Bosco Catholic University, Brazil
Isabel N. Figueiredo–Universidade de Coimbra, Portugal
Jaime S. Cardoso–Universidade do Porto, Portugal
Javier Melenchón–Universitat Oberta de Catalunya, Spain
Jeffrey A. Weiss–University of Utah, USA
João Abrantes–Universidade Lusófona, Portugal
João Paulo Papa–Universidade Estadual Paulista, Brazil
João Santos Baptista–Universidade do Porto, Portugal
João Vilaça–Instituto Politécnico do Cávado e do Ave, Portugal
Joaquim Mendes–Universidade do Porto, Portugal
Jorge Barbosa–Universidade do Porto, Portugal
Jorge Belinha–Universidade do Porto, Portugal
Jorge Miranda Dias–Universidade de Coimbra, Portugal
Jorge Salvador Marques–Universidade de Lisboa, Portugal
José Augusto Ferreira–Universidade de Coimbra, Portugal
Laurent Cohen–Universite Paris Dauphine, France
Luís Alexandre Rocha–Universidade do Minho, Portugal
Luís Amaral–Instituto Politécnico de Coimbra, Portugal
Luís Paulo Reis–Universidade do Minho, Portugal
Luísa Sousa–Universidade do Porto, Portugal
Lyuba Alboul–Sheffield Hallam University, UK
M. Emre Celebi–Louisiana State University in Shreveport, USA
Mahmoud El-Sakka–The University of Western Ontario, Canada
Manuel González-Hidalgo–Universidad de las Islas Baleares, Spain
Marc Thiriet–Universite Pierre et Marie Curie, France
Maria Helena Moreira–Universidade de Trás-os-Montes e Alto Douro, Portugal
Mario Forjaz Secca–Universidade Nova de Lisboa, Portugal
Miguel Velhote Correia–Universidade do Porto, Portugal
Mislav Grgic–University of Zagreb, Croatia
Nguyen Dang Binh–Hue University, Vietnam
Nuno Rocha–Instituto Politécnico do Porto, Portugal
Paola Lecca–University of Trento, Italy
Paolo Di Giamberardino–Università degli Studi di Roma "La Sapienza", Italy
Petia Radeva–Universitat Autònoma de Barcelona, Spain
Reneta Barneva–State University of New York at Fredonia, USA
Ricardo Simões–Universidade do Minho, Portugal
Roger Kamm–Massachusetts Institute of Technology, USA
Ronaldo Eugenio Gabriel–Universidade de Trás-os-Montes e Alto Douro, Portugal

Rui B. Ruben–Instituto Politécnico de Leiria, Portugal
Sabina Tangaro–Instituto Nazionale di Fisica Nucleare, Italy
Sanderson L. Gonzaga de Oliveira–Universidade Federal de Lavras, Brazil
Sandra M. Rua Ventura–Instituto Politécnico do Porto, Portugal
Shuo Li–University of Western Ontario, Canada
Sophia Ananiadou–University of Manchester, UK
Susana Oliveira Branco–Instituto Politécnico de Lisboa, Portugal
Teresa Mascarenhas–Universidade do Porto, Portugal
Valentin Brimkov–State University of New York, USA
Xiongbiao Luo–Nagoya University, Japan
Xue-Cheng Tai–University of Bergen, Norway
Yongjie (Jessica) Zhang–Carnegie Mellon University, USA
Zeyun Yu–University of Wisconsin-Milwaukee, USA
Zhen Ma–Universidade do Porto, Portugal

Acknowledgments

The editors and conference co-chairs wish to acknowledge:

- Direção Regional do Turismo dos Açores
- Governo Regional dos Açores (Programa Operacional dos Açores / Apoio do Fundo Europeu de Desenvolvimento Regional - PROCONVERGÊNCIA)
- Universidade do Porto
- Faculdade de Engenharia da Universidade do Porto
- Instituto de Engenharia Mecânica e Gestão Industrial
- Instituto de Engenharia Mecânica
- Fundação para a Ciência e a Tecnologia
- Associação Portuguesa de Mecânica Teórica, Aplicada e Computacional (APMTAC)
- Springer

for the support given in the organization of this *ICCEBS 2013–1st International Conference on Computational and Experimental Biomedical Sciences*.

Contents

Structural Shear Stress Evaluation of Triple Periodic Minimal Surfaces

H.A. Almeida and P.J. Bártolo

Abstract Tissue engineering represents a new, emerging interdisciplinary field involving combined efforts of several scientific domains towards the development of biological substitutes to restore, maintain, or improve tissue functions. Scaffolds provide a temporary mechanical and vascular support for tissue regeneration while shaping the in-growth tissues. These scaffolds must be biocompatible, biodegradable, with appropriate porosity, pore structure and pore distribution and optimal structural and vascular performance, having both surface and structural compatibility. Surface compatibility means a chemical, biological and physical suitability to the host tissue. Structural compatibility corresponds to an optimal adaptation to the mechanical behaviour of the host tissue. The design of optimised scaffolds based on the fundamental knowledge of its macro microstructure is a relevant topic of research. This research proposes the use of geometric structures based on Triple Periodic Minimal Surfaces for Shear Stress applications. Geometries based on these surfaces enables the design of vary high surface-to-volume ratio structures with high porosity and mechanical/vascular properties. Previous work has demonstrated the potential of Schwartz and Schoen surfaces in tensile/compressive solicitations, when compared to regular geometric based scaffolds. The main objective is to evaluate the same scaffold designs under shear stress solicitations varying the thickness and radius of the scaffold's geometric definition.

Keywords Tissue engineering · Scaffold design · Computational mechanics · Structural shear stress · Triple periodic minimal surfaces

H.A. Almeida (✉)
School of Technology and Management, Polytechnic Institute of Leiria, Leiria, Portugal
e-mail: henrique.almeida@ipleiria.pt

P.J. Bártolo
Institute of Biotechnology, School of Mechanical, Aerospace and Civil Engineering, University of Manchester, Manchester, UK

© Springer International Publishing Switzerland 2015
J.M.R.S. Tavares and R.M. Natal Jorge (eds.), *Computational and Experimental Biomedical Sciences: Methods and Applications*, Lecture Notes in Computational Vision and Biomechanics 21, DOI 10.1007/978-3-319-15799-3_1

1

1 Introduction

Tissue engineering is a multidisciplinary field that requires the combined effort of cell biologists, engineers, material scientists, mathematicians, geneticists, and clinicians toward the development of biological substitutes that restore, maintain, or improve tissue function. Initially defined by Skalak and Fox [18] as "the application of principles and methods of engineering and life sciences toward the fundamental understanding of structure-function relationships in normal and pathological mammalian tissues and the development of biological substitutes to restore, maintain, or improve tissue function" is a major component of regenerative medicine. Diseases such as Parkinson, Alzheimer, osteoporosis, spine injuries or cancer, might in the near future be treated with methods that aim at regenerating diseased or damaged tissues.

Tissue engineering comprises three main strategies [6, 15, 16]:

- Cell self-assembly, which corresponds to the direct in vivo implantation of isolated cells or cell substitutes and it is based on cells synthesizing their own matrix. This approach avoids the complications of surgery and allows replacement of only those cells that supply the needed function. The main limitations include immunological rejection and failure of the infused cells.
- Acellular scaffold, which is based on the ingrowth of tissue cells into a porous material, loaded with growth factors or any other therapeutic agent.
- Cell-seeded temporary scaffolds, which is based on the use of a temporary scaffold that provides a substrate for the implanted cells and a physical support to organize the formation of the new tissue. In this approach, transplanted cells adhere to the scaffold, proliferate, secrete their own extracellular matrices and stimulate new tissue formation.

The third therapeutic strategy, the most important one, involves cellular implantation. Cells derived from an endogenous source in the patient or from a donor are either injected into the damaged tissue or are combined in vitro with a degradable scaffold (Fig. 1) and then implanted. Cell seeding depends on fast attachment of cell to scaffold, high cell survival and uniform cell distribution. The seeding time is

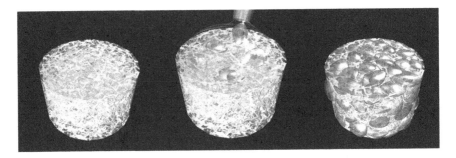

Fig. 1 Cell deposition and cellular proliferation in scaffolds

Table 1 Biological, mechanical and physical requirements [7]

Biological requirements	
Biocompatibility	The scaffold material must be non-toxic and allow cell attachment, proliferation and differentiation
Biodegradability	The scaffold material must degrade into non-toxic products
Controlled degradation rate	The degradation rate of the scaffold must be adjustable in order to match the rate of tissue regeneration
Porosity	Appropriate macro and microstructure porosity and pore shape to allow tissue in-growth and vascularisation
Mechanical and physical requirements	
Strength and stiffness	Sufficient strength and stiffness to withstand stresses in the host tissue environment
Surface finish	Adequate surface finish to guarantee that a good biomechanical coupling is achieved between the scaffold and the tissue
Sterilised	Easily sterilised either by exposure to high temperatures or by immersing in a sterilisation agent remaining unaffected by either of these processes

strongly dependent on the scaffold material and architecture. Scaffolds are critical bioactive structural elements serving the following purposes [11, 12]:

- Allow cell attachment, proliferation and differentiation;
- Deliver and retain cells and growth factors;
- Enable diffusion of cell nutrients and oxygen;
- Enable an appropriate mechanical and biological environment for tissue regeneration in an organised way.

To achieve these goals, an ideal scaffold must satisfy some biological and mechanical requirements as shown in Table 1. Table 2 illustrates the relationship between the scaffold's characteristics and its biological effect. In order to meet the requirements stated for biomimicry, strategies are developed to optimize the control in the scaffold architecture design, in terms of macro- and microstructure [20, 21].

Table 2 Relationship between scaffold characteristics and the corresponding biological effect [14]

Scaffold characteristics	Biological effect
Biocompatibility	Cell viability and tissue response
Biodegradability	Aids tissue remodelling
Porosity	Cell migration inside the scaffold
	Vascularisation
Chemical properties of the material	Aids in cell attachment and signalling in cell environment
	Allows release of bioactive substances
Mechanical properties	Affects cell growth and proliferation response
	In vivo load bearing capacity

The prediction of the effective optimal properties of tissue scaffolds is very important for tissue engineering applications, either regarding mechanical, vascular or topological [1, 2, 4] properties. To aid this specific issue of the design process of scaffolds, a computational tool, Computer-Aided Design of Scaffolds (CADS) [3], is been developed which enables to quantify the structural heterogeneity and mechanical and vascular properties of a scaffold with a designed macro and microstructure [7–9].

The design of optimised scaffolds for tissue engineering is a relevant topic of research. Previous work [1–3], developed a strategy to optimize both mechanical and vascular behaviour of both polymeric and ceramic scaffolds. The evaluation of the scaffold's porosity, mechanical properties and vascularisation properties was performed for a wide range of regular geometries. In this paper, triple periodic minimal surfaces are explored bearing in mind the mechanical performance under shear solicitations in order to design optimised biomimetic scaffolds for tissue engineering applications.

2 Triply Periodic Minimal Surfaces

2.1 Definition

Hyperbolic surfaces have attracted the attention of physicists, chemists and biologists as they commonly exist in natural structures. Amongst various hyperbolic surfaces, minimal surfaces (those with mean curvature of zero) are the most studied. If a minimal surface has space group symmetry, it is periodic in three independent directions. These surfaces are known as Triply Periodic Minimal Surfaces (TPMS) (Fig. 2).

In nature, TPMS are found in lyotropic liquid crystals, zeolite sodalite crystal structures, diblock polymers, soluble proteins in lipid-protein water phases and certain cell membranes [5, 10, 17]. TPMS allow very high surface-to-volume ratios and provide good analytic description of highly porous structures.

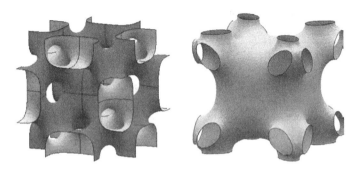

Fig. 2 Examples of TPMS geometries [13]

2.2 Periodic Surface Modelling

A periodic surface can be generally defined as:

$$\phi(\mathbf{r}) = \sum_{k=1}^{K} A_k \cos[2\pi(\mathbf{h}_k \cdot \mathbf{r})/\lambda_k + p_k] = C \tag{1}$$

where r is the location vector in the Euclidean space, hk is the kth lattice vector in the reciprocal space, Ak is the magnitude factor, λk is the wavelength of periods, pk is the phase shift, and C is a constant. Specific periodic structures and phases can be constructed based on this implicit form [19].

In the case of TPMS, the Weierstrass formula describes their parametric form as follows:

$$\begin{cases} x = \text{Re} \int_{\omega_0}^{\omega_1} e^{i\theta}(1 - \omega^2)R(\omega)d\omega \\ y = \text{Im} \int_{\omega_0}^{\omega_1} e^{i\theta}(1 + \omega^2)R(\omega)d\omega \\ z = -\text{Re} \int_{\omega_0}^{\omega_1} e^{i\theta}(2\omega)R(\omega)d\omega \end{cases} \tag{2}$$

where ω is a complex variable, θ is the so-called Bonnet angle, and $R(\omega)$ is a function which varies for different surfaces.

From a multi-dimensional control parameter space point of view, the geometric shape of a periodic surface is specified by a periodic vector, such as [19]:

$$\mathbf{V} = \langle \mathbf{A}, \mathbf{H}, \mathbf{P}, \mathbf{\Lambda} \rangle_{K \times 6} \tag{3}$$

where:

$$\mathbf{A} = [A_k]_{K \times 1}$$
$$\mathbf{H} = [\mathbf{h}_k]_{K \times 3}$$
$$\mathbf{P} = [p_k]_{K \times 1}$$
$$\mathbf{\Lambda} = [\lambda_k]_{K \times 1}$$

are row concatenations of magnitudes, reciprocal lattice matrix, phases, and period lengths respectively.

2.3 Schwartz TPMS Primitives

An important sub-class of triply periodic minimal surfaces are those that partition space into two disjoint but intertwining regions that are bi-continuous. An example of such surfaces includes the so-called Schwartz primitives (Fig. 3) for which, each disjoint region has a volume fraction equal to ½.

Fig. 3 Schwartz TPMS
primitive

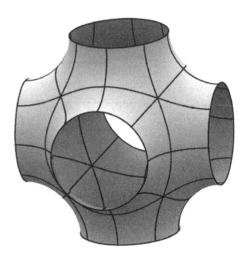

The periodic Schwartz primitive surface is given by [19]:

$$\phi(\mathbf{r}) = A_P\left[\cos(2\pi x/\lambda_x) + \cos(2\pi y/\lambda_y) + \cos(2\pi z/\lambda_z)\right] = 0 \qquad (4)$$

The concatenations of magnitudes vector, reciprocal lattice matrix and phase vector are given by [19]:

$$\mathbf{A}^T = \begin{bmatrix} 1 & 1 & 1 \end{bmatrix}$$
$$\mathbf{H}^T = \begin{bmatrix} 1 & 0 & 0 \\ 0 & 1 & 0 \\ 0 & 0 & 1 \end{bmatrix} \qquad (5)$$
$$\mathbf{P}^T = \begin{bmatrix} 0 & 0 & 0 \end{bmatrix}$$

Two important parameters can be used as modelling control constraints: thickness and radius. Figures 4 and 5 illustrate the effect of these parameters on the Schwartz primitives (P-minimal surfaces) obtained structures.

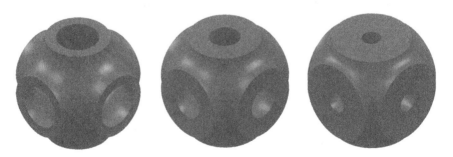

Fig. 4 P-minimal surfaces obtained through thickness variation with constant surface radius

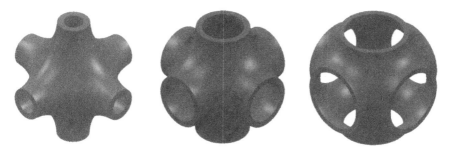

Fig. 5 P-minimal surfaces obtained through radius variation with constant surface thickness

2.4 Schoen TPMS Primitives

Another important sub-class of triply periodic minimal surfaces are the Schoen surfaces (Fig. 6).

The periodic Schoen primitive surface is given by [19]:

$$\phi(\mathbf{r}) = A_I \begin{bmatrix} 2\cos(2\pi x/\lambda_x) + \cos(2\pi y/\lambda_y) + 2\cos(2\pi z/\lambda_y)\cos(2\pi z/\lambda_z) \\ +2\cos(2\pi z/\lambda_z)\cos(2\pi x/\lambda_x) \\ -\cos(4\pi x/\lambda_x) - \cos(4\pi y/\lambda_y) - \cos(4\pi z/\lambda_z) \end{bmatrix} = 0 \qquad (6)$$

Fig. 6 Schoen TPMS primitive

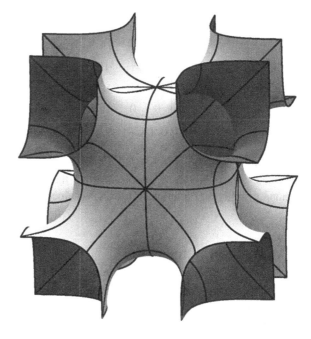

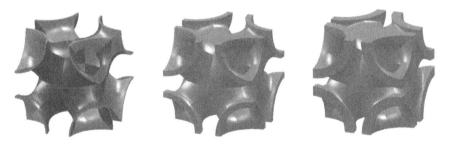

Fig. 7 P-minimal surfaces obtained through thickness variation with constant surface radius

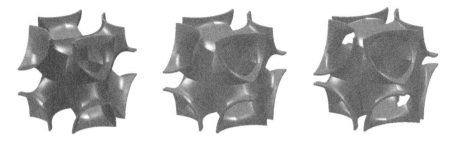

Fig. 8 P-minimal surfaces obtained through radius variation with constant surface thickness

The concatenations of magnitudes vector, reciprocal lattice matrix and phase vector are given by [19]:

$$
\begin{aligned}
\mathbf{A}^\mathrm{T} &= \begin{bmatrix} 1 & 1 & 1 & 1 & 1 & 1 & -1 & -1 & -1 \end{bmatrix} \\
\mathbf{H}^\mathrm{T} &= \begin{bmatrix} 1 & 1 & 0 & 0 & 1 & 1 & 2 & 0 & 0 \\ -1 & 1 & 1 & 1 & 0 & 0 & 0 & 2 & 0 \\ 0 & 0 & -1 & 1 & -1 & 1 & 0 & 0 & 2 \end{bmatrix} \\
\mathbf{P}^\mathrm{T} &= \begin{bmatrix} 0 & 0 & 0 & 0 & 0 & 0 & 0 & 0 & 0 \end{bmatrix}
\end{aligned}
\tag{7}
$$

Two important parameters can be used as modelling control constraints: thickness and radius. Figures 7 and 8 illustrate the effect of these parameters on the Schoen primitives (P-minimal surfaces) obtained structures.

3 Mechanical Simulation

The main goal for simulating the scaffold mechanical behaviour is to evaluate the porosity dependence on the shear modulus. For a given unit block with a specific open pore architecture, boundary and loading conditions considered for evaluating

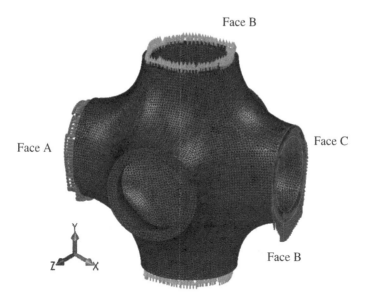

Fig. 9 Loads and constraints for the numerical analysis of scaffolds under a shear solicitation

the mechanical shear properties are shown in Fig. 9. For the numerical computation of the shear modulus, a uniform displacement in a single direction is considered (the Y direction), which is equivalent to the strain on the same direction (γxy), imposed to a face of the block (Face C). The opposite face (Face A) of the scaffold unit is constrained and unable to have any displacement. The two lateral faces (Faces B) are also constrained and unable to have any displacement in the X direction. The average reaction force produced on Face A is used to determine the shear modulus, due to the imposed displacement.

3.1 Results

Mechanical computer simulations were carried out to evaluate the effect of both the P-minimal surface thickness and radius variation. The material considered for simulation purposes is Polycaprolactone (PCL), that is a semicrystalline biodegradable polymer having a melting point of $\sim 60\ °C$ and a glass transition temperature of $\sim -60\ °C$. The elastic modulus and shear modulus of PCL was considered to be 400 and 150 MPa respectively. The results will be displayed in function of the Scaffold's Shear Ratio: quantified scaffold shear modulus/material reference shear modulus (G/G0).

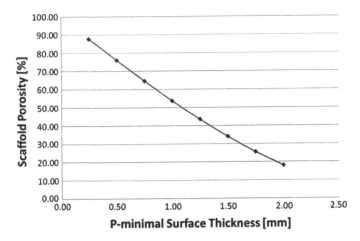

Fig. 10 Variation of the scaffold porosity with the P-minimal surface thickness

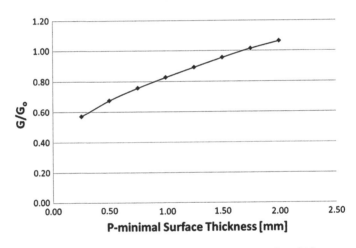

Fig. 11 Variation of the shear modulus ratio with the P-minimal surface thickness

Results for the Schwartz geometries, considering both the thickness and radius variations, are shown in Figs. 10, 11, 12, 13, 14 and 15.

As illustrated in Fig. 10, porosity decreases with the P-minimal surface thickness. Figure 11 shows that the shear modulus ratio increases with thickness. This figure also demonstrates that the P-minimal surface presents a higher shear modulus behaviour compared to the materials reference shear modulus. In other words, the P-minimal surface increases the shear performance above reference for high thickness values. A linear dependence between the scaffold porosity and the shear modulus ratio was obtained as observed in Fig. 12.

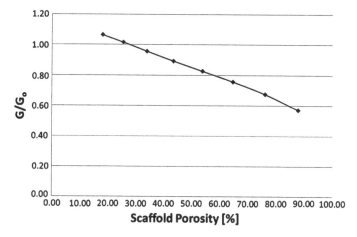

Fig. 12 Variation of the shear modulus ratio with porosity

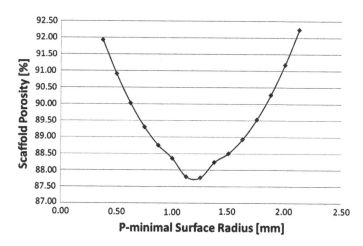

Fig. 13 Variation of the scaffold porosity with the P-minimal surface radius

Regarding the effect of the P-minimal surface radius variations, Fig. 13 shows that porosity decreases till a threshold value for the surface radius from which starts to increase. The shear modulus ratio increases then begins to decrease as the P-minimal surface radius increases, as shown by Fig. 14.

In spite of the porosity and the radius having a hyperbolic behaviour, the shear modulus ratio with the P-minimal surface radius has a sinusoidal behaviour, while the shear modulus ratio with the porosity has an approximated hyperbolic behaviour (Fig. 15). In this case, we may decrease or increase the shear modulus of the scaffold while maintaining high porosity values.

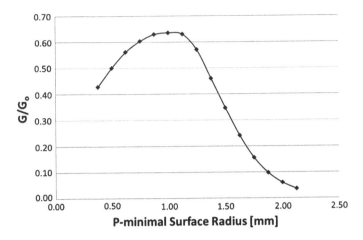

Fig. 14 Variation of the shear modulus ratio with the P-minimal surface radius

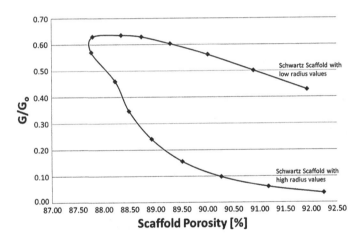

Fig. 15 Variation of the shear modulus ratio with the porosity

Regarding then Schoen geometries, Figs. 16, 17, 18, 19, 20 and 21, present the results considering both the thickness and radius variations.

As illustrated in Fig. 16, porosity decreases with the P-minimal surface thickness. Figures 17 and 18 shows that the shear modulus ratio increases with thickness and decreases with porosity.

Concerning the effect of the P-minimal surface radius variations, Fig. 19 shows that porosity increases with the increase of the surface radius. The shear modulus ratio decreases by increasing either the surface radius (Fig. 20) or the porosity (Fig. 21).

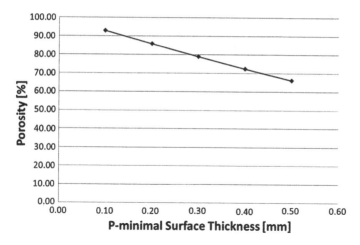

Fig. 16 Variation of the scaffold porosity with the P-minimal surface thickness

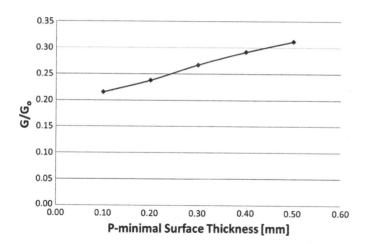

Fig. 17 Variation of the shear modulus ratio with the P-minimal surface thickness

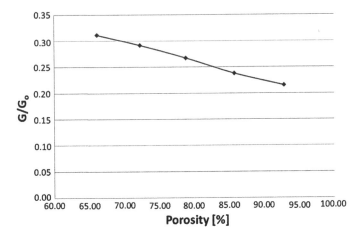

Fig. 18 Variation of the shear modulus ratio with the porosity

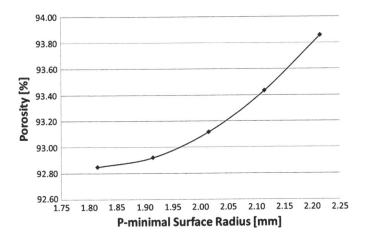

Fig. 19 Variation of the scaffold porosity with the P-minimal surface radius

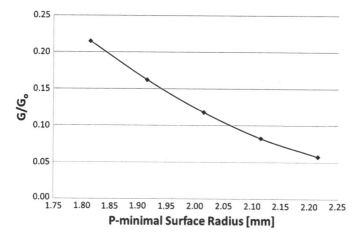

Fig. 20 Variation of the shear modulus ratio with the P-minimal surface radius

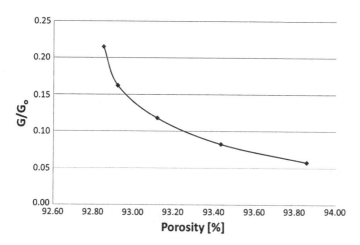

Fig. 21 Variation of the shear modulus ratio with the porosity

4 Conclusions

Understanding the mechanical and transport properties of highly porous scaffolds from a knowledge of its microstructure is a problem of great interest in tissue engineering. In this paper, porous scaffolds are designed and its shear mechanical behaviour simulated using Triple P-minimal surfaces, namely Schwartz and Schoen geometries.

Regarding the Schwartz geometries, the results show that porosity decreases with the P-minimal surface thickness, decreasing also till a threshold value for the

P-minimal surface radius. From this threshold value, the porosity then starts to increase. The shear modulus ratio increases with the P-minimal surface thickness and presents an approximated hyperbolic behaviour by increasing the P-minimal surface radius.

Regarding the Schoen geometries, the results show that porosity decreases and the shear modulus ratio increases with the P-minimal surface thickness. On the other hand, the porosity increases and the shear modulus decreases with the P-minimal surface radius. In both cases, the shear modulus ratio decreases with the porosity.

When comparing both geometries, concerning the thickness variation, Schoen geometries present both lower values of porosity and lower values of shear modulus ratio. Regarding the radius variations, Schoen geometries present slightly higher porosity levels but still lower values of shear modulus ratio when compared to the Schwartz geometries. Schwartz geometries present a more versatile behaviour, for one given porosity, you may have a structure with a lower or higher shear modulus, and they also present a higher range of values for both shear modulus ratio and porosity levels, when compared to Schoen geometries.

By using triple periodic surfaces in scaffold design for tissue engineering applications, it is possible to use highly porous structures with optimum mechanical properties.

Acknowledgments The authors acknowledge the support of the Strategic Project (PEST-OE/EME/UI4044/2013) funded by the Portuguese Foundation for Science and Technology. Authors also acknowledge the support of the European Commission through the Marie Curie Project International Research Exchange for Biomedical Devices Design and Prototyping IREBID.

References

1. Almeida, H.A, Bártolo, P.J. and Ferreira, J., 2007a. Design of Scaffolds Assisted by Computer, in Modelling in Medicine and Biology VII, edited by C.A. Brebbia, Wit Press, 157-166.
2. Almeida, H.A, Bártolo, P.J. and Ferreira, J., 2007b. Mechanical Behaviour and Vascularisation Analysis of Tissue Engineering Scaffolds, in Virtual and Rapid Manufacturing, edited by P.J. Bártolo et al, Taylor&Francis, 73-80.
3. Almeida, H.A. and Bártolo, P.J., 2008. Computer Simulation and Optimisation of Tissue Engineering Scaffolds: Mechanical and Vascular Behaviour, 9th Biennial ASME Conference on Engineering Systems Design and Analysis (ESDA2008).
4. Almeida, H.A. and Bártolo, P.J., 2010. Topological optimization of scaffolds for rapid prototyping, Medical Engineering & Physics, 32:775-783.
5. Andersson S., 1983. On the description of complex inorganic crystal structures, Angew Chem Int Edit; 22(2):69-81.
6. Bártolo P.J., Almeida H.A., Rezende R.A., Laoui T. and and Bidanda B., 2007. Advanced processes to fabricate scaffolds for tissue engineering. In: B. Bidanda and P. Bártolo, ed. Virtual prototyping & bio manufacturing in medical applications. Springer Verlag, 299.
7. Bártolo, P.J., Almeida H. and Laoui, T., 2007. Rapid prototyping & manufacturing for tissue engineering scaffolds, International Journal of Computer Applications in Technology, 36(1):1-9.

8. Chua, C.K., Yeong, W.Y. and Leong, K.F., 2005. Development of scaffolds for tissue engineering using a 3D inkjet model maker, Virtual modelling and rapid manufacturing, edited by P.J. Bártolo et al, Taylor&Francis, London.
9. Hutmacher, D.W., Sittinger, M. and Risbud, M.V., 2004. Scaffold-based tissue engineering: rationale for computer-aided design and solid free-form fabrication systems, Trends in Biotechnology, 22(7), pp. 354-362.
10. Larsson M, Terasaki O, Larsson K., 2003. A solid state transition in the tetragonal lipid bilayer structure at the lung alveolar surface, Solid State Sci, 5(1):109-14.
11. Leong K.F., Cheah C.M. and Chua, C.K., 2003. Solid freeform fabrication of three-dimensional scaffolds for engineering replacement tissues and organs, Biomaterials, 24 (13):2363-2378.
12. Leong, K.F., Chua, C.K., Sudarmadjia, N. and Yeong, W.Y. 2008, Engineering functionally graded tissue engineering scaffolds. Journal of Mechanical Behaviour of Biomedical Materials 1: 140-152.
13. Lord, E.A. and Mackay, A.L., 2003. Periodic minimal surfaces of cubic symmetry, Current Science, 85(3):346-362.
14. Mahajan, H. P. 2005, Evaluation of chitosan gelatine complex scaffolds for articular cartilage tissue engineering. MSc Thesis, Mississipi State University, USA.
15. Matsumoto, T. and Mooney, D.J., 2006. Cell instructive polymers. Adv Biochem Eng Biotechnol, 102 113-137.
16. Mistry, A.S. and Mikos, A.G., 2005. Tissue engineering strategies for bone regeneration. Adv Biochem Eng Biotechnol, 94 1-22.
17. Scriven LE., 1976. Equilibrium bicontinuous structure, Nature, 263(5573):123-5.
18. Skalak, R. and Fox, C.F. 1988, Tissue Engineering, New York: Alan R. Liss.
19. Wang, Y., 2007. Periodic surface modeling for computer aided nano design, Computer-Aided Design, 39:179-189.
20. Yang, S., Leong, K.F., Du, Z. and Chua, C.K., 2001. The design of scaffolds for use in tissue engineering. Part I. Traditional factors. Tissue Eng, 7(6), 679-689.
21. Yeong, W.Y., Chua, C.K., Leong, K.F. and Chandrasekaran, M., 2004. Rapid prototyping in tissue engineering: challenges and potential. Trends Biotechnol, 22(12), 643-652.

On the Microstructural Modeling of Vascular Tissues

Estefania Peña

Abstract Accurate determination of the biomechanical implications of vascular surgeries or pathologies on patients requires developing patient-specific models of the organ or vessel under consideration. In this regard, combining the development of advanced constitutive laws that mimic the behaviour of the vascular tissue with advanced computer analysis provides a powerful tool for modelling vascular tissues on a patient-specific basis. Collagen is the most abundant protein in mammals and provides soft biological tissue, like the vasculature, with mechanical strength, stiffness and toughness. In several tissues there is a strong alignment of the collagen fibres with little dispersion in their orientation, but in other cases, such as the artery wall, there is significant dispersion in the orientation, which has a significant influence on the mechanical response. Proposed structure-based models was used by taking into account the spatial dispersion or waviness of collagen fiber directions. Vascular tissues exhibits simultaneously elastic and viscous material response. The rate-dependent material behavior of this kind of materials has been well-documented and quantified in the literature. Furthermore, non-physiological loads drive soft tissue to damage that may induce a strong reduction of the stiffness. In this chapter, we have provided a critical review of the fundamental aspects in modeling this kind of the materials. The application of these constitutive relationships in the context of vascular system has been presented.

E. Peña (✉)
Applied Mechanics and Bioengineering Group,
Aragón Institute of Engineering Research (I3A), University of Zaragoza,
María de Luna s/n, Edif. Betancourt, 50018 Zaragoza, Spain
e-mail: fany@unizar.es

E. Peña
Centro de Investigación Biomédica en Red en Bioingeniería, Biomateriales
y Nanomedicina (CIBER-BBN), Zaragoza, Spain

© Springer International Publishing Switzerland 2015
J.M.R.S. Tavares and R.M. Natal Jorge (eds.), *Computational and Experimental Biomedical Sciences: Methods and Applications*, Lecture Notes in Computational Vision and Biomechanics 21, DOI 10.1007/978-3-319-15799-3_2

1 Introduction

The arterial wall is composed of three distinct elements: the vascular smooth muscles (VSM) that form the cellular part of the vessel, and the extracellular matrix major components elastin and collagen. Collagen is the main load-bearing component within the tissue, while the elastin provides elasticity to the tissue. Identification of an appropriate strain energy function (SEF) is the preferred method to describe the complex nonlinear elastic properties of vascular tissues [31]. An ideal SEF should be based on histological analysis to provide a better description of wall deformation under load [33, 54]. Early SEFs were purely phenomenological functions where parameters involved in the mathematical expression are not physiological meaning [17, 56]. Later, structure-based or constituent-based SEF were developed, where the parameters means some physical and structural properties of the different components of the vessel wall [26, 63]. In several tissues there is a strong alignment of the collagen fibres with little dispersion in their orientation, but in other cases, such as the artery wall, there is significant dispersion in the orientation, which has a significant influence on the mechanical response. Proposed structure-based models was used by taking into account the spatial dispersion or distribution or waviness of collagen fiber directions [2, 23, 33, 58, 62].

Collagen is the most abundant protein in mammals and provides soft biological tissue, like the vasculature, with mechanical strength, stiffness and toughness. Roach and Burton suggested that collagen had a main impact on the mechanical properties of arterial tissue at higher strain levels, i.e. where mechanical failure is supposed to appear. Vascular tissues exhibits simultaneously elastic and viscous material response. The rate-dependent material behavior of this kind of materials has been well-documented and quantified in the literature [21, 27, 41]. Furthermore, non-physiological loads drive soft tissue to damage that may induce a strong reduction of the stiffness [19, 35, 39, 41]. Damage may arise from two possible mechanisms: tear or plastic deformation of the fibers, or biochemical degradation of the extracellular matrix from protease release associated with the observed cellular necrosis.

Since the main modelling effort in the literature has been on the passive response of arteries, this is also the concern of the major part of this chapter. Taken all this into account, this chapter is focused on the development of microstructural constitutive models for vascular tissues and organized as follows. In Sect. 2 the constitutive equations of anisotropic hyperelastic materials are reviewed. In Sect. 3, we present the elastic micro-structurally based models. Section 4 considered a microstructural anisotropic damage and softening model for vessel tissues. Finally, Sect. 5 includes some concluding remarks.

2 Hyperelastic Behavior

This section deals with the formulation of standard finite strain material models for soft biological tissues. To clarify the framework it is necessary to summarize the formulation of finite strain hyperelasticity in terms of invariants with uncoupled volumetric/deviatoric responses, first suggested by Flory [16], generalized in [52] and employed for anisotropic soft biological tissues in [26, 59] among others.

Let $\mathcal{B}_0 \subset \mathbb{E}^3$ be a reference or rather material configuration of a body of interest. The notation $\varphi : \mathcal{B}_0 \times \mathcal{T} \rightarrow \mathcal{B}_t$ represents the one to one mapping, continuously differentiable, transforming a material point $\mathbf{X} \in \mathcal{B}_0$ to a position $\mathbf{x} = \varphi(\mathbf{X}, t) \in \mathcal{B}_t \subset \mathbb{E}^3$, where $\mathcal{B}_t$ represents the deformed configuration at time $t \in \mathcal{T} \subset \mathbb{R}$. The mapping φ represents a motion of the body that establishes the trajectory of a given point when moving from its reference position $\mathbf{X}$ to $\mathbf{x}$. The two-point deformation gradient tensor is defined as $\mathbf{F}(\mathbf{X}, t) := \nabla_{\mathbf{X}} \varphi(\mathbf{X}, t)$, with $J(\mathbf{X}) = \det(\mathbf{F}) > 0$ the local volume variation.

The direction of a fiber at a point $\mathbf{X} \in \mathcal{B}_0$ is defined by a unit vector field $\mathbf{m}_0(\mathbf{X})$, $|\mathbf{m}_0| = 1$. It is usually assumed that, under deformation, the fiber moves with the material points of the continuum body, that is, it follows an affine deformation. Therefore, the stretch λ of the fiber defined as the ratio between its lengths at the deformed and reference configurations can be expressed as

$$\lambda \mathbf{m}(\mathbf{x}, t) = \mathbf{F}(\mathbf{X}, t) \mathbf{m}_0(\mathbf{X}), \qquad (1)$$

where $\mathbf{m}$ is the unit vector of the fiber in the deformed configuration and

$$\lambda^2 = \mathbf{m}_0 \cdot \mathbf{F}^T \mathbf{F} \cdot \mathbf{m}_0 = \mathbf{m}_0 \cdot \mathbf{C} \mathbf{m}_0 \qquad (2)$$

stands for the stretch along the fiber direction at point $\mathbf{X}$ (Fig. 1). In (2) $\mathbf{C} = \mathbf{F}^T \mathbf{F}$ is the standard deformation gradient and the corresponding right Cauchy-Green strain measure. The introduced kinematics for one family of fibers can be applied to a second fiber family in an analogous manner. We shall denote a second preferred fiber orientation by the unit vector field $\mathbf{n}_0(\mathbf{X})$.

It is sometimes useful to consider the multiplicative decomposition of $\mathbf{F}$

$$\mathbf{F} := J^{1/3} \mathbf{I} \cdot \bar{\mathbf{F}}. \qquad (3)$$

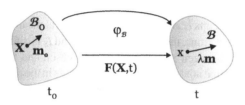

Fig. 1 Kinematics of a unit vector field $\mathbf{m}_0(\mathbf{X})$

Hence, deformation is split into a dilatational part, $J^{1/3}\mathbf{I}$, where $\mathbf{I}$ represents the second-order identity tensor, and an isochoric contribution, $\bar{\mathbf{F}}$, so that $\det(\bar{\mathbf{F}}) = 1$ [16]. With these quantities at hand, the isochoric counterparts of the right Cauchy-Green deformation tensors associated with $\bar{\mathbf{F}}$ are defined as $\bar{\mathbf{C}} := \bar{\mathbf{F}}^{\mathrm{T}} \cdot \bar{\mathbf{F}} = J^{-2/3}\mathbf{C}$.

The free energy function (SEF) is given by a scalar-valued function Ψ defined per unit reference volume in the reference configuration and for isothermal processes. Flory [16] postulated the additive decoupled representation of this SEF in volumetric and isochoric parts. To differentiate between the isotropic and the anisotropic parts, the free energy density function can be split up again as

$$\Psi = \Psi_{\mathrm{vol}} + \bar{\Psi} = \Psi_{\mathrm{vol}} + \bar{\Psi}_{\mathrm{iso}} + \bar{\Psi}_{\mathrm{ani}}, \tag{4}$$

where Ψ_{vol} describes the free energy associated to changes of volume, $\bar{\Psi}_{\mathrm{iso}}$ is the isochoric isotropic contribution of the free energy (usually associated to the ground matrix) and $\bar{\Psi}_{\mathrm{ani}}$ takes into account the isochoric anisotropic contribution (associated to the fibers) [55].

This strain-energy density function must satisfy the principle material frame invariance $\Psi(\mathbf{C}, \mathbf{M}, \mathbf{N}) = \Psi(\mathbf{Q} \cdot \mathbf{C}, \mathbf{Q} \cdot \mathbf{M}, \mathbf{Q} \cdot \mathbf{N})$ for all $[\mathbf{C}, \mathbf{Q}] \in [\mathbb{S}_+^3 \times \mathbb{Q}_+^3]$. Because of the directional dependence on the deformation, we require that the function Ψ explicitly depends on both the right Cauchy-Green tensor $\mathbf{C}$ and the fibers directions in the reference configuration ($\mathbf{m}_0$ and $\mathbf{n}_0$ in the case of two fiber families). Since the sign of $\mathbf{m}_0$ and $\mathbf{n}_0$ is not significant, Ψ must be an even function of $\mathbf{m}_0$ and $\mathbf{n}_0$ and so it may be expressed by $\Psi = \Psi(\mathbf{C}, \mathbf{M}, \mathbf{N})$ where $\mathbf{M} = \mathbf{m}_0 \otimes \mathbf{m}_0$ and $\mathbf{N} = \mathbf{n}_0 \otimes \mathbf{n}_0$ are structural tensors [55]. In terms of the strain invariants [55], Ψ can be written as

$$\Psi = \Psi_{\mathrm{vol}}(J) + \bar{\Psi}_{\mathrm{iso}}(\bar{I}_1, \bar{I}_2) + \bar{\Psi}_{\mathrm{ani}}(\bar{I}_4, \bar{I}_5, \bar{I}_6, \bar{I}_7, \bar{I}_8, \bar{I}_9) \tag{5}$$

with $\bar{I}_1$ and $\bar{I}_2$ the first two modified strain invariants of the symmetric modified Cauchy-Green tensor $\bar{\mathbf{C}}$ (note that $I_3 = J^2$). Finally, the anisotropic invariants $\bar{I}_4, \ldots, \bar{I}_9$ characterize the constitutive response of the fibers [55]:

$$\begin{aligned}
\bar{I}_4 &= \bar{\mathbf{C}} : \mathbf{M} = \bar{\lambda}_m^2, \quad \bar{I}_5 = \bar{\mathbf{C}}^2 : \mathbf{M} \\
\bar{I}_6 &= \bar{\mathbf{C}} : \mathbf{N} = \bar{\lambda}_n^2, \quad \bar{I}_7 = \bar{\mathbf{C}}^2 : \mathbf{N} \\
\bar{I}_8 &= [\mathbf{m}_0 \cdot \mathbf{n}_0]\mathbf{m}_0 \cdot \bar{\mathbf{C}}\mathbf{n}_0 \quad \bar{I}_9 = [\mathbf{m}_0 \cdot \mathbf{n}_0]^2.
\end{aligned} \tag{6}$$

Remark While the invariants $\bar{I}_4$ and $\bar{I}_6$ have a clear physical meaning, the square of the stretch λ in the fibers directions, the influence of $\bar{I}_5$, $\bar{I}_7$ and $\bar{I}_8$ is difficult to evaluate due to the high correlation between them [28]. For this reason and the lack of sufficient experimental data it is usual not to include these invariants in the definition of Ψ for soft biological tissues. Finally, $\bar{I}_9$ does not depend on the deformation.

The second Piola-Kirchhoff stress tensor is obtained by derivation of (4) with respect to the right Cauchy-Green tensor [37]. Thus, the stress tensor consists of a purely volumetric and a purely isochoric contribution, i.e. $\mathbf{S}_{\text{vol}}$ and $\bar{\mathbf{S}}$, so the total stress is

$$
\mathbf{S} = \mathbf{S}_{\text{vol}} + \bar{\mathbf{S}} = 2\frac{\partial \Psi_{\text{vol}}(J)}{\partial \mathbf{C}} + 2\frac{\partial \bar{\Psi}(\bar{\mathbf{C}}, \mathbf{M}, \mathbf{N})}{\partial \mathbf{C}} = \left[\frac{\partial \Psi_{\text{vol}}(J)}{\partial J} \frac{\partial J}{\partial \mathbf{C}} + \frac{\partial \bar{\Psi}(\bar{\mathbf{C}}, \mathbf{M}, \mathbf{N})}{\partial \bar{\mathbf{C}}} \frac{\partial \bar{\mathbf{C}}}{\partial \mathbf{C}} \right]
$$

$$
= Jp\mathbf{C}^{-1} + \sum_{j=1,2,4,6} \mathsf{P} : 2\frac{\partial \bar{\Psi}}{\partial \bar{I}_j} \frac{\partial \bar{I}_j}{\partial \bar{\mathbf{C}}} = Jp\mathbf{C}^{-1} + \mathsf{P} : \tilde{\mathbf{S}}, \tag{7}
$$

where the second Piola-Kirchhoff stress $\mathbf{S}$ consists of a purely volumetric contribution and a purely isochoric one. Moreover, one obtains the following noticeable relations $\partial_{\mathbf{C}} J = \frac{1}{2} J \mathbf{C}^{-1}$ and $\mathsf{P} = \partial_{\mathbf{C}} \bar{\mathbf{C}} = J^{-2/3}[\mathsf{I} - \frac{1}{3}\mathbf{C} \otimes \mathbf{C}^{-1}]$. P is the fourth-order projection tensor and I denotes the fourth-order unit tensor, which, in index notation, has the form $\mathsf{I}_{IJKL} = \frac{1}{2}[\delta_{IK}\delta_{JL} + \delta_{IL}\delta_{JK}]$. The projection tensor P furnishes the physically correct deviatoric operator in the Lagrangian description, i.e. $DEV[\cdot] = (\cdot) - 1/3(\bar{\mathbf{C}} : (\cdot))\bar{\mathbf{C}}^{-1}$.

Note that it is possible to obtain the Cauchy stress tensor by applying the push-forward operation to (7) $\sigma = J^{-1}\chi_*(\mathbf{S})$ [37]. Hence:

$$
\sigma = \sigma_{\text{vol}} + \bar{\sigma} = p\mathbf{1} + \frac{1}{J}dev\left[\bar{\mathbf{F}}\tilde{\mathbf{S}}\bar{\mathbf{F}}^{\mathbf{T}}\right] = p\mathbf{1} + \frac{1}{J}dev[\tilde{\sigma}] = p\mathbf{1} + \mathsf{p} : \tilde{\sigma}, \tag{8}
$$

where we have introduced the projection tensor $\mathsf{p} = J^{-1}[\mathsf{I} - \frac{1}{3}\mathbf{1} \otimes \mathbf{1}]$ which furnishes the physically correct deviatoric operator in the Eulerian description, i.e. $dev[\cdot] = (\cdot) - \frac{1}{3}tr[\cdot]\mathbf{1}$.

Based on the kinematic decomposition of the deformation gradient tensor, the tangent operator, also known as the elasticity tensor when dealing with elastic constitutive laws, is defined in the reference configuration as

$$
\mathsf{C} = 2\frac{\partial \mathbf{S}(\mathbf{C}, \mathbf{M}, \mathbf{N})}{\partial \mathbf{C}} = \mathsf{C}_{\text{vol}} + \bar{\mathsf{C}} = 2\frac{\partial \mathbf{S}_{\text{vol}}}{\partial \mathbf{C}} + 2\frac{\partial \bar{\mathbf{S}}}{\partial \mathbf{C}}
$$

$$
= 4\left[\frac{\partial^2 \Psi_{\text{vol}}(J)}{\partial \mathbf{C} \otimes \partial \mathbf{C}} + \frac{\partial^2 \bar{\Psi}(\bar{\mathbf{C}}, \mathbf{M}, \mathbf{N})}{\partial \mathbf{C} \otimes \partial \mathbf{C}}\right], \tag{9}
$$

where

$$
\mathsf{C}_{\text{vol}} = 2\mathbf{C}^{-1} \otimes \left(p\frac{\partial J}{\partial \mathbf{C}} + J\frac{\partial p}{\partial \mathbf{C}} + 2Jp\frac{\partial \mathbf{C}^{-1}}{\partial \mathbf{C}}\right) = J\tilde{p}\mathbf{C}^{-1} \otimes \mathbf{C}^{-1} - 2J\mathsf{I}_{\mathbf{C}^{-1}}, \tag{10}
$$

with $(I_{C^{-1}})_{IJKL} = -(C^{-1} \odot C^{-1})_{IJKL} = -\frac{1}{2}(C_{IK}^{-1}C_{JL}^{-1} + C_{IL}^{-1}C_{JK}^{-1})$, and $\tilde{p} = p + J\frac{dp}{dJ}$.
The term $\bar{C}$ corresponding to the deviatoric part is given by:

$$\bar{C} = -\frac{4}{3}J^{-\frac{4}{3}}\left(\frac{\partial\bar{\Psi}}{\partial\bar{C}}\otimes\bar{C}^{-1} + \bar{C}^{-1}\otimes\frac{\partial\bar{\Psi}}{\partial\bar{C}}\right) + \frac{4}{3}J^{-\frac{4}{3}}\left(\frac{\partial\bar{\Psi}}{\partial\bar{C}}:\bar{C}\right)$$
$$\times\left(\mathbb{I}_{\bar{C}^{-1}} - \frac{1}{3}\bar{C}^{-1}\otimes\bar{C}^{-1}\right) + J^{-\frac{4}{3}}\bar{C}_{\bar{w}}, \tag{11}$$

where term $\bar{C}_{\bar{w}}$ is defined as:

$$\bar{C}_{\bar{w}} = 4\frac{\partial^2\bar{\Psi}}{\partial\bar{C}\partial\bar{C}} - \frac{4}{3}\left[\left(\frac{\partial^2\bar{\Psi}}{\partial\bar{C}\partial\bar{C}}:\bar{C}\right)\otimes\bar{C}^{-1} + \bar{C}^{-1}\otimes\left(\frac{\partial^2\bar{\Psi}}{\partial\bar{C}\partial\bar{C}}:\bar{C}\right)\right]$$
$$+ \frac{4}{9}\left(\bar{C}:\frac{\partial^2\bar{\Psi}}{\partial\bar{C}\partial\bar{C}}:\bar{C}\right)\bar{C}^{-1}\otimes\bar{C}^{-1}. \tag{12}$$

Note that its spatial counterpart of (9) is obtained from the application of the push-forward operation to (9) $c = J^{-1}\chi_*(C)$ [8]. Hence:

$$c = c_{vol} + \bar{c}, \tag{13}$$

where:

$$c_{vol} = (\tilde{p}\mathbf{1}\otimes\mathbf{1} - 2p\mathsf{I}). \tag{14}$$

The deviatoric term, $\bar{c}$, can be obtained using the expression

$$\bar{c} = \frac{2}{3}tr(\tilde{\sigma})\mathsf{P} - \frac{2}{3}(\mathbf{1}\otimes dev(\bar{\sigma}) + dev(\bar{\sigma})\otimes\mathbf{1}) + \bar{c}_{\bar{w}}, \tag{15}$$

where $\bar{c}_{\bar{w}}$ in (15) is the weighted push forward of $\bar{C}_{\bar{w}}$

$$\bar{c}_{\bar{w}} = \mathsf{P}:\bar{c}:\mathsf{P}. \tag{16}$$

For a more detailed derivation of the material and spatial elasticity tensors for fully incompressible or compressible fibered hyperelastic materials and their explicit expressions, see i.e. [26] or [42].

The assumption that the anisotropic terms only contribute to the global mechanical response of the tissue when fibers are stretched, that is, $\bar{I}_i > \bar{I}_{i_0}$ is related to the waving of the collagen fibers [39] and represents a very simple framework to consider this waving. However, from a continuum mechanics point of view, a more elegant formulation to consider the waving is the dual mechanism constitutive theory initially proposed for polymeric and elastomeric materials by Tobolsky et al. [57] and Wineman and Rajagopal [60], respectively, and for biological tissues by Wulandana and Robertson [61]. The first mechanism is associated to the matrix

Fig. 2 Schematic of relevant
reference configurations for
the dual mechanism
constitutive model [40]

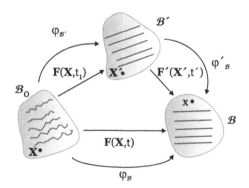

tissue and the second mechanism, associated to the fibers, has a different unloaded
configuration, corresponding to non-zero loading of the original material.

A brief discussion of the kinematics necessary for the dual mechanism constitutive equation is given below. A schematic of relevant reference configurations is
given in Fig. 2. The section of fibred tissue will be represented by a three-dimensional body B which initially, say at time $t = t_0$, is stress free and occupies a region
that will be referred to as the undeformed reference configuration $\mathscr{B}_0$. We consider
a typical material particle, $\mathbf{X} \in \mathscr{B}_0$, in the body B. Using this notation, the motion of
an arbitrary material particle can be described through the relationship
$\mathbf{x} = \boldsymbol{\varphi}_{\mathscr{B}}(\mathbf{X}, t)$. The deformation gradient $\mathbf{F}$ at time t for an arbitrary material particle
relative to the reference configuration $\mathscr{B}_0$ is given by $\mathbf{F}(\mathbf{X}, t) = \mathbf{F}_{\mathscr{B}}(\mathbf{X}, t) := \frac{\partial \boldsymbol{\varphi}_{\mathscr{B}}(\mathbf{X},t)}{\partial \mathbf{X}}$.
The mechanical response of the first mechanism (matrix) will only be a function of
$\mathbf{F}$. At some critical level of deformation, the second mechanism (fibers) is presumed
to commence load bearing. The contribution of the second mechanism to load
bearing is presumed to be a function of the deformation relative to $\mathscr{B}'$. Let $\mathbf{X}'$
denote the coordinates of the particle that was in position $\mathbf{X}$ in $\mathscr{B}_0$. If the config-
uration $\mathscr{B}'$ is reached at some time $t = t_1$, then $\mathbf{X}' = \boldsymbol{\varphi}_{\mathscr{B}}(\mathbf{X}, t_1)$. The motion of an
arbitrary material particle may then be described relative to the $\mathscr{B}_0$ configuration in
standard form or $\mathscr{B}'$ as $\mathbf{x} = \boldsymbol{\varphi}'_{\mathscr{B}}(\mathbf{X}', t')$ with $t' = t - t_1$. The deformation gradient $\mathbf{F}'$,
relative to the reference configuration $\mathscr{B}'$ is given by $\mathbf{F}'(\mathbf{X}', t') =$
$\mathbf{F}'_{\mathscr{B}}(\mathbf{X}_1, t') := \frac{\partial \boldsymbol{\varphi}'_{\mathscr{B}}(\mathbf{X}',t')}{\partial \mathbf{X}'}$. After operations, we obtain that $\mathbf{F}'(\mathbf{X}', t') = \mathbf{F}_{\mathscr{B}}(\mathbf{X}, t) \cdot$
$\mathbf{F}_{\mathscr{B}}^{-1}(\mathbf{X}, t_1)$. The fiber activation occurs (second mechanism) when $\lambda_i = \lambda_{i_0}$ and both
mechanisms will be active as load bearing components.

By particularization of this framework to fibred soft biological tissues, we have
that the matrix is associated to the first mechanics and collagen fibers with the
second and deform with $\mathbf{F}(\mathbf{X}, t)$ and $\mathbf{F}'(\mathbf{X}', t')$ respectively. In this context, the SEF
presented in (4) is

$$\bar{\Psi}\big(\bar{\mathbf{C}}(\mathbf{X},t),\mathbf{M},\mathbf{N}\big) = \bar{\Psi}_{\mathrm{iso}}\big(\bar{\mathbf{C}}(\mathbf{X},t)\big) + \bar{\Psi}_{\mathrm{ani}}\big(\bar{\mathbf{C}}'(\mathbf{X}',t'),\mathbf{M},\mathbf{N}\big)$$

$$= \mu_1[\bar{I}_1(\mathbf{X},t) - 3] + \mu_2[\bar{I}_2(\mathbf{X},t) - 3]$$

$$+ \frac{\gamma}{a\eta}\big[\exp\big(\eta[\bar{I}_1(\mathbf{X},t) - 3]^a\big) - f(\bar{I}_1(\mathbf{X},t),a)\big]$$

$$+ \sum_{i=4,6} \frac{c_{i-3}}{bc_{i-2}}\big[\exp\big(c_{i-2}[\bar{I}_i(\mathbf{X}',t') - 1]^b\big) - g(\bar{I}_i(\mathbf{X}',t'),b)\big],$$

$$(17)$$

where $\quad \bar{I}_i(\mathbf{X}',t') = \bar{\lambda}_i^2(\mathbf{X}',t') \quad$ and $\quad \bar{\lambda}_i(\mathbf{X}',t') = \bar{\lambda}_i(\mathbf{X},t)/\bar{\lambda}_i(\mathbf{X},t_1) = \lambda_i(\mathbf{X},t)/\bar{\lambda}_{i_0}.$
Finally, $\bar{\lambda}_{i_0} \geq 1$ is regarded as the initial crimping of the fibers. From the next and for simplicity of the nomenclature, we denote $\bar{I}_i(\mathbf{X},t) = \bar{I}_i$ and $\bar{I}_i(\mathbf{X}',t') = \bar{I}_{i'}$, so $\bar{\lambda}_{i'} = \bar{\lambda}_i/\bar{\lambda}_{i_0}$ and

$$\bar{\Psi}\,(\bar{\mathbf{C}}_1,\mathbf{M},\mathbf{N}) = \mu_1[\bar{I}_1 - 3] + \mu_2[\bar{I}_2 - 3] + \frac{\gamma}{a\eta}\big[\exp\big(\eta[\bar{I}_1 - 3]^a\big) - f(\bar{I}_1,a)\big]$$

$$+ \sum_{i=4,6} \frac{c_{i-3}}{bc_{i-2}}\big[\exp\big(c_{i-2}[\bar{I}_i' - 1]^b\big) - g(\bar{I}_i',b)\big]. \qquad (18)$$

3 Micro-Structurally Based Models: Elastic Behavior

The models proposed for soft tissues could be classified into two groups. The first comprises the macroscopic models previously presented, in which a SEF is obtained disregarding the nature of the micro-structural components of the tissue. Second, a group of micro-structurally based models are presented in this section, in which the macroscopic mechanical properties are obtained by assuming a constitutive relation for the microscopic components along each direction, whereas the macroscopic behaviour is obtained by integration of the contributions in all directions of space.

Gasser et al. [23] proposed the SEF

$$\bar{\Psi}(\mathbf{C},\mathbf{M},\mathbf{N}) = \mu[\bar{I}_1 - 3] + \frac{k_1}{2k_2}[\exp(k_2[\kappa\bar{I}_1 + [1 - 3\kappa]\bar{I}_4 - 1]^2) - 1] \qquad (19)$$

$$+ \frac{k_3}{2k_4}[\exp(k_4[\kappa\bar{I}_1 + [1 - 3\kappa]\bar{I}_6 - 1]^2) - 1], \qquad (20)$$

where $\kappa \in [0,1/3]$ is a measure of the dispersion of the fibers around the preferred orientations. This parameter is a result of considering the fibers oriented following the von Mises orientation density function. Thus, $\kappa = 1/3$ means isotropy and $\kappa = 0$ no fiber dispersion.

Anisotropy can straightfordwardly introduced in micro-structurally based models by considering an orientation density function, ρ, weighting the contribution of the fibers in space

$$\bar{\Psi} = \frac{3}{4\pi} \int_{\mathbb{U}^2} \rho \bar{\Psi} \mathrm{d}A. \tag{21}$$

First contributions considering this approach are due to Lanir [33], who proposed a structural model for planar tissues assuming that fibers are arranged in three-dimensional but almost planar wavy array. Thus, collagen fibers were restricted to a plane in which they were oriented following a Gaussian distribution around a mean preferred direction. The same assumption was adopted for the elastin fibers, which were oriented following a different distribution.

More recently, Alastrue et al. [1] proposed a hyperelastic microsphere-based model with statistically distributed fibers. In that model, it is assumed the existence of a uniaxial orientation distribution function $\rho(\mathbf{r}; \mathbf{a}) = \rho(-\mathbf{r}; \mathbf{a})$ for $\mathbf{r} \in \mathbb{U}^2$ a referential unit vector and $\mathbb{U}^2$ the unit sphere surface. The macroscopic strain energy density corresponding to one family of fibers associated with the so-called preferred direction $\mathbf{a}$ and with n fibers per unit volume is then defined as

$$\bar{\Psi}_f = \sum_{i=1}^{n} \rho(\mathbf{r}^i; \mathbf{a}) \bar{\Psi}_f^i, \tag{22}$$

where $\mathbf{r}^i$ are referential unit vectors associated with the direction of the ith fiber, and Ψ_f^i is the fiber's strain energy according to the deformation in the direction of $\mathbf{r}^i$. When expanding this expression in order to account for N preferred orientations $\mathbf{a}_I$ related to different families of fibers one obtains

$$\bar{\Psi}_{\mathrm{ani}} = \sum_{I=1}^{N} \bar{\Psi}_f^I = \sum_{I=1}^{N} \langle n\rho_I \bar{\Psi}_f(\bar{\lambda}) \rangle = \frac{1}{4\pi} \int_{\mathbb{U}^2} n\rho_I \bar{\Psi}_f \mathrm{d}A. \tag{23}$$

Apart from the symmetry condition $\rho(\mathbf{r}; \mathbf{a}) = \rho(-\mathbf{r}; \mathbf{a})$ it was considered that fibers are rotationally symmetrically distributed with respect to the preferred mean orientation $\mathbf{a}$—in other words, $\rho(\mathbf{Q} \cdot \mathbf{r}; \mathbf{a}) = \rho(\mathbf{r}; \mathbf{a}) \; \forall \; \mathbf{Q} \in \mathbb{Q}_+^3$ with rotation axis $\mathbf{a}$. As a consequence of the uniaxial distribution assumed for the one family of fibers considered, ρ can be defined as a function of the so-called mismatch angle $\omega = \arccos(\mathbf{a} \cdot \mathbf{r})$.

In Alastrue et al. [1], it was adopted the frequently applied π-periodic von Mises orientation distribution function (ODF)

$$\rho(\theta) = 4\sqrt{\frac{b}{2\pi}} \frac{\exp(b[\cos(2\theta)+1])}{\mathrm{erfi}(\sqrt{2b})}, \tag{24}$$

where the positive concentration parameter b constitutes a measure of the degree of anisotropy. Moreover, $\mathrm{erfi}(x) = -i\mathrm{erf}(x)$ denotes the imaginary error function with $\mathrm{erf}(x)$ given by

$$\mathrm{erf}(x) = \sqrt{\frac{2}{\pi}} \int_0^x \exp(-\xi^2)\mathrm{d}\xi. \tag{25}$$

Recently, the ODF Bingham [7] was proposed by Alastrue et al. [5] to account for the dispersion of the collagen fibrils with respect to their preferential orientation. That function is expressed as

$$\rho(r;A)\frac{\mathrm{d}A}{4\pi} = [K(A)]^{-1}\exp(r^{\mathrm{t}} \cdot A \cdot r)\frac{\mathrm{d}A}{4\pi}, \tag{26}$$

where A is a symmetric 3×3 matrix, $\mathrm{d}A$ is the Lebesgue invariant measure on the unit sphere, $r \in \mathbb{U}^2$ and $K(A)$ is a normalizing constant. As its main features, it is worth noting that this distribution always exhibits antipodal symmetry, but not rotational symmetry for the general case.

Applying straightforward transformations, Eq. (26) can be rewritten as

$$\rho(r;Z,Q)\frac{\mathrm{d}A}{4\pi} = [F_{000}(Z)]^{-1}\mathrm{etr}(Z \cdot Q^{\mathrm{t}} \cdot r \cdot r^{\mathrm{t}} \cdot Q)\frac{\mathrm{d}A}{4\pi}, \tag{27}$$

where $\mathrm{etr}(\cdot) \equiv \exp(\mathrm{tr}(\cdot))$, Z is a diagonal matrix with eigenvalues $\kappa_{1,2,3}$, $Q \in \mathbb{Q}^3$ such that $A = Q \cdot Z \cdot Q^{\mathrm{T}}$ and $F_{000}(Z)$ may be written as

$$F_{000}(Z) = [4\pi]^{-1}\int_{\mathbb{U}^2} \mathrm{etr}(Z \cdot r \cdot r^{\mathrm{t}})\mathrm{d}A = {}_1F_1(\frac{1}{2};\frac{3}{2};Z), \tag{28}$$

with ${}_1F_1$ a confluent hypergeometric function of matrix argument as defined by Herz [25].

Thus, the probability concentration is controlled by the eigenvalues of Z, which might be interpreted as concentration parameters. Specifically, the difference between pairs of $\kappa_{1,2,3}$—i.e., $[\kappa_1 - \kappa_2]$, $[\kappa_1 - \kappa_3]$ and $[\kappa_2 - \kappa_3]$—determines the shape of the distribution over the surface of the unit sphere, Fig. 3. Therefore, the value of one of these three parameters may be fixed to a constant value without reducing the versatility of (27). In fact, setting two of the parameters equal to zero the Von Mises ODF is obtained and when two parameters come close up, a rotational symmetry is achieved.

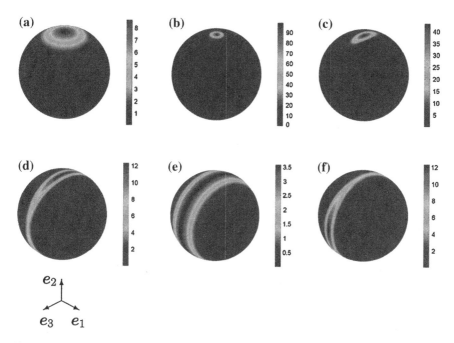

Fig. 3 Representation of the Bingham ODF for different sets of parameters with $\kappa_1 = 0.0$ [5]. **a** $\kappa_2 = 0.0, \kappa_3 = 5.0$. **b** $\kappa_2 = 0.0, \kappa_3 = 50.0$. **c** $\kappa_2 = 40.0, \kappa_3 = 50.0$. **d** $\kappa_2 = 49.0, \kappa_3 = 50.0$. **e** $\kappa_2 = 10.0, \kappa_3 = 10.0$. **f** $\kappa_2 = 50.0, \kappa_3 = 49.0$

Measurements of 3D organization of the collagen fibers, which are birefringent, can be made with the universal stage, an attachment to the polarizing microscope. The calibrated rotational movement, in three dimensions, of the inner stage of the universal stage permits the measurement of directional alignment of individual fibers, relative to the reference plane of the section [11, 12, 15, 53]. The experimental data obtained by Garcia [18] was fitted using the ODF Bingham, Table 1.

Once the ODF is fitted by means of microstructural observations [18, 22], it is necessary to fit the rest of the material constitutive parameters. For the isotropic component of elastin, we use two different SEF for $\bar{\Psi}_{\text{iso}}$, the classical Neo-Hookean model

$$\bar{\Psi}_{\text{iso}} = \mu[\bar{I}_1 - 3],$$

(29)

and the Demiray's SEF [13]

$$\bar{\Psi}_{\text{iso}} = \frac{c_1}{c_2}\left[\exp\left(\frac{c_2}{2}[\bar{I}_1 - 3]\right) - 1\right].$$

(30)

Table 1 Bingham distribution parameters that determine the collagen orientation density in the porcine wall [18]

	Family 1			Family 2		
	κ_1	κ_2	κ_3	κ_1	κ_2	κ_3
All proximal	9.6	0.0	22.4	18.6	0.0	30.3
All distal	18.6	0.0	30.6	15.5	0.0	28.4

Finally, phenomenological strain energy density function proposed by Holzapfel et al. [26] was used to approach the fiber response

$$n\bar{\psi}_f^i(\bar{\lambda}_i) = \frac{k_1}{2k_2}(e^{k_2((\bar{\lambda}_i)^2-1)^2} - 1) \qquad if \qquad \bar{\lambda}_i \geq 1 \qquad (31)$$

where $\bar{\lambda}_i = \left\|\bar{\mathbf{t}}^i\right\|$ defines the isochoric stretch in the fiber direction $\mathbf{r}^i$ and assuming $n\bar{\psi}_f^i(\bar{\lambda}_i) = 0$ when $(\bar{\lambda}_i) < 1$, since it is known that collagen fibers only affects to the global mechanical behavior in tensile states. Basically the parameters μ or c_1 and c_2 corresponding to the mechanical behavior of the isotropic part (Neo-Hookean or Demiray's SEF) and k_1 and k_2 for anisotropic one.

Due to lack of experimental data of the specimens analyzed in this work, experimental uniaxial tension tests previously developed in our group for porcine carotids in a proximal and distal regions were fitted [20]. The fitting of the experimental mechanical data was developed by using a Levenberg-Marquardt type minimization algorithm [36], by defining the objective function considering an isochoric tissue, Eq. (32). In this function, $\sigma_{\theta\theta}$ and σ_{zz} are the Cauchy (true) stress data obtained from the tests, $\sigma_{\theta\theta}^{\Psi}$ and σ_{zz}^{Ψ} are the Cauchy stresses for the ith point computed following Eq. (33), and n is the number of data points.

$$\chi^2 = \sum_{i=1}^n \left[(\sigma_{\theta\theta} - \sigma_{\theta\theta}^{\Psi})_i^2 + (\sigma_{zz} - \sigma_{zz}^{\Psi})_i^2 \right], \qquad (32)$$

where

$$\sigma_{\theta\theta}^{\Psi} = \lambda_\theta \frac{\partial \Psi}{\partial \lambda_\theta} \qquad \sigma_{zz}^{\Psi} = \lambda_z \frac{\partial \Psi}{\partial \lambda_z}. \qquad (33)$$

The goodness of the fitting was measured by computing the coefficient of determination of the normalized mean square root error ε was computed for each fitting $\varepsilon = \frac{\sqrt{\frac{\chi^2}{n-q}}}{\mu}$. In this equation μ the mean value of the measured stresses $\mu = \frac{\Sigma_{i=1}^n (\sigma)_i}{n}$, q is the number of parameters of the SEF, so $n - q$ is the number of degrees of freedom, and μ the mean stress already defined above.

Figure 4 illustrates the results of the mean of the proximal and distal specimens which was fitted based on the isotropic Neo-Hookean or Demiray SEFs. In this

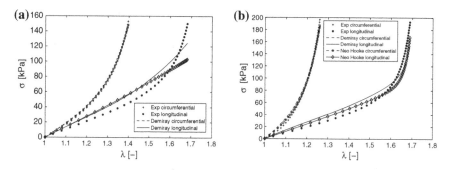

Fig. 4 Stress-stretch curves fitting [18] of the uniaxial tension tests from [20]. **a** Proximal specimens. **b** Distal specimens

Table 2 Structural material coefficients for the both SEF considered [18]

Neo-Hookean SEF	Specimen	μ (kPa)	k_1 (kPa)	$k_2(-)$	ε	
	Proximal	46	5.1	1.42	0.145	
	Distal	40	20	3.2	0.1574	
Demiray' SEF	Specimen	c_1 (kPa)	$c_2(-)$	k_1 (kPa)	k_2 (−)	ε
	Proximal	7.640	1.250	5.910	1.955	0.095
	Distal	14.98	0.830	21.04	2.995	0.124

case, the Neo-Hookean model resulted in an excellent fit for the distal specimen, showing a $\varepsilon = 0.110$. However, it substantially underestimated the proximal results in the longitudinal curve with a $\varepsilon = 0.145$. This shows that although the linear model of the isotropic part can very well describe the distal, it falls when proximal data is considered. The nonlinear model for the isotropic part improve the numerical fitting. It can be seen that the proposed nonlinear model can describe both proximal and distal data. The fit based on the Demiray SEF for elastin gave smaller normalized mean square root error ($\varepsilon = 0.124$ and $\varepsilon = 0.095$). The material coefficients corresponding to the fitting results are shown in the Table 2.

4 Micro-structurally Based Models: Softening and Damage Behavior

4.1 Probabilistic Damage Model

Histological studies performed in a number of soft tissues [14, 30] have shown that elastic fibers appear to be wavy and distributed about preferential directions [34]. Thus, as the load is applied, more and more fibers start to bear load. However, the degree of straightening of each fiber will also depend upon its orientation relative to the loading and the interstitial matter which might avoid its complete straightening. A model that consider the wavy nature of elastic fibers was proposed by Rodriguez et al. [45, 46]. Each bundle of fibers is assumed to behave following the worm-like eight-chain model proposed by Arruda and Boyce [6]

$$
n\bar{\Psi}_f(\bar{\lambda}) = \begin{cases} 0 & \text{if } \bar{\lambda} < 1 \\ B[2\frac{\bar{r}^2}{L^2} + \frac{1}{1-\bar{r}/L} - \frac{\bar{r}}{L} \\ \quad - \frac{\ln(\bar{\lambda}^4 r_0)}{4r_0 L}[4\frac{r_0}{L} + \frac{1}{[1-r_0/L]^2} - 1] - \Psi_r] & \text{if } \bar{\lambda} \le 1 \end{cases}, \tag{34}
$$

with $B = \frac{1}{4}nK\Theta r_0/A$ a stress-like material parameter, L the maximum fiber length, r_0 the fiber length in the undeformed configuration, $\bar{r} = \bar{\lambda} r_0 < L$ the actual fiber length, $\bar{\lambda}$ the actual isochoric fiber stretch, and

$$
\Psi_r = 2\frac{r_0^2}{L^2} + \frac{1}{1 - r_0/L} - \frac{r_0}{L}, \tag{35}
$$

being a repository constant accounting for a zero strain energy at $\bar{\lambda} = 1$. This model considers the maximum fiber length, L, as a Beta random variable, and assumes the same average orientation for all fibers within the bundle as well as that fibers do not bear compressive loads. Hence, the strain energy density function for a bundle of fibers is given by

$$
\bar{\Psi}_{bun}(\bar{\lambda}, \bar{\lambda}_{t^*}) = \begin{cases} 0, & \bar{\lambda} < 1, \\ \int_1^{\bar{\lambda}} \int_{a(r_0\bar{\lambda}_{t^*})}^{\iota} \bar{\Psi}'_f(\xi, x)\ell_L(x)\mathrm{d}x\mathrm{d}\xi, & \bar{\lambda} \ge 1, \end{cases} \tag{36}
$$

where $a(r_0\bar{\lambda}_{t^*})$ is a monotonically increasing function that determines the minimal fiber length within the bundle for which failure has not yet occurred,[1] $\Psi'_f = n\partial\Psi_f/\partial\bar{\lambda}$, and $\ell_L(x)$ is a Beta probability density function with parameters γ and η

$$
\ell_L(x) = \frac{1}{\iota - r_0}\frac{\Gamma(\eta + \gamma)}{\Gamma(\eta)\Gamma(\gamma)}\left[\frac{x - r_0}{\iota - r_0}\right]^{\gamma-1}\left[1 - \frac{x - r_0}{\iota - r_0}\right]^{\eta-1}, \quad x \in [r_0, \iota]. \tag{37}
$$

The parameter $\bar{\lambda}_{t^*}$ in (36) corresponds to the maximum isochoric fiber stretch attained by the bundle over the past history up to time $t \in \mathcal{T}_+$. Therefore, the damage of the fiber bundle increases whenever $\bar{\lambda}_t - \bar{\lambda}_{t^*} \ge 0$ and, therefore, it is strain driven. On the other hand, function $a(r_0\bar{\lambda}_{t^*})$ determines the minimum fiber length within the bundle for which failure has not yet occurred, and is given by

---

[1] Notice that x is a dummy variable used for integration purposes.

$$a(r_0\bar{\lambda}_{t^*}) = \exp\left(\left[\frac{r_0\bar{\lambda}_{t^*}}{\delta}\right]^{\varpi}\right) r_0\bar{\lambda}_{t^*}, \tag{38}$$

where ϖ and δ are dimensionless model parameters. Note that with this form of $a(r_0\bar{\lambda}_{t^*})$, the bundle will degrade faster as the deformation gets larger (i.e., longer fiber will fail at a smaller fraction of their maximum length).

With these considerations at hand, fiber damage is quantified as

$$D_{\mathrm{f}} = \frac{1}{1 - r_0}\frac{\Gamma(\eta + \gamma)}{\Gamma(\eta) + \Gamma(\gamma)} \int_{r_0}^{a(r_0\bar{\lambda}_t)} \left[\frac{x - r_0}{1 - r_0}\right]^{\gamma-1} \left[1 - \frac{x - r_0}{1 - r_0}\right]^{\eta-1} \mathrm{d}x$$

$$= \mathrm{Beta}\left(\frac{a(r_0\bar{\lambda}_t)}{1 - r_0}, \gamma, \eta\right). \tag{39}$$

Rodriguez et al. [45] used the damage model to study the balloon inflation of a coronary artery 40 mm long, with an inner diameter of 2.7 mm and a thickness of 1.8 mm. The artery has been simulated as a multi-layer composite material by considering the media, and adventitia layers and included the residual stresses. Figure 5 shows the damage distributions in the arterial wall under balloon inflation. The balloon induces large longitudinal and circumferential stretching in the artery which causes larger fiber deformation in the adventitia than in the media leading to larger stresses and more rapid damage of this layer.

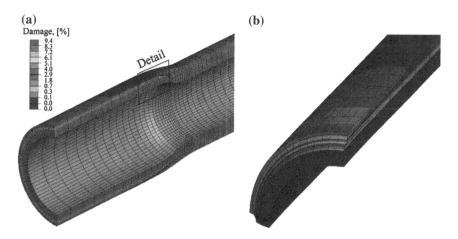

Fig. 5 Damage distribution in the arterial wall under balloon inflation from [45]

4.2 Deterministic Damage Model

If an uniaxial tension is developed six distinct stages A-H should be considered, Fig. 6—for clarity only one family of fibers is considered when furnished with matrix (light grey background) and fibers (wavy dark solid lines)—. Stage A is defined by $\lambda = 1$. After that, stage B, the uniaxial loading is small and the collagen fibers to become less wavy without contributing significantly to load bearing—only first mechanism—$(\lambda < \lambda_o)$. When $\lambda \geq \lambda_o$, the tissue has been loaded just to the level where the fibers have straightened and will resist further extension—both mechanism are bearing load (stage C). If the strip of fibred tissue is unloaded, the fibers had not returned to the original unstrained wave pattern but remained in a straightened state—this fact means that the reference configuration for the second mechanism has changed (λ_o^*)—a softened behavior until free-stress state (stage D)—. Subsequent reloading follows the former unloading curve until the previous maximum stretch is reached. However, during stage E the fibers are less wavy, so critical level of deformation for the second mechanism to start load bearing has also change and this stage D is characterized by $\lambda < \lambda_o^*$. When $\lambda \geq \lambda_o^*$ fibers again resist further extension, however if loading level λ_{min} is reached some fibers are disrupted, stage G, with partial collagen disruption. Upon further loading, only some fibers will resist stretch until $\lambda = \lambda_{max}$ where bond rupture and complete damage is produced (stage H).

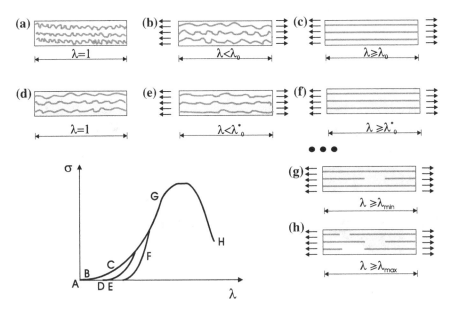

Fig. 6 Schematic representation of stages of tissue deformation. **a** Initial unloaded tissue. **b** Only matrix load bearing $\left(l_{io} = \lambda_o^2\right)$. **c** Fibers load bearing. **d** Initial state after unloading. **e** Only matrix load bearing after unloading $\left(w_i \lambda_i = \lambda_o^*\right)$. **f** Fibers load bearing after unloading. **g** Partial disruption of fibers. **h** Total disruption of the fibers, [40]

The experimental results suggest that just like the elastic properties, the inelastic behavior of soft tissues is also characterized by anisotropy [3, 41, 43, 44]. Accordingly, a suitable constitutive model should account for this directional dependence and take into account the different alteration mechanisms associated with this anisotropy. The phenomenological inelastic model should include the Mullins effect, the permanent set resulting from the residual strains after unloading, and the fibre and matrix disruption associated to supraphysiological loads or strains [9].

To model these inelastic processes, we apply the following considerations:

- We have introduced the $\bar{\lambda}_{i_0}(i = 4, 6)$ parameter that governs the anisotropic contribution to the global mechanical response of the tissue only when stretched, that is, $\bar{\lambda}'_i = \bar{\lambda}_i/\bar{\lambda}_{i_0} \geq 1$. We modified this parameter by a weight factor w_i associated to $\bar{\lambda}_{i_0}$ that changes independently from each direction to take into account structural alterations along the fibers direction, that is, $\lambda^*_o = w_i \cdot \bar{\lambda}_{i_0}$. With this modification, we can reproduce at the same time the softening behavior and the permanent set presented in this kind of tissue.

- The preconditioning until "saturated" state is modelled using a continuous damage model that accumulates within the whole strain history of the deformation process by a weight factor $D_{r_k}(k = m, 4, 6)$ associated to the matrix ($\bar{I}_1$ and $\bar{I}_2$) and the fibers ($\bar{I}_i$) [44].

- Finally, the softening as a result of the bond rupture and complete damage is accomplished by using the classical Continuum Damage Mechanics (CDM) theory using the well-known reduction factors [50], $D_{s_k}(k = m, 4, 6)$, associated to the matrix ($\bar{I}_1$ and $\bar{I}_2$) and the fibers (I_i) [10].

With these considerations, the free energy for the fibers is assumed to be of the form

$$
\begin{aligned}
\bar{\Psi}_{\text{ani}}\langle n\rho\bar{\psi}_f(\lambda)\rangle &= [1 - D]\frac{1}{4\pi}\int_{\mathbb{U}^2} n\rho\bar{\psi}_0(\bar{\lambda}^i)\mathrm{d}A \\
&\approx \sum_{j=1}^{N}[1 - D_j]\left[\sum_{i=1}^{m} n\rho_i w^i \bar{\psi}^i_{j,0}(\bar{\lambda}^i)\right]
\end{aligned}
\tag{40}
$$

with $D_j = D^\alpha_j + D^\beta_j$ the normalized scalars referred to as the damage, $D^\alpha_j : \mathbb{R}_+ \to \mathbb{R}_+$ and $D^\beta_j : \mathbb{R}_+ \to \mathbb{R}_+$ are monotonically increasing smooth functions with the following properties $D^\alpha_j(0) = 0$, $D^\beta_j(0) = 0$ and $D^\alpha_j + D^\beta_j \in [0, 1]$ and $\bar{\psi}_0(\bar{\lambda}^j)$ the effective strain energy density functions of each j family of fibers.

The second law of thermodynamics asserts a non-negative rate of entropy production. Using standard arguments based on the Clausius-Duhem inequality [37]

$$\mathscr{D}_{int} = -\dot{\Psi} + \frac{1}{2}\mathbf{S} : \dot{\mathbf{C}} \geq 0 \qquad (41)$$

yields

$$\mathscr{D}_{int} = -\sum_{j=1}^{N}\left[\frac{\partial\bar{\psi}_{j,0}}{\partial D_j^{\alpha}}\dot{D}_j^{\alpha} + \frac{\partial\bar{\psi}_{j,0}}{D_j^{\beta}}\dot{D}_j^{\beta} + \frac{\partial\bar{\psi}_{j,0}}{\partial w_j}\dot{w}_j\right] \geq 0 \qquad (42)$$

where the thermodynamic forces are

$$f_j^{\alpha} = -\frac{\partial\bar{\psi}_{j,0}(\bar{\lambda}^i)}{D_j^{\alpha}} = \bar{\psi}_{j,0}(\bar{\lambda}^i) \quad f_j^{\beta} = -\frac{\partial\bar{\psi}_{j,0}(\bar{\lambda}^i)}{D_j^{\beta}} = \bar{\psi}_{j,0}(\bar{\lambda}^i)$$

$$f_{w_j} = -\frac{\partial\bar{\psi}_{j,0}(\bar{\lambda}^i)}{\partial w_j} = \partial\bar{\psi}_{j,0}(\bar{\lambda}^i) \qquad (43)$$

The thermodynamic forces f_{α}, f_{β} and f_{w_j} are conjugated to the internal variables D_j^{α}, D_j^{β} and w_j respectively.

4.2.1 Evolution of the Internal Variables

Continuous damage variables $\left(D_j^{\alpha}\right)$

The continuous damage D_j^{α} is assumed that accumulate within the whole strain history of the deformation process which is also governed by the local effective strain energy and have the form

$$D_j^{\alpha} = d_{\infty}^j\left[1 - \exp\left(-\frac{\alpha}{\zeta_j}\right)\right]$$

where

$$\alpha \doteq \int_0^t |\dot{f}_j(s)|ds \qquad \dot{r}_j = |\dot{f}_j| = \text{sign}(\dot{\bar{\Psi}}_{j,0}^0) \qquad (44)$$

with the initial condition $\alpha(0) = 0$. Finally, ζ_j is the damage saturation parameters and the parameters d_{∞}^j describe the maximum possible continuous damage, thus we have the constraint $d_{\infty}^j \in [0, 1]$ [44].

Discontinuous damage variables $\left(D_j^{\beta}\right)$

We define a damage criterion in the strain space by the condition that, at any time t of the loading process, the following expression is fulfilled [49]

$$\Phi_j(\overline{\lambda}(s), \Xi_{s,j}^*) = \Xi_j - \Xi_j^* = \sqrt{2\overline{\psi}_{j,0}(\overline{\lambda}^i(s))} - \Xi_j^* \leq 0, \tag{45}$$

where $\Xi_j^* = \max_{s\varepsilon(-\infty,t]} \left(\sqrt{2\overline{\psi}_{j,0}(\overline{\lambda}^i(s))} \right)$ signifies damage threshold (energy barrier) at current time t (i.e. the radius of the damage surface). If $\Phi_j < 0$, no damage occurs while $\Phi_j = 0$ defines the damage surface. Note that $\Phi_j > 0$ is an impossible situation. Update of this surface is needed when the free energy density of a material point or fiber goes up over Ξ_j^*

$$\Xi_j^* = \begin{cases} \dot{f}_j^\beta = \dot{\overline{\psi}}_{j,0}(\overline{\lambda}^i) & \text{if } \Phi_j = 0 \text{ and } \dot{f}_j^\beta > 0 \\ 0 & \text{otherwise} \end{cases} \tag{46}$$

The last equation needed for a complete definition of the model is the irreversible rate of the damage variable D_i^β

$$\frac{dD_j^\beta}{dt} = \begin{cases} h_j(\Xi_j)\dot{\Xi}_j & \text{if } \Phi_j = 0 \text{ and } \dot{f}_j^\beta > 0 \\ 0 & \text{otherwise} \end{cases} \tag{47}$$

where $h_j(\Xi_j) = dD_j^\beta/d\Xi_j$ are the functions that characterize the damage evolution in the material.

Following previous work [38], we consider the discontinuous damage evolution equation

$$D_j^\beta = \frac{1}{1 + \exp(-\varpi_j[\Xi_j - \gamma_j])}, \tag{48}$$

where the parameter ϖ_j controls the slope and γ_j defines the value Ξ such that $D_j^\beta = 0.5$.

Softening variables (w_j)

For the softening variables w_j, we consider the following criteria

$$\Upsilon_j(\mathbf{C}(t), \Gamma_{j_t}) = \frac{\partial \psi_{j,0}(\overline{\lambda}^i)}{\partial \overline{\lambda}^i} - \Gamma_{j_t} = \Gamma_j - \Gamma_{j_t} \leq 0 \tag{49}$$

where $\Gamma_j = \frac{\partial \psi_{j,0}(\overline{\lambda}^i)}{\partial \overline{\lambda}^i}$ is the softening stress release rate at time $t \in \mathbb{R}_+$ and Γ_{j_t} signifies the softening threshold (stress barrier) at current time t for matrix and fibers

$$\Gamma_{j_t} = \max_{sr\in(-\infty,t)} \frac{\partial \psi_{j,0}(\overline{\lambda}^i)}{\partial \overline{\lambda}^i} \tag{50}$$

The equation $\Upsilon_j(\mathbf{C}(t), \Gamma_{j_t}) = 0$ defines a softening surface in the strain space. With these means at hand, we finally propose the following set of rate equations for an evolution of the softening variables

$$\dot{w}_j \doteq \begin{cases} \kappa_j \dot{\Gamma}_{j_t}, & \text{if } \quad \Upsilon = 0 \quad \text{and} \quad \mathbf{N}_j : \dot{\mathbf{C}} > 0 \\ 0 & \text{otherwise} \end{cases} \tag{51}$$

Let us now consider softening functions of the simple form

$$w_j = \kappa_j \Gamma_{j_t} + 1 \tag{52}$$

where κ_j is the only parameter to define the softening mechanism in each fiber direction.

4.2.2 Computational Aspects

If the material state is known at a time t_n and the deformation is known at a time $t_{n+1} = t_n + \Delta t$, we may write [32]

$$\mathbf{S}_{n+1} = J_{n+1} p_{n+1} \mathbf{C}_{n+1}^{-1} + J_{n+1}^{-\frac{2}{3}} \sum_{k=m,f_1,f_2} [1 - D_{j_{n+1}}] \bar{\mathbf{S}}_{(j)n+1}^0, \tag{53}$$

where the subscripts n and $n+1$ denote quantities evaluated at times t_n and t_{n+1}.

The iterative Newton procedure to solve a nonlinear finite element problem requires the determination of the consistent tangent material operator. This can be derived analytically for the given material Eq. (53). The symmetric algorithmic material tensor is expressed as [49, 51]

$$\begin{aligned}
\mathbf{C}_{n+1} &= 2 \frac{\partial \mathbf{S}_{n+1}(\mathbf{C}_{n+1}, \mathbf{M}, \mathbf{N}, D_{(j)n+1}, w_{(j)n+1})}{\partial \mathbf{C}_{n+1}} = \mathbf{C}_{\mathrm{vol}_{n+1}} + \bar{\mathbf{C}}_{n+1} \\
&= 4 \left[\frac{\partial^2 \Psi_{\mathrm{vol}_{n+1}}(J_{n+1})}{\partial \mathbf{C}_{n+1} \otimes \partial \mathbf{C}_{n+1}} + \frac{\partial^2 \bar{\Psi}_{n+1}(\bar{\mathbf{C}}_{n+1}, \mathbf{M}, \mathbf{N}, D_{(j)n+1}, w_{(j)n+1})}{\partial \mathbf{C}_{n+1} \otimes \partial \mathbf{C}_{n+1}} \right] \\
&= \mathbf{C}_{\mathrm{vol}_{n+1}} + \sum_{j=m,f_1,f_2} \left[[1 - D_{(j)n+1}] \bar{\mathbf{C}}_{(j)n+1}^0 - \bar{\mathbf{S}}_{(j)n+1} \right]
\end{aligned} \tag{54}$$

where

$$\bar{\mathbf{S}}_{(j)n+1} = \begin{cases} \left[D_{(j)n+1}'^{\alpha} + D_{(j)n+1}'^{\beta} \operatorname{sign}(\dot{f}_{(j)n+1}) \right] \bar{\mathbf{S}}_{(j)n+1} \otimes \bar{\mathbf{S}}_{(j)n+1} - & \text{if} \quad \phi = 0 \\ -4J^{-\frac{2}{3}} \frac{\kappa_j}{I_{j0}} \tilde{\Gamma}_j \frac{\partial^2 \bar{\Psi}_{n+1}}{\partial \Gamma_{j n+1}^2} \tilde{\mathbf{M}} \otimes \tilde{\mathbf{M}} & \text{and} \quad \mathbf{N}_{(j)n+1} : \dot{\mathbf{C}}_{n+1} > 0 \\ D_{(j)n+1}'^{\beta} \operatorname{sign}(\dot{f}_{(j)n+1}) \bar{\mathbf{S}}_{(j)n+1} \otimes \bar{\mathbf{S}}_{(j)n+1} & \text{otherwise} \end{cases} \tag{55}$$

where $\tilde{\mathbf{M}} = \mathbf{P} : \mathbf{M}$. Note that the present formulation results in a symmetric algorithmic tangent modulus Eq. (54) with a low computational cost [49].

Following plasticity nomenclature, further examination of Eqs. (45–49) results in the observation that if $\Phi_j < 0$ or $\Lambda_j < 0$, then no damage or softening evolution takes place with respect to the jth damage or softening surface. Algorithmically, this motivates the notation of a "trial" elastic predictor state defined by $\dot{r}_{j_t} = 0$ for all k or $\dot{\Gamma}_{j_t} = 0$ for all j [24]. The trial stress is given by

$$\sigma_{n+1}^{trial} = p_{n+1}\mathbf{1} + \sum_{j=m,f_1,f_2} \left[1 - D_{j_n} \right] \bar{\sigma}_{(j)n+1}^0 \tag{56}$$

the trial damage is given by

$$D_{j_{n+1}}^{\alpha\ trial} = D_{j_n}^\alpha \quad \text{and} \quad w_{j_{n+1}}^{trial} = w_{j_n} \tag{57}$$

and the symmetric algorithmic material tensor

$$\mathbf{C}_{n+1}^{trial} = \mathbf{C}_{vol\,n+1}^0 + \sum_{j=m,f_1,f_2} \left[1 - D_{j_n} \right] \mathbf{C}_{(j)n+1}^0 \tag{58}$$

A predictor-corrector type algorithmic can now be defined as follows:

1. For each j check whether $\Phi_{j_{n+1}} \leq 0$. If so, then assume the surface is inactive, so $D_{(j)n+1}^\alpha = D_{(j)n+1}^{\alpha\ trial}$.
2. If $\Phi_{j_{n+1}} > 0$, then assume that the surface is active and update $D_{(j)n+1}^\alpha$ using Eq. (48).
3. For each j check whether $\Lambda_{(j)n+1} \leq 0$. If so, then assume the surface is inactive, so $w_{j_{n+1}} = w_{j_{n+1}}^{trial}$.
4. If $\Lambda_{(j)n+1} > 0$, then assume that the surface is active and update w_j using Eq. (52).

To update softening and damage variables, we summarize the computational algorithm for the case of $\Gamma_{i_{n+1}} = \frac{\partial \Psi_{ich(i)n+1}}{\partial \Gamma_i}$ and explicit actualization of $w_{i_{n+1}}$ in Table 3.

In this example, we compare the model here presented with experimental stress-stretch data from uniaxial cyclic loading tests on vein tissue [3]. These experiments were developed in our laboratory in order to study the properties of ovine vena cava tissue. Two families of fibers oriented in circumferential (collagen) and longitudinal (elastin) directions were considered. The material is treated as incompressible $\left(\mathbf{C} = \bar{\mathbf{C}} \right)$, with the matrix modelled using the following strain energy

Table 3 Algorithmic procedure and explicit actualization of damage and softening variables

1. Database at each Gaussian point D_{skn}, $\Xi_{(k_t)n}$, D_{rkn}, $\bar{\Psi}^0_{(k)n}$, w_{in}, $\Gamma_{i_t n}$
2. Compute the initial elastic stress tensors $(\sigma^0_{(k)n+1})$ and the initial elastic modulus $(\mathbf{c}^0_{n+1})$
3. Compute the current equivalent measures

   $\Xi_{k_{n+1}} = \sqrt{2\bar{\Psi}^0_{(k)n+1}}$ and $\Gamma_{i_{n+1}} = \dfrac{\partial \bar{\Psi}_{(i)n+1}}{\partial I'_i}$
4. Check the discontinuous damage criterion

   $\Phi_{k_{n+1}}(\bar{\mathbf{C}}_{n+1}, \Xi_{(k_t)n}) = \sqrt{2\bar{\Psi}^0_{(k)n+1}} - \Xi_{(k_t)n} = \Xi_{k_{n+1}} - \Xi_{(k_t)n} > 0$

   YES: update discontinuous damage internal variables

   $D_{sk_{n+1}} = \dfrac{1}{1+\exp(-\alpha_k[\Xi_{k_{n+1}} - \gamma_k])}$

   $\bar{\mathbf{S}}^{sk}_{(k)n+1} = D'_{sk_{n+1}} \bar{\mathbf{S}}^0_{(k)n+1} \otimes \bar{\mathbf{S}}^0_{(k)n+1}$

   $\Xi_{(k_t)n+1} = \Xi_{k_{n+1}}$

   NO: no additional damage $D_{sk_{n+1}} = D_{skn}$ and $\bar{\mathbf{S}}^{sk}_{(k)n+1} = 0$.
5. Update continuous damage internal variables

   $r_{k_{n+1}} = r_{kn} + |\bar{\Psi}^0_{(k)n+1} - \bar{\Psi}^0_{(k)n}|$.

   $D_{rk_{n+1}} = d^{rk}_\infty \left[1 - \exp\left(-\dfrac{r_{k_{n+1}}}{\zeta_k}\right)\right]$

   $\bar{\mathbf{S}}^{rk}_{(k)n+1} = D'_{(rk)n+1} \operatorname{sign}(\dot{f}_{(k)n+1}) \bar{\mathbf{S}}^0_{(k)n+1} \otimes \bar{\mathbf{S}}^0_{(k)n+1}$
6. Check the softening criterion

   $\Lambda_i(\mathbf{C}(t), \Gamma_{i_t}) = \dfrac{\partial \bar{\Psi}_{(i)}}{\partial I'_i}(\bar{\mathbf{C}}(t), \mathbf{M}, \mathbf{N}) - \Gamma_{i_t} = \Gamma_i - \Gamma_{i_t} \leq 0$

   YES: update softening internal variables

   $w_{i_{n+1}} = \dfrac{\kappa_i}{I_{i0}} \Gamma_{i_{n+1}} + 1$

   $\bar{\mathbf{S}}^{wi}_{(i)n+1} = -4J^{-\frac{2}{3}} \dfrac{\kappa_i}{I_{i0}} \bar{\Gamma}_i \dfrac{\partial^2 \bar{\Psi}_{n+1}}{\partial I'^2_{i\,n+1}} \tilde{\mathbf{M}} \otimes \tilde{\mathbf{M}}$

   $\Gamma_{i_t n+1} = \Gamma_{i_{n+1}}$

   NO: no additional damage $w_{i_{n+1}} = w_{in}$ and $\bar{\mathbf{S}}^{wi}_{(i)n+1} = 0$.
7. Compute the Cauchy stress tensor

   $p_{n+1} = \dfrac{d\Psi_{vol}(J_{n+1})}{dJ}\big|_{n+1}$

   $\sigma_{n+1} = p_{n+1}\mathbf{1} + \sum_{k=m, f_1, f_2}[1 - D_{k_{n+1}}]\operatorname{dev}(\sigma^0_{(k)n+1})$
8. Compute the extra term of the elastic modulus

   $\bar{\mathbf{S}}_{(k,i)n+1} = \bar{\mathbf{S}}^{sk}_{(k)n+1} + \bar{\mathbf{S}}^{rk}_{(k)n+1} + \bar{\mathbf{S}}^{wi}_{(i)n+1}$
9. Compute the elastic modulus

   $\mathbf{c}_{n+1} = \mathbf{c}^0_{vol\,n+1} + \sum_{k=m, f_1, f_2}[1 - D_{k_{n+1}}]\bar{\mathbf{c}}^0_{(k)n+1} - \bar{\mathbf{s}}_{(k)n+1}$ with $\bar{\mathbf{s}}_{(k)n+1} = J^{-1}\chi_*(\bar{\mathbf{S}}_{(k)n+1})$

$$\bar{\Psi}(\bar{\mathbf{C}}, \mathbf{M}, \mathbf{N}, D_j, w_j) = \mu[1 - D_m][\bar{I}_1 - 3] + [1 - D_{f4}]\frac{k_1}{2k_2}\left[\exp\left(k_2[\bar{I}'_4 - 1]^2\right) - 1\right]$$

$$+ [1 - D_{f6}]\frac{k_3}{2k_4}\left[\exp\left(k_4[\bar{I}'_6 - 1]^2\right) - 1\right]. \tag{59}$$

Table 4 Material, damage and softening parameters for uniaxial simple tension. μ, k_1, k_3 and ζ_j are in MPa, γ_j is in $MPa^{1/2}$ and other parameters are dimensionless [40]

I	μ	k_1	k_2	λ_{4_0}	k_3	k_4	λ_{6_0}								
	0.029	0.013	7.760	1.0	0.010	0.972	1.0								
	ϖ_m	γ_m	ϖ_{f_4}	γ_{f_4}	κ_{f_4}	ϖ_{f_6}	γ_{f_6}	κ_{f_6}	$d^{I_m}_\infty$	ζ_m	$d^{f_4}_\infty$	ζ_{f_4}	$d^{f_6}_\infty$	ζ_{f_6}	R^2
	33.443	0.149	0.816	9.313	0.026	5.491	0.285	1.372	7.242	0.0	0.100	4.645	0.673	0.182	0.979
II	μ	k_1	k_2	λ_{4_0}	k_3	k_4	λ_{6_0}								
	0.01	0.662	1.295	1.0	0.049	0.036	1.0								
	ϖ_m	γ_m	ϖ_{f_4}	γ_{f_4}	κ_{f_4}	ϖ_{f_6}	γ_{f_6}	κ_{f_6}	$d^{I_m}_\infty$	ζ_m	$d^{f_4}_\infty$	ζ_{f_4}	$d^{f_6}_\infty$	ζ_{f_6}	R^2
	3.45	0.68	0.93	19.3	0.08	0.9	12.23	0.3	0.3	1.0	0.3	1.0	0.3	1.0	0.874

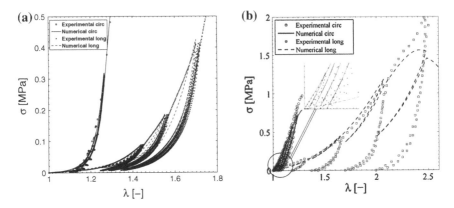

Fig. 7 Experimental and numerical simulation of loading and unloading curves at different load limits in cava tissue [40]. **a** Individual I. **b** Individual II

Table 5 Elastic and damage parameters for the uniaxial test from [47]

μ (kPa)	k_1 (kPa)	k_2 (−)	b (−)	ϖ (−)	γ (kPa)	α (deg)
1.051	286.36	1.40	10.62	0.41	20.10	47.77

μ, k_1 and γ are in MPa, and other parameters are dimensionless

Both pairs of curves—circumferential and longitudinal direction tests for Individuals I and II—were fitted using the representative set of uniaxial data in both axial and circumferential directions with the optimization procedure previously described. The optimized parameters obtained are included in Table 4 and experimental and numerical results for loading and unloading are shown in Fig. 7.

The purpose of this simulation was to present a numerical example of arterial angioplasty with relevance to modeling vascular tissue to demonstrate the capabilities of the model. The model consists of a 10 (mm) length phantom with an external diameter of $D_e = 5$ (mm) and an internal diameter of $D_i = 3.7$ (mm) corresponding to coronary arteries. Only one layer was considered since no experimental data were available for the separates layers and the material parameters are presented in Table 5. The load steps were applied sequentially as follows: (i) Imposition of an initial deformation gradient [4], (ii) Application of an internal pressure of 13.3 (kPa) in the vessel assuming this as the average physiological hemodynamic pressure and (iii) Imposition of pressure to the internal face of the balloon [47] (Fig. 8).

(a) **(b)**

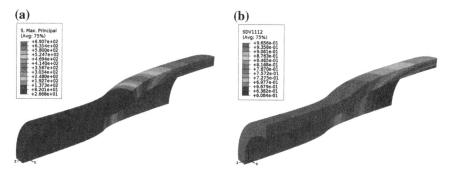

Fig. 8 Stress and average damage at the end of the analysis [47]. **a** Maximal principal Cauchy stress map. **b** Average damage map

5 Conclusions

It is well known that vascular tissues are subject to finite deformations and that their mechanical behavior is highly nonlinear, anisotropic and essentially incompressible with non-zero residual stress and in the non-physiological domain presents viscous and damage behavior and there is significant dispersion in the orientation, which has a significant influence on the mechanical response. The high complexity of biological tissues requires mechanical models that include information of the underlying constituents and look for the physics of the whole processes within the material. This behavior of the micro-constituents can be taken into macroscopic models by means of computational homogenization. It is in this context where the microsphere-based approach acquires high relevance.

In this chapter, we have provided a critical review of the fundamental aspects in modeling this kind of the materials. The application of these constitutive relationships in the context of vascular system has been presented. The increasing effort devoted to studies of mechanical models for soft fibred tissues and the applications aimed at refining basic and clinical analysis demonstrates the vitality of the field of biomechanics [29]. With this approach, a more realistic response of the inelastic evolution is expected due to a smoother transition of the damage in the micro scale. We have limited ourself to an affine model, without taking into account the existing cross-links between fibrils nor the sliding between fibers and matrix [48]. Models presented herein are based on purely passive baseline elasticity. Smooth muscle cells display an important active response, the myogenic tone, which allows the arterial wall to contract or expand acutely to maintain a baseline lumen.

Computational models can help to understand the underlying mechanochemical processes and provide a framework for biological and clinical researchers to jointly enhance the pharmagolocial or surgical management.

Acknowledgments This work was supported by the Spanish Ministry of Economy and Competitiveness (DPI2010-20746-C03-01 and PRI-AIBDE-2011-1216) and the Instituto de Salud Carlos III (ISCIII) through the CIBER initiative and the Plataform for Biological Tissue Characterization of CIBER-BBN. CIBER-BBN is an initiative funded by the VI National R&D&i Plan 2008–2011, Iniciativa Ingenio 2010, Consolider Program, CIBER Actions and financed by the Instituto de Salud Carlos III with assistance from the European Regional Development Fund.

References

1. V. Alastrué, M. A. Martinez, A. Menzel, and M. Doblare. On the use of non-linear transformations for the evaluation of anisotropic rotationally symmetric directional integrals. application to the stress analysis in fibred soft tissues. *Int J Numer Meth Biom Eng*, 79:474–504, 2009.
2. V. Alastrué, M. A. Martínez, M. Doblaré, and A. Menzel. Anisotropic micro-sphere-based finite elasticity applied to blood vessel modelling. *J Mech Phys Solids*, 57:178–203, 2009.
3. V. Alastrué, E. Peña, M. A. Martínez, and M. Doblaré. Experimental study and constitutive modelling of the passive mechanical properties of the ovine infrarenal vena cava tissue. *J Biomech*, 41:3038–3045, 2008.
4. V. Alastrué, J. F. Rodríguez, B. Calvo, and M. Doblaré. Structural damage models for fibrous biological soft tissues. *Int J Solids Struc*, 44:5894–5911, 2007.
5. V. Alastrué, P. Saez, M. A. Martínez, and M. Doblaré. On the use of bingham statistical distribution in microsphere-based constitutive models fo arterial tissue. *Mech Res Commun*, 37:700–706, 2010.
6. E. M. Arruda and M. C. Boyce. A three-Ddimensional constitutive model for the large stretch behavior of rubber elastic materials. *J Mech Phys Solids*, 41:389–412, 1993.
7. C. Bingham. An antipodally summetric distribution on the sphere. *Ann Stat*, 2:1201–1225, 1974.
8. J. Bonet and R. D. Wood. *Nonlinear Continuum Mechanics for Finite Element Analysis*. Cambridge University Press, Cambridge, 2008.
9. B. Calvo, E. Peña, P. Martins, T. Mascarenhas, M. Doblare, R. Natal, and A. Ferreira. On modelling damage process in vaginal tissue. *J Biomech*, 42:642–651, 2009.
10. B. Calvo, E. Peña, M. A. Martínez, and M. Doblaré. An uncoupled directional damage model for fibered biological soft tissues. Formulation and computational aspects. *Int J Numer Meth Engng*, 69:2036–2057, 2007.
11. P. B. Canham, H. M. Finlay, and D. R. Boughner. Contrasting structure of the saphenous vein and internal mammary artery used as coronary bypass vessels. *Cardiovasc Res*, 34:557–567, 1997.
12. P. B. Canham, H. M. Finlay, J. G. Dixon, D. R. Boughner, and A. Chen. Measurements from light and polarised light microscopy of human coronary arteries fixed at distending pressure. *Cardiovasc Res*, 23:973–982, 1989.
13. H. Demiray, H. W. Weizsacker, K. Pascale, and H. Erbay. A stress-strain relation for a rat abdominal aorta. *J Biomech*, 21:369–374, 1988.
14. K.P. Dingemans, P. Teeling, J. H. Lagendijk, and A. E. Becker. Extracellular matrix of the human aortic media: an ultrastructural histochemical and immunohistochemical study of the adult aortic media. *Anat Rec*, 258:1–14, 2000.
15. H. M. Finlay, L. McCullough, and P. B. Canham. Three-dimensional collagen organization of human brain arteries at different transmural pressures. *J Vasc Res*, 32:301–312, 1995.
16. P. J. Flory. Thermodynamic relations for high elastic materials. *Trans Faraday Soc*, 57:829–838, 1961.

17. Y. C. Fung, K. Fronek, and P. Patitucci. Pseudoelasticity of arteries and the choice of its mathematical expression. *Am J Physiol*, 237:H620–H631, 1979.

18. A. García. *Experimental and numerical framework for modelling vascular diseases and medical devices*. PhD thesis, University of Zaragoza, Spain, Division of Solids and Structural Mechanics, 2012.

19. A. García, M. A. Martínez, and E. Peña. Determination and Modeling of the Inelasticity Over the Length of the Porcine Carotid Artery. *ASME J Biomech Eng*, 135:031004–1, 2013.

20. A. García, E. Peña, A. Laborda, F. Lostalé, M. A. De Gregorio, M. Doblaré, and M. A. Martínez. Experimental study and constitutive modelling of the passive mechanical properties of the porcine carotid artery and its relation to histological analysis. Implications in animal cardiovascular device trials. *Med Eng Phys*, 33:665–676, 2011.

21. A. García, E. Peña, and M. A. Martínez. Viscoelastic properties of the passive mechanical behavior of the porcine carotid artery: Influence of proximal and distal positions. *Biorheology*, 49:271–288, 2012.

22. P. Sáez, A. García, E. Peña, T.C. Gasser and M. A. Martínez. Microstructural analysis of fiber orientation in swine carotid artery: structural quantification and constitutive modelling. *Submitted*, 2015.

23. T. C. Gasser, R. W. Ogden, and G. A. Holzapfel. Hyperelastic modelling of arterial layers with distributed collagen fibre orientations. *J R Soc Interface*, 3:15–35, 2006.

24. S. Govindjee, G. J. Kay, and J. C. Simo. Anisotropic modelling and numerical simulation of brittle damage in concrete. *Int J Numer Meth Engng*, 38:3611–3633, 1995.

25. C. S. Herz. Bessel functions of matrix argument. *Ann Math*, 61:474–523, 1955.

26. G. A. Holzapfel, T. C. Gasser, and R. W. Ogden. A new constitutive framework for arterial wall mechanics and a comparative study of material models. *J Elasticity*, 61:1–48, 2000.

27. G. A. Holzapfel, T. C. Gasser, and M. Stadler. A structural model for the viscoelastic behaviour of arterial walls: Continuum formultaion and finite element analysis. *Eur J Mech A/ Solids*, 21:441–463, 2002.

28. G. A. Holzapfel and R. W. Ogden. Constitutive modelling of passive myocardium: a structurally based framework for material characterization. *Phil Trans R Soc A*, 367:3445–3475, 2009.

29. G. A. Holzapfel and R. W. Ogden. Constitutive modelling of arteries. *Phil Trans R Soc A*, 466:1551–1597, 2010.

30. E. W. Hsu, A. L. Muzikant, S. A. Matulevicius, R. C. Penland, and C. S. Henriquez. Magnetic resonance myocardial fiber-orientation mapping with direct histological correlation. *Am J Physiol HeartCirc Physiol*, 274:H1627–H1634, 1998.

31. J. D. Humphrey. Mechanics of the arterial wall: Review and directions. *Crit Rev Biomed Eng*, 23:1–162, 1995.

32. J. W. Ju. On energy-based coupled elastoplastic damage theories: Constitutive modeling and computational aspects. *Int J Solids Struct*, 25:803–833, 1989.

33. Y. Lanir. A structural theory for the homogeneous biaxial stress-strain relationship in flat collageneous tissues. *J Biomech*, 12:423–436, 1979.

34. Y. Lanir. Constitutive equations for fibrous connective tissues. *J Biomech*, 16:1–12, 1983.

35. E. Maher, M. Early, A. Creane, C Lally, and D. J. Kelly. Site specific inelasticity of arterial tissue. *J Biomech*, 45:1393–1399, 2012.

36. D. W. Marquardt. An algorithm for least-squares estimation of nonlinear parameters. *Siam J Appl Math*, 11:431–441, 1963.

37. J. E. Marsden and T. J. R. Hughes. *Mathematical Foundations of Elasticity*. Dover, New York, 1994.

38. E. Peña. ". Application to soft biological tissues. *Comp Mech*, 48:407–420, 2011.

39. E. Peña. Prediction of the softening and damage effects with permanent set in fibrous biological materials. *J Mech Phys Solids*, 59:1808–1822, 2011.

40. E. Peña. Computational aspects of the numerical modelling of softening, damage and permanent set in soft biological tissues. *Comput Struct*, 130:57–72, 2014.

41. E. Peña, V. Alastrue, A. Laborda, M. A. Martínez, and M. Doblare. A constitutive formulation of vascular tissue mechanics including viscoelasticity and softening behaviour. *J Biomech*, 43:984–989, 2010.

42. E. Peña, A. Pérez del Palomar, B. Calvo, M. A. Martínez, and M. Doblaré. Computational modelling of diarthrodial joints. Physiological, pathological and pos-surgery simulations. *Arch Comput Method Eng*, 14(1):47–91, 2007.

43. E. Peña, P. Martins, T. Mascarenhas, R. M. Natal-Jorge, A. Ferreira, M. Doblaré, and B. Calvo. Mechanical characterization of the softening behavior of human vaginal tissue. *J Mech Behav Biomed*, 4:275–283, 2011.

44. E. Peña, J. A. Peña, and M. Doblaré. On the Mullins effect and hysteresis of fibered biological materials: A comparison between continuous and discontinuous damage models. *Int J Solids Struct*, 46:1727–1735, 2009.

45. J. F. Rodríguez, V. Alastrue, and M. Doblaré. Finite element implementation of a stochastic three dimensional finite-strain damage model for fibrous soft tissue. *Comput Methods Appl Mech Engrg*, 197:946–958, 2008.

46. J. F. Rodríguez, F. Cacho, J. A. Bea, and M. Doblaré. A stochastic-structurally based three dimensional finite-strain damage model for fibrous soft tissue. *J Mech Phys Solids*, 54:564–886, 2006.

47. P. Sáez, V. Alastrué, E. Peña, M. Doblaré, and M. A. Martínez. Anisotropic microsphere-based approach to damage in soft fibered tissue. *Biomechan Model Mechanobiol*, 11:595–608, 2012.

48. P. Sáez, E. Peña, and M. A. Martínez. A structural approach including the behavior of collagen cross-links to model patient-specific human carotid arteries. *Ann Biomed Eng*, 42:1158–1169, 2014.

49. J. C. Simo. On a fully three-dimensional finite-strain viscoelastic damage model: Formulation and computational aspects. *Comput Methods Appl Mech Engrg*, 60:153–173, 1987.

50. J. C. Simo and J. W. Ju. Strain- and stress-based continuum damage models. I. Formulation. *Int J Solids Struct*, 23:821–840, 1987.

51. J. C. Simo and J. W. Ju. Strain- and stress-based continuum damage models. II. Computational aspects. *Int J Solids Struct*, 23:841–870, 1987.

52. J. C. Simo, R. L. Taylor, and K. S. Pister. Variational and projection methods for the volume constraint in finite deformation elasto-plasticity. *Comput Methods Appl Mech Engrg*, 51:177–208, 1985.

53. J. F. Smith, P. B. Canham, and J. Starkey. Orientation of collagen in the tunica adventitia of the human cerebral artery measured with polarized light and the universal stage. *J Ultrastruct Res*, 77:133–45, 1981.

54. D. P. Sokolis. A passive strain-energy function for elastic and muscular arteries: correlation of material parameters with histological data. *Med Biol Eng Comput*, 48:507–518, 2010.

55. A. J. M. Spencer. Theory of Invariants. In *Continuum Physics*, pages 239–253. Academic Press, New York, 1971.

56. K. Takamizawa and K. Hayashi. Strain-Energy Density-Function and Uniform Strain Hypothesis for Arterial Mechanics. *J Biomech*, 20:7–17, 1987.

57. A. Tobolsky, I. Prettyman, and J Dillon. Stress relaxation of natural and synthetic rubber stocks. *J Appl Phys*, 15:380–395, 1944.

58. C.N. van den Broek, A. van der Horst, M. C. M. Rutten, and F. N. van de Vosse. A generic constitutive model for the passive porcine coronary artery. *Biomech Mod Mechanobiol*, 10:249–258, 2011.

59. J. A. Weiss, B. N. Maker, and S.Govindjee. Finite element implementation of incompressible, transversely isotropic hyperelasticity. *Comput Methods Appl Mech Engrg*, 135:107–128, 1996.

60. A. S. Wineman and K. R. Rajagopal. On a constitutive theory for materials undergoing microstructural changes. *Arch Mech*, 42:53–75, 1990.

61. R. Wulandana and A. M. Robertson. An inelastic multi-mechanism constitutive equation for cerebral arterial tissue. *Biomech Model Mechanbiol*, 4:235–248, 2005.

62. M. Zullinger, P. Fridez, K. Hayashi, and N. Stergiopulos. A strain energy function for arteries accounting for wall composition and structure. *J Biomech*, 37:989–1000, 2004.
63. M. Zullinger, A. Rachev, and N. Stergiopulos. A constitutive formulation of arterial mechanics including vascular smooth muscle tone. *Am J Physiol Heart Circ Physiol*, 287:H1335–H1343, 2004.

What Exists in the Scientific Literature About Biomechanical Models in Pelvic Floor?—a Systematic Review

Renato Andrade, Rui Viana, Sara Viana, Thuane da Roza,
Teresa Mascarenhas and R.M. Natal Jorge

Abstract To date, several relevant models to the female pelvic support system have been built. Recently, scientific literature has demonstrated biomechanical models as an alternative to better understand and assess the pelvic floor muscles. Biomechanical modelling is a useful approach for investigate the association between pelvic floor defects and stress urinary incontinence or prolapse. Computational models are already a reality and in the future may represent a significant tool for the study of pelvic floor pathophysiology. However, only a few studies used biomechanical models to assess the pelvic floor muscles.

Keywords Pelvic floor · Computational models · Biomechanical model · Female

1 Introduction

Recently, scientific literature has demonstrated biomechanical models as an alternative to better understand and assess the pelvic floor muscles (PFM). Janda et al. [1] conducted an important research which used magnetic resonance imaging and

R. Andrade (✉) · R. Viana · S. Viana
UFP—University of Fernando Pessoa, Porto, Portugal
e-mail: 23781@ufp.edu.pt

R. Viana · S. Viana
CHSJ:EPE, Porto, Portugal

T. da Roza · R.M. Natal Jorge
IDMEC-Polo FEUP, Faculty of Engineering of University of Porto,
Porto, Portugal
e-mail: rnatal@fe.up.pt

T. da Roza
CIAFEL—Faculty of Sport of University of Porto, Research Centre
in Physical Activity, Health and Leisure, Porto, Portugal

T. Mascarenhas
Faculty of Medicine, University of Porto, Porto, Portugal

© Springer International Publishing Switzerland 2015
J.M.R.S. Tavares and R.M. Natal Jorge (eds.), *Computational and Experimental Biomechanical Sciences: Methods and Applications*, Lecture Notes in Computational Vision and Biomechanics 21, DOI 10.1007/978-3-319-15799-3_3

3D-palpator measurements on a cadaver specimen to collect data for studying the PFM behavior using a computer model based on the Finite Element Model (FEM) theory.

The FEM method is a tool of mathematic simulation consisting in discretization of a continuous model in small pieces, preserving their properties of the original model. This method has the advantage of being able to model structures and indirectly quantify their mechanical behavior under any theoretical conditions [2]. The FEM of the pelvic floor shows to have several applications: (1) allows making hypothesis about the anatomical and physiological pelvic supporting system. These hypotheses can be introduced in the FEM system and can be validated when compared to the evolution of the normal and pathological patient; (2) could help to understand the pelvic organ prolapsed and the incontinence mechanism. The model can be developed for a single patient with their anatomy, vaginal forces and pelvic tissues for a generalised global approach; (3) the models also could be useful to develop special tools for diagnosis of patients with risk of genital prolapse and therefore develop prevention strategies in case of pregnancy or pelvic surgery; (4) the simulation results of patients will allow offering an individual optimized therapeutic strategy [3].

Therefore, biomechanical modelling can be a useful approach for investigate the pelvic floor dysfunctions, the vaginal birth and how the PFM function. The main objective of this study was to systematize the information concerning biomechanical models of the PMF.

2 Methods

A search strategy was developed to search the electronic databases of Pubmed to look for published studies involving biomechanical models of the PFM. These electronic databases were searched between 2000 and 2013. The key-words used were: pelvic floor; computational models; biomechanical model; female; the logic operators used were (AND, OR). Our search strategy followed the PRISMA Flow Diagram (Fig. 1).

The inclusion criteria were: human studies; written in English language and biomechanical models to the PFM. The exclusion criteria were: reviews and meta-analyzes; PFM studies using ultra-sound and magnetic resonance images instead of biomechanical models. After selection, studies were analyzed based on their protocol, results and findings.

3 Results

Were included 14 studies that investigated the biomechanical models of the PFM. From the studies, 6 concerned about the vaginal birth, 3 analyzed the PFM function and 5 explored the PFM disorders (Table 1). Three studies were excluded once they

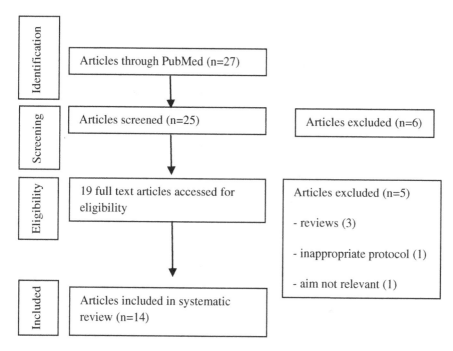

Fig. 1 PRISMA flow diagram

were reviews; one because its aim was not analyze vaginal birth, PFM function or PFM disorders; and another because used ultrasound and magnetic resonance images to asses PFM instead of 3D models.

The ones that investigated the vaginal birth shown that pubococcygeus and levantor ani muscles had the greatest risk for stretch-related injury. Flexion of the fetal head during vaginal delivery may facilitate and protect the PFM during birth. Also the "peak push" reduced energy expenses when compared to "triple push" [2, 4, 5, 7–9].

Regarding PFM function, studies demonstrated that due to the geometry of PFM fibers, these muscles could increase the stiffness of the pelvic ring [1, 11, 12].

The studies concerning PFM disorders reported the significance of PFM strength in vaginal support, mainly related to urinary (in) continence. Prolapse results shown an impairment of the muscular and apical supports of the anterior vaginal wall. The models also illustrate the repartitioning of different stress, strain and intra-abdominal pressure either in pelvic organs or in the ligaments [3, 13–16].

Table 1 Study characteristics

Ref.	Issue	Objective	Data source	Protocol	Results	Findings
Lien et al. [4]	Vaginal birth	Develop a 3D computer model to predict LA muscle stretch during vaginal birth	Serial MRI from a healthy nulliparous 34-year-old woman, published anatomic data, and engineering graphics software	Construction of a structural model of the LA muscles along with related passive tissues. The model was used to quantify PMF stretch induced during the second stage of labor as a model fetal head progressively engaged and then stretched the iliococcygeus, pubococcygeus, and puborectalis muscles	The largest tissue strain reached a stretch ratio (tissue length under stretch/original tissue length) of 3.26 in medial pubococcygeus muscle, the shortest, most medial and ventral LA muscle. Regions of the ileococcygeus, pubococcygeus, and puborectalis muscles reached maximal stretch ratios of 2.73, 2.50, and 2.28, respectively. Tissue stretch ratios were proportional to fetal head size: For example, increasing fetal head diameter by 9 % increased medial pubococcygeus stretch by the same amount	The medial pubococcygeus muscles undergo the largest stretch of any LA muscles during vaginal birth. They are therefore at the greatest risk for stretch-related injury
Parente et al. [5]	Vaginal birth	Represent the effects that the passage of the fetal head can induce on PFM	Experimental data produced by Janda et al. [1, 6]	Modified form of a incompressible transversely isotropic hyperelastic model	The logarithmic maximum principal strain along the curve is approximately the same for the three different PFM behaviors	Non-invasive procedure which can estimate the damage that a vaginal delivery can induce on a specific PF

(continued)

Table 1 (continued)

Ref.	Issue	Objective	Data source	Protocol	Results	Findings
Parente et al. [2]	Vaginal birth	Investigate the influence of the fetal head flexion during a vaginal delivery with a 3D FEM	Data was obtained from Janda et al. [1], Martins et al. [16]. Parente et al. [5, 7, 10]	FEM of the pelvic skeletal structure, PF, and fetus was developed. The movements of the fetus during birth were simulated in engagement, descent flexion, internal rotation, and extension of the fetal head. The opposite forces against the fetal descent and the stress of the PFM were obtain on simulations with different degrees of head flexion	The simulated increase in fetal head flexion is associated with lower values of opposite forces against the fetal descent. The descending fetus with abnormal flexion head meets resistance in later stations. Lower stress in the PF was demonstrated with simulated increase in fetal head flexion during vaginal delivery	The analytic evidence suggests that the fetal head flexion during vaginal delivery may facilitate birth and protect the PF
Parente et al. [7]	Vaginal birth	Contribute to the clarification of the mechanisms behind PF disorders related to a vaginal delivery and verify the effect values when compared to the normal occipito-anterior position	Data obtained from cadaver measurements conducted by Janda et al. [1]	A FEM representing the effects of the fetal head passage induced on the PFM, from a mechanical point of view. The model represents the pelvic bones, with PFM attached and the fetus. It was also simulated the movements of the fetus during birth, in vertex position, with the fetus presenting in an occipito-posterior malposition	A maximum stretch value of 1.73 was obtained in the numerical simulation, where the occipito-posterior malposition was simulated	During a vaginal delivery, the LA and the pubococcygeus muscle are the ones subjected to the largest values of stretch and strain. They are at greater risk for a stretch related injury. The occipito-posterior malposition produces substantially higher values for the PFM, increasing the risk for a stretch related injury

(continued)

Table 1 (continued)

Ref.	Issue	Objective	Data source	Protocol	Results	Findings
Li et al. [8]	Vaginal birth	Investigate the effects of anisotropy by varying the relative stiffness between the fiber and the matrix components, whilst maintaining the same overall stress–strain response in the fiber direction	Data used from Kruger et al. [18, 19]	A foetal skull was passed through two PF models, which incorporated the LA muscle with different anisotropy ratios	Substantial decrease in the magnitude of the force required for delivery as the fibre anisotropy was increased. The anisotropy ratio markedly affected the mechanical response of the LA muscle during a simulated vaginal delivery	The presented models may advance our understanding of the injury mechanisms of PF during childbirth
Lien et al. [9]	Vaginal birth	Develop and use a biomechanical computer model to simulate the effect of varying the timing of voluntary maternal pushes during uterine contraction on second-stage labor duration	The initial geometry of female PF at the beginning of the second stage of labor was based on MRI of a healthy woman taken from Lien et al. [4]	A simplified 3D biomechanical model with six representative viscoelastic LA muscle bands interconnected by a hyperelastic iliococcygeal raphé. An incompressible sphere simulated the molded fetal head. Forces from uterine contraction and voluntary expulsive efforts were summed to push the model fetal head along the Curve of Carus opposed by the resistance of the PF structures to stretch	Calculated second stage durations ranged from 57.5 min ("triple" or Pre-Peak- Post pattern) to 75.8 min ("pre-push" and "post-push" patterns). Delivery with the "triple push" pattern required 59 voluntary pushes, while the "peak push" pattern required 23 voluntary pushes, a 61 % reduction. The corresponding reduction for the "pre-and-peak push" pattern was 29 %, the "peak-and-post push" pattern was 30 %, the "pre-push" pattern was 54 %, and the "post-push" pattern was 56 %	Although the "triple push" pattern resulted in a 16 % shorter second stage, this came at the energetic expense of a 61 % increase in the number of pushes required

(continued)

Table 1 (continued)

Ref.	Issue	Objective	Data source	Protocol	Results	Findings
Janda et al. [1]	PFM	Obtain a complete data set needed for studying the complex biomechanical behaviour of the PFM using a FEM	A 3D geometric data set of the PF including muscle fibre directions was obtained using a palpator device. Apart from these measurements they obtained a data set of the PF structures based on nuclear MRI on the same cadaver specimen	Semi-automated gradient-oriented segmentation of the MRI scans. A 3D reconstruction of the PMF. Mostly sarcomere lengths were at or just below the optimal muscle length. Numerical comparison of two triangle model meshes	A set of MRI measurements, cadaver measurements and a model comparison. Mean surface-to-surface distance square error is 3.9 mm	The produced data set is not only important for biomechanical modelling of the PFM, but it also describes the geometry of muscle fibres and is useful for functional analysis of the PF in general
Pool-Goudzwaard et al. [11]	PFM	To gain insight into the effect of tension in the PMF on stiffness of the pelvic ring	Data recoiled from dissection of 18 embalmed specimens	Assessment of the relationship between rotation angle and moment. Application of springs to the pelvis to simulate tension in PFM	In females, simulated tension in the PFM stiffened the sacroiliac joints with 8.5 % ($p < 0.05$). In males, no significant changes occurred. In both sexes a backward rotation of the sacrum occurred due to simulated tension in the PFM ($p < 0.05$). The sacroiliac joints of female specimens were more mobile comparing to the male specimens ($p < 0.05$)	In females, PFM have the capacity to increase the stiffness of the pelvic ring. Furthermore, these muscles can generate a backward rotation of the sacrum in both sexes

(continued)

Table 1 (continued)

Ref.	Issue	Objective	Data source	Protocol	Results	Findings
Noakes et al. [12]	PFM	Present simulation results of LA function using FEM on computational meshes based on live subject data	An anatomically realistic female PF model, based on live subject MRI data [17]	The LA muscle mesh was used as the domain over which the governing equations of finite elasticity were solved using the FEM with a Mooney-Rivlin material law. Deformation of the LA was simulated during a 'bear down' maneuver in order to visualize the way this muscle group functions in an asymptomatic subject. A pressure of 4 kPa was imposed on the mesh and the computed mesh displacements were compared to those obtained from dynamic MRI	The RMS error for this movement was 0.7 mm equating to a percentage error of 2.6 % in the supero-inferior direction and 13.7 mm or 74.5 % in the antero-posterior direction	The functional simulation performed produced promising results which were consistent with live experimental data taken from the subject. The benefits of the inclusion of a detailed anisotropic material laws and more realistic boundary conditions are unknown at this stage, but may enable improved simulation accuracy

(continued)

Table 1 (continued)

Ref.	Issue	Objective	Data source	Protocol	Results	Findings
Rao et al. [3]	PF disorders	Establish a geometrical 3D model, characterizing the mechanical behaviour of tissues and ligaments implied in pelvic static, the definition of the boundary conditions in displacement and numerical loading of the model	The model comes from a single patient without genital prolapse but who was presented with a fibroid of the uterus that explains the lateral deviation of the uterus	An FEM mesh is generated for all the individual parts and then reassembled. The geometric model is meshed with shell elements with different wall thickness for various subregions of each organ	The bladder, vagina, uterus and rectum move down as the load increases, except for the top portion of the rectum. The maximum strain occurs at the boundary of vagina and rectum and is found to be in the order of 0.2 MPa with five pairs of ligaments and 0.5 MPa with eight ligaments. The maximum strain seems to occur in the upper anterior part of the vagina	The presented model is found to be very important for a better understanding of pelvic disorders, as it allows understanding more accurately the repartitioning of the different stress and strain in either organs or in the ligaments
Noakes et al. [13]	PF disorders	Provide a framework with which to examine the mechanics of normal function and stability in the PF, and abnormalities associated with the defecation disorders fecal incontinence and obstructed defecation	Anatomical data from the Visible Human Project was used to provide the anatomical positioning of each model component within the region of interest	Creation of a 3D cubic Hermite FEM mesh using an iterative linear fitting procedure (RMS error of fit <2 mm)	Results for each PF component in the Visible Man gave a RMS error less than 2 mm	These models will provide a framework with which to examine the mechanics of normal function and the abnormalities associated with the defecation disorders fecal incontinence and obstructed defecation

(continued)

Table 1 (continued)

Ref.	Issue	Objective	Data source	Protocol	Results	Findings
Yip et al. [14]	PF disorders	Explore the contribution of PFM defect to the development of SUI	From a pool of 135 patients, clinical data of 26 patients with pelvic muscular defect were used in modelling	The model was employed to estimate the parameters that describe the stiffness properties of the vaginal wall and ligament tissues for individual patients. The parameters were then implemented into the model to evaluate for each patient the impact of PFM defect on the vaginal apex support and the bladder neck support	For the modelling analysis, the compromise of pelvic muscular support was demonstrated to contribute to vaginal apex prolapse and bladder neck prolapse, a condition commonly seen in SUI patients, while simulated conditions of restored muscular support were shown to help. reestablish both vaginal apex support and bladder neck supports	The findings illustrate the significance of PFM strength to vaginal support and urinary continence; therefore, the clinical recommendation of pelvic muscle strengthening, such as Kegel exercises, has been shown to be an effective treatment for patients with SUI symptoms
Chen et al. [15]	PF disorders	Use a biomechanical model to explore how impairment of the pubovisceral portion of the LA muscle and/ or the apical vaginal suspension might interact to affect anterior vaginal wall prolapse severity	The dimensions and orientation of the anterior vaginal wall and its support system were measured from mid-sagittal plane MRI scans of 10 healthy volunteers with no symptoms of incontinence or prolapse	The anterior vaginal wall and main muscular and connective tissue support elements, namely the levator plate, pubovisceral muscle, cardinal and uterosacral ligaments, were included and their geometry based on mid-sagittal plane MRIs. The change in the sagittal profile of the anterior vaginal wall during a maximum Valsalva was then simulated when different combinations of muscle and connective tissue impairment were present	A 90 % impairment of apical support led to an increase in anterior wall prolapse from 0.3 to 1.9 cm (a 530 % increase) at 60 % pubovisceral muscle impairment, and from 0.7 to 2.4 cm (a 240 % increase) at 80 % pubovisceral muscle impairment	The presented results suggest that a prolapse can develop as a result of impairment of the muscular and apical supports of the anterior vaginal wall

Table 1 (continued)

Ref.	Issue	Objective	Data source	Protocol	Results	Findings
Martins et al. [16]	PF disorders	Evaluate the PF tension response during simulated increased intra-abdominal pressure and the vaginal biomechanical properties	Development of a FEM based on MRIs from a nulliparous healthy volunteer without urinary incontinence or genital prolapse. Fifteen female cadavers were evaluated to assess the biomechanical properties of vaginal tissue	FEM of PMF was created from 20 MRIs. The MRIs was used to drawn manually the PFM and then the 3D model were generate. Using the software *Abaqus*, the FEM model composed by tetrahedral elements and with the appropriate boundary conditions were used to simulate an IAP of 1×10^{-1} MPa (90 cm H_2O), applied to the inner surface of the PFM. The stresses in the PFM were evaluated in the longitudinal and transversal axes	Inter-rater correlations of the pubovisceral muscle cross-section area measurements were excellent for the anterior (ICC 0.9413, 95 % CI 0.7068–0.9882), middle (ICC 0.9562, 95 % CI 0.8263–0.9930) and posterior (ICC 0.9518, 95 % CI 0.7594–0.9904) compartments of the FE model. There was no difference between the longitudinal and transversal axes PF state stress under simulated IAP ($p = 0.891$). There was a great variability in the measurements of stiffness and maximum stress in vaginal tissues. The stiffness ranged from 2.7 to 15.7 MPa, with a mean of 6.6 ± 0.9 MPa. The mean maximum stress was 2.6 ± 0.4, ranging from 0.9 to 6.4 MPa. The vaginal tissue presented an isotropic biomechanical behavior	Isotropic biomechanical behavior of the vagina is in agreement with the PF stress state during conditions with increased IAP

Legend 3D—Three dimensional; LA—Levantor ani muscle; MRI—Magnetic resonance image; PFM—Pelvic floor muscle; PF—Pelvic floor; FEM—Finite element model; RMS—Root mean square; SUI—Stress urinary incontinence; ICC—Intraclass correlation coefficient; CI—Confidence interval; IAP—Intra-abdominal pressure; MPa—Megapascal

4 Discussion

The FEM of the pelvic floor are useful to understand the PFM function, their disorders and to study the implications of the vaginal birth on it.

The biomechanical studies concerning the vaginal birth shown that the medial pubococcygeus muscles are the ones that undergo the largest stretch and strain of any *levantor ani* muscles during vaginal birth. They are therefore at the greatest risk for stretch-related to injury [4, 7]. Parente et al., demonstrated that fetal head flexion during vaginal delivery can may facilitate the birth and protect the PFM [6]. When compared to the normal occipito-anterior position, the occipito-posterior malposition produces substantially higher values for the PFM, increasing the risk for a stretch related injury [7]. Although the "triple push" pattern resulted in a 16 % shorter second stage, this came at the energetic expense of a 61 % increase in the number of pushes required [9].

The utilization of different material parameters to simulate the PFM behavior is essential to obtain the correct results. The computer model presented in Parente et al. [5] is the first step in understanding how obstetrical factors and interventions might influence *levator ani* injury risk, since experimental measurements of *levator ani* stretch in laboring women are not currently feasible for many clinician, technical and ethical reasons. Using different measuring techniques, like magnetic resonance imaging, the model presented in this study can also be applied to women in reproductive age. Therefore, their work shown a non-invasive procedure which can estimate the damage that a vaginal delivery can induce on a specific PFM. The models may advance our understanding of the injury mechanisms on pelvic floor during childbirth [8].

Studies exploring the geometry of PFM fibers shown that the increase of tension in PFM, viz. the combination of pubococcygeus, iliococcygeus and coccygeus muscles, stiffens the female sacroiliac joints and hence the pelvic ring. Furthermore, these muscles can generate a backward rotation of the sacrum in both sexes [11]. The produced data set on Janda et al. study [1] is not only important due to the PFM biomechanical modelling, but it also describes the geometry of muscle fibers that is useful for functional analysis of the PFM. The PFM simulation reproduced, demonstrated promising results which were consistent with live experimental data taken from the individual. The benefits of the inclusion of a detailed anisotropic material laws and more realistic boundary conditions are unknown at this stage, but may enable improved simulation accuracy [12].

The biomechanical models shown to be useful to better understand the pelvic floor disorders. In particular the model presented by Rao et al. [3] appears to be very important, as it allows understanding more accurately the repartitioning of the different stress and strain in either organs or in the ligaments. Isotropic biomechanical behavior of the vagina is in agreement with the pelvic floor stress state during conditions with increased intra-abdominal pressure [16]. A prolapse can develop as a result of impairment of the muscular and apical supports of the anterior vaginal wall [15]. The components (puborectalis, *levantor ani*, rectum, internal and external sphincters, obturator internus, vagina, uterus, bladder, pubis, coccyx, transverse perineae, perineal body and the bulbospongiosus muscle) appear clearer in the female images which consequently improves the accuracy of digitization and hence the female model. In addition, the rectum and anal canal in the male data set appear to be squashed and do not lie in normal orientation that is expected in live subjects—caused by the post-mortem perineal pressure—that does not allow an accurate representation of the pelvic floor region [13]. The findings illustrate the significance of PFM strength to vaginal support and urinary continence. Therefore, the clinical recommendation of pelvic muscle strengthening, such as Kegel exercises, has been shown to be an effective treatment for patients with urinary incontinence symptoms [14].

5 Conclusion

From this systematic review it can be concluded that biomechanical models of the PFM it is helpful to better understand the PFM functions, it behavior and how we can manage their disorders. Computational models are already a reality and in the future may represent a significant tool for the study of pelvic floor pathophysiology. However, until now, few studies used biomechanical models to assess the PFM. Therefore, we suggest more investigation, through well-designed studies with a larger data sample to better standardize the values, to assess the PFM behavior on vaginal birth and also their role to prevent and restore the normality from pelvic floor dysfunctions. The studies should also include ligaments, fascial and pelvic organs, once it is important to assess the pelvic floor complex as a whole and build a biotensegrity model.

Acknowledgments The authors gratefully acknowledge to the funding by CNPq—from Brazil government and the project Pest-OE/EME/LA0022/2013 and also to the project "Biomechanics: contributions to the healthcare", reference NORTE-07-0124-FEDER-000035 co-financed by Programa Operacional Regional do Norte (ON.2—O Novo Norte), through the Fundo Europeu de Desenvolvimento Regional (FEDER).

References

1. Janda, Š., van der Helm, F. C., & de Blok, S. B. (2003). Measuring morphological parameters of the pelvic floor for finite element modelling purposes. *Journal of biomechanics 36*(6):749-757.
2. Parente, M. P., Natal Jorge, R. M., Mascarenhas, T., Fernandes, A. A., & Silva-Filho, A. L. (2010). Computational modeling approach to study the effects of fetal head flexion during vaginal delivery. *American journal of obstetrics and gynecology 203*(3):217-e1.
3. Venugopala Rao, G., Rubod, C., Brieu, M., Bhatnagar, N., & Cosson, M. (2010). Experiments and finite element modelling for the study of prolapse in the pelvic floor system. *Computer methods in biomechanics and biomedical engineering, 13*(3), 349-357.

4. Lien, K. C., Mooney, B., DeLancey, J. O., & Ashton-Miller, J. A. (2004). Levator ani muscle stretch induced by simulated vaginal birth. *Obstetrics and gynecology, 103*(1), 31.

5. Parente, M. P. L., Natal Jorge, R. M., Mascarenhas, T., Fernandes, A. A., & Martins, J. A. C. (2009). The influence of the material properties on the biomechanical behavior of the pelvic floor muscles during vaginal delivery. *Journal of biomechanics, 42*(9), 1301-1306.

6. Janda, S. (2006). Biomechanics of the pelvic floor musculature (Vol. 55, pp. 367-381).

7. Parente, M. P. L., Jorge, R. M., Mascarenhas, T., Fernandes, A. A., & Martins, J. A. C. (2009). The influence of an occipito-posterior malposition on the biomechanical behavior of the pelvic floor. *European Journal of Obstetrics & Gynecology and Reproductive Biology, 144*, S166-S169.

8. Li, X., Kruger, J. A., Nash, M. P., & Nielsen, P. M. (2011). Anisotropic effects of the levator ani muscle during childbirth. *Biomechanics and modeling in mechanobiology, 10*(4), 485-494.

9. Lien, K. C., DeLancey, J. O., & Ashton-Miller, J. A. (2009). Biomechanical analyses of the efficacy of patterns of maternal effort on second-stage progress.*Obstetrics and gynecology, 113* (4), 873.

10. Parente, M. P. L., Jorge, R. N., Mascarenhas, T., Fernandes, A. A., & Martins, J. A. C. (2008). Deformation of the pelvic floor muscles during a vaginal delivery. International Urogynecology Journal, 19(1), 65-71.

11. Pool-Goudzwaard, A., Hoek van Dijke, G., van Gurp, M., Mulder, P., Snijders, C., & Stoeckart, R. (2004). Contribution of pelvic floor muscles to stiffness of the pelvic ring. *Clinical Biomechanics, 19*(6), 564-571.

12. Noakes, K. F., Pullan, A. J., Bissett, I. P., & Cheng, L. K. (2008). Subject specific finite elasticity simulations of the pelvic floor. *Journal of biomechanics,41*(14), 3060-3065.

13. Noakes, K. F., Bissett, I. P., Pullan, A. J., & Cheng, L. K. (2006). Anatomically based computational models of the male and female pelvic floor and anal canal. In *Engineering in Medicine and Biology Society, 2006. EMBS'06. 28th Annual International Conference of the IEEE* (pp. 3815-3818). IEEE.

14. Yip, C., Kwok, E., Sassani, F., Jackson, R., & Cundiff, G. (2012). A biomechanical model to assess the contribution of pelvic musculature weakness to the development of stress urinary incontinence. *Computer Methods in Biomechanics and Biomedical Engineering*, (ahead-of-print), 1-14.

15. Chen, L., Ashton-Miller, J. A., Hsu, Y., & DeLancey, J. O. (2006). Interaction between Apical Supports and Levator Ani in Anterior Vaginal Support: Theoretical Analysis. *Obstetrics and gynecology, 108*(2), 324.

16. Martins, P. A., Jorge, R. M. N., Ferreia, A. J., Saleme, C. S., Roza, T., Parente, M. M., ... & Silva-Filho, A. L. (2010). Vaginal Tissue Properties versus Increased Intra-Abdominal Pressure: A Preliminary Biomechanical Study. *Gynecologic and obstetric investigation, 71*(3), 145-150.

17. Noakes, K. F., Bissett, I. P., Pullan, A. J., & Cheng, L. K. (2008). Anatomically realistic three-dimensional meshes of the pelvic floor & anal canal for finite element analysis. Annals of biomedical engineering, 36(6), 1060-1071.

18. Kruger, J. A., Murphy, B. A., & Heap, S. W. (2005). Alterations in levator ani morphology in elite nulliparous athletes: a pilot study. Australian and New Zealand journal of obstetrics and gynaecology, 45(1), 42-47.

19. Kruger, J. A., Heap, S. W., Murphy, B. A., & Dietz, H. P. (2008). Pelvic floor function in nulliparous women using three-dimensional ultrasound and magnetic resonance imaging. Obstetrics & Gynecology, 111(3), 631-638.

The Impairment of Female Pelvic Ligaments and Its Relation With Pelvic Floor Dysfunction: Biomechanical Analysis

Sofia Brandão, Marco Parente, Ana Rita Silva, Thuane Da Roza, Teresa Mascarenhas, Isabel Ramos and R.M. Natal Jorge

Abstract Computational simulation of degeneration or damage on the structures that sustain the female pelvic organs may point to how they behave in real-life conditions. This work evaluated the effect of the impairment of female pelvic ligaments by means of numerical simulation considering rest and valsalva maneuver conditions. The model included the pelvic organs and several support structures, identified on magnetic resonance images from a young healthy female. For each tissue, material properties were obtained in the literature, and the best constitutive model was chosen for each structure. The displacement of the pelvic organs was assessed for normal ligaments, and also when their impairment was simulated by individually reducing their stiffness. The pelvic organs evidenced increased displacement when considering the damaged ligaments, similarly to what was found in previous imaging evidence. This model was suited for assessing ligaments damage. This is an important issue when simulating aging or trauma of the pelvic support structures.

Keywords Biomechanical simulation · Pelvic floor dysfunction · Ligament impairment

S. Brandão (✉) · T. Mascarenhas · I. Ramos
Centro Hospitalar de São João – EPE, Faculty of Medicine, University of Porto, Porto, Portugal
e-mail: sofia.brand@gmail.com

M. Parente · A.R. Silva · T. Da Roza · R.M. Natal Jorge
IDMEC-Pólo FEUP, Faculty of Engineering, University of Porto, Porto, Portugal
e-mail: rnatal@fe.up.pt

T. Da Roza
CIAFEL (Research Centre in Physical Activity, Health and Leisure), Faculty of Sport, University of Porto, Porto, Portugal

© Springer International Publishing Switzerland 2015
J.M.R.S. Tavares and R.M. Natal Jorge (eds.), *Computational and Experimental Biomedical Sciences: Methods and Applications*, Lecture Notes in Computational Vision and Biomechanics 21, DOI 10.1007/978-3-319-15799-3_4

1 Introduction

Female pelvic organs are grouped into anterior (bladder and urethra), central (vagina and uterus), and posterior (or anorectal) compartments. The spectrum of pelvic floor dysfunction depends on the compartment involved, and includes urinary incontinence (UI), constipation, and pelvic organ prolapse (POP), occurring in varying combinations. These are major issues among urologists and gynecologists. Farther, as they are also related with damage or weakness of the supports for the pelvic organs —provided by muscles, ligaments and fascia—its biomechanical analysis is also of interest to better understand the overall model of the disease.

The position and mobility of the structures of the anterior compartment are important to the study of UI. Loss of anterior vaginal support may result in urethral hypermobility, cystocele or anterior vaginal wall prolapse. The pubovesical, the pubourethral (PUL), and the uterosacral-cardinal muscles complex uphold the vesical and vaginal positions, as they stabilize the distal urethra, and maintain the cervix and the bladder base attached to the connective tissue of the fascia in the pelvic bones [1–4]. Damage or degradation of these apical supports is common in women with stress UI (SUI) and vaginal prolapse [5]. The normal position of the rectum is also maintained by the rectal fascia and the *levator ani* musculature [6]. Increased pressure in the proximal portion of the anal canal is supported by the puborectal muscle through vigorous contraction. To strengthen this effect, the iliococcygeal muscle firms the *levator plate* and the lateral ligaments of the rectum [7].

While physical examination, standardized questionnaires and imaging studies are the usual tools to assess pelvic floor dysfunction, computer simulation may also be used to learn and predict the biomechanical behavior of the pelvic structures under stress or after damage [8–10]. This is important in a clinical perspective, because the biomechanics involved in pelvic organ support is very difficult to evaluate experimentally. The finite element method (FEM) can be used to simulate pelvic floor muscles contraction against downward pressures that simulate intra-abdominal pressure or straining, as performed on dynamic magnetic resonance imaging (MRI) acquisitions. It allows testing pelvic floor muscles performance and compartmental stability when subjected to complex multidirectional forces. A study of Saleme et al. showed that a contraction intensity of 50 % would be necessary to avoid urine loss [11]. In addition, FEM can be used to mimic and predict vaginal delivery features and effects on pelvic floor muscles, illustrating true mechanical phenomena of one of the main causes of pelvic floor dysfunction. Interesting findings have been reproduced and reported, including that there is a mechanical response of the *levator ani* during the second stage of labor; muscle activation during vaginal delivery may represent an obstacle to fetal descent and increase the risk for pelvic floor injuries [12]; the shape of the head influences the mechanical response of the muscle; fetal head flexion during vaginal delivery may facilitate birth and protect the pelvic floor [13]; and increased fetal head diameter can influence medial *levator ani* portion to overstretch and injure, predicting injury patterns on predisposed women [14].

Few previous works focused the modeling of pelvic floor dysfunction in relation to damage in the support structures. Yip et al. [8] found that impaired pelvic floor muscles lead to vaginal and bladder neck prolapse. Additionally, Chen et al. reproduced anterior vaginal prolapse as related with progressive muscle and uterine ligaments damage [15, 16]. However, these studies focused on the middle compartment, but the whole pelvic cavity may suffer from ligament damage. Accordingly, this work evaluated the displacement of the pelvic organs considering the effect of the impairment on the pelvic ligaments. It was performed based on MRI of a healthy volunteer and numerical simulation using the FEM.

2 Method

The numerical model was built along several steps. The geometry of the pelvic organs and bones was obtained from MR images.

Some anatomical features of the PUL, uterosacral, cardinal and lateral rectal ligaments were confirmed in the literature [17]. The surfaces were meshed by rendering techniques using the software Inventor® (Autodesk, San Raphael, CA, USA) (Fig. 1).

A FE model (Fig. 2) was developed in Abaqus/CAE® software v. 6.12 (Dassault Systèmes Simulia Corp., Providence, RI, USA) (Fig. 2). The pelvic floor muscles were considered as a single mesh, while respecting its average 3-mm thickness. Material properties [18–20] and constitutive models were defined for each structure according to previous work, using the curve-fitting algorithms from the Abaqus®. The bones were fixed and considered as rigid, while the supportive structures were attached to the organs and bone using multi-point constrains (Abaqus® tie).

Fig. 1 3D model of the pelvis

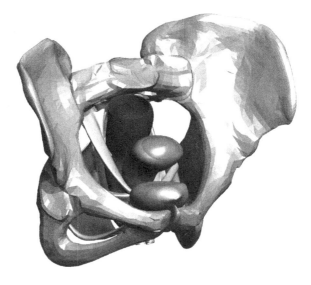

(a)   **(b)**

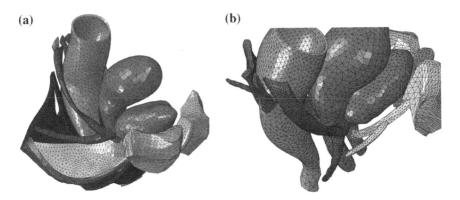

Fig. 2 Finite element model of the pelvis. The pelvic floor muscles and the pelvic fascia were excluded to better visualize the position of the pelvic ligaments

For the constitutive equation adopted in this work for the 3D passive and active behaviour of the pelvic floor muscles, a modified form of the incompressible transversely isotropic hyperelastic model used by Parente et al. [20], based on the work of Humphrey and Yin for passive cardiac tissues.

In the constitutive model, the strain energy per unit volume of the reference configuration can be written in the following form:

$$U = U_I\left(\overline{I}_1^C\right) + U_J(J) + U_f\left(\overline{\lambda}_f, \alpha\right) \tag{1}$$

where U_I,

$$U_I = c\left[e^{b\left(\overline{I}_1^C - 3\right)} - 1\right] \tag{2}$$

is the strain energy stored in the isotropic matrix, embedding the muscle fibres,

$$U_J = \frac{1}{D}(J - 1)^2 \tag{3}$$

is the portion of the strain energy associated with the volume change and

$$U_f\left(\overline{\lambda}_f, \alpha\right) = U_{pas}\left(\overline{\lambda}_f\right) + U_{act}\left(\overline{\lambda}_f, \alpha\right) \tag{4}$$

is the strain energy stored in each muscle fibre, which can be divided into a passive elastic part and an active part due to the contraction. The passive elastic part U_{pas} is given by:

$$U_{pas} = A\left\{\exp\left[a(\bar{\lambda}_f - 3)^2\right] - 1\right\} \tag{5}$$

when $\bar{\lambda}_f > 1$, otherwise we consider the strain energy to be zero, assuming that the fibres offer no resistance to compression. The active part U_{act} is given by:

$$U_{act} = \alpha\, T_0^M \int\limits_1^{\bar{\lambda}_f} 1 - 4(\bar{\lambda} - 1)^2 d\bar{\lambda} \tag{6}$$

where α is the activation level, ranging from 0 to 1. When $0.5 < \bar{\lambda}_f < 1.5$, U_{act} is larger than 0, for other values of $\bar{\lambda}_f$ the muscle produces no force and, therefore, the strain energy is zero. The constant T_0^M is the maximum tension produced by the muscle at resting length $(\bar{\lambda}_f = 1)$.

In the above equation, T_0^M, c, b, A, a and D are constants [20], $\bar{I}_1^C$ is the first invariant of the right Cauchy-Green strain tensor with the volume change eliminated, i.e.

$$\bar{I}_1^C = \text{tr}\,\bar{\mathbf{C}} = \text{tr}\left(\bar{\mathbf{F}}^T\bar{\mathbf{F}}\right) = J^{-2/3}\text{tr}\,\mathbf{C} \tag{7}$$

where $\bar{\mathbf{F}}$ is the deformation gradient with the volume change eliminated (Eq. 8)

$$\bar{\mathbf{F}} = J^{-1/3}\mathbf{F} \tag{8}$$

$\mathbf{F}$ is the deformation gradient and

$$J = \det \mathbf{F} \tag{9}$$

the volume change. Eq. (10) illustrates the fibre stretch ratio in the direction N of the undeformed fibre, given by:

$$\bar{\lambda}_f = \sqrt{\mathbf{N}^T\bar{\mathbf{C}}\mathbf{N}} = \sqrt{\bar{\mathbf{C}} : (\mathbf{N} \otimes \mathbf{N})} \tag{10}$$

where $\otimes$ denotes the tensor product.

The 2nd Piola-Kirchhoff stress tensor S can be obtained by the strain energy density given in Eq. (1), as:

$$\mathbf{S} = \frac{\partial U}{\partial \mathbf{E}} = \frac{\partial U_I}{\partial \mathbf{E}} + \frac{\partial U_f}{\partial \mathbf{E}} + \frac{\partial U_J}{\partial \mathbf{E}} \tag{11}$$

The Cauchy stress tensor σ is related to the 2nd Piola-Kirchhoff stress tensor S by

$$\sigma = J^{-1}\mathbf{F}\mathbf{S}\mathbf{F}^T \tag{12}$$

The material version of the tangent operator is defined as

$$\mathbf{H} = \frac{\partial^2 U}{\partial \mathbf{E}\, \partial \mathbf{E}} = \frac{\partial \mathbf{S}}{\partial \mathbf{E}} \tag{13}$$

and the spatial version can be obtained through a push-forward transformation

$$h_{ijkl} = \frac{1}{J} F_{im} F_{jn} F_{kp} F_{lp} H_{mnpq} \tag{14}$$

Muscles were assumed as having isotropic behavior, and the direction of the muscle fibers was assumed as being coincident with the direction of the maximum stress lines during deformation. Accordingly, a pressure of 1 kPa was applied in the inner surface of the pelvic cavity in order to obtain the direction of the fibers. Afterwards, the model was tested for supine rest (0.50 kPa) and supine valsava maneuver (4.00 kPa) conditions [10]. Mean values of magnitude displacement of the pelvic organs and pelvic floor muscles were evaluated when simulating healthy and progressive impaired support structures, by reducing material stiffness by 25, 50 and 75 %.

3 Results

The results from the magnitude displacement of the pelvic organs and pelvic floor muscles are presented on Table 1, and are illustrated on Figs. 3 and 4. The subtle pressure induced by the organs at rest lead to minor displacement of the pelvic floor muscles, upper portion of the bladder and uterus. When simulating valsalva maneuver, all the structures exhibited posterior and downward movement (Fig. 3b).

Table 1 Results from mean magnitude displacement from numerical simulation of rest, valsalva maneuver (VM) with healthy ligaments, and VM with different degrees of ligament impairment

Structure	Displacement (mm)	Rest	VM	VM, 25 % impairment	VM, 50 % impairment	VM, 75 % impairment
Uterus	min	0.48	1.86	3.61	4.54	6.16
	max	4.92	20.1	29.04	29.73	30.17
Bladder	min	0.61	2.6	4.8	5.5	6.59
	max	5.89	10.13	15.85	16.75	17.71
Rectum	min	0.11	0.34	0.53	0.66	0.98
	max	1.92	5.58	8.34	8.63	8.97
Pelvic floor	min	0	0	0	0	0
	max	4.25	11.65	17.14	17.42	17.41

(a)   (b)

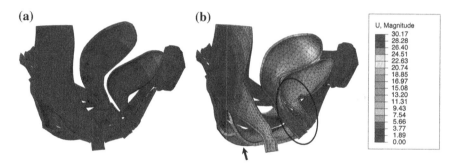

Fig. 3 Numerical simulation of valsalva maneuver. The basal pressure from the organ load was simulated on **a**, while the magnitude of the displacements for valsalva are illustrated on **b**

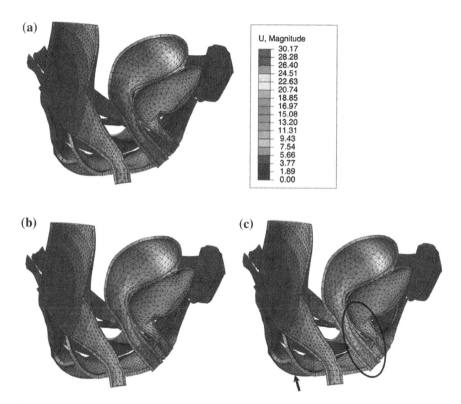

Fig. 4 Numerical simulation of Valsava Manuever, assuming 25 **a**, 50 **b**, and 75 % **c** reduction in ligament stiffness

The rectal portion of the pelvic floor muscles evidenced higher displacement than the anterior region, which was still not very evident when the support from the pelvic ligaments failed (Fig. 4c). Accordingly, the maximum displacement of the rectum was less than 4 mm from rest to valsalva maneuver, and 7.05 mm when almost total damage of the pelvic ligaments was simulated. When considering the middle and anterior compartments, organs were more prone to descend, as indicated by the results on Table 1. The bladder and the uterus descended 11.82 and 25.25 mm, which is considerably more than the rectum. These results are in agreement with previous studies that evaluated the position of the pelvic organs for different stages of organ prolapse [21] and SUI [22] through MRI.

4 Discussion

UI requires integration of central and peripheral nervous systems, bladder wall and detrusor muscle, bladder neck, urethra, and pelvic support structures. Anteriorly, the PUL insert on the *arcus tendineus levator fascia* and in the inferior aspect of the pubic bone, assisting bladder neck opening during voiding [23]. The bladder neck position is influenced by connections between the puborectal muscle, vagina and proximal urethra. Additionally, the lateral ligaments of the bladder, and attachments to the cervix and anterior vagina provide postero-inferior support to the trigone.

SUI is characterized by involuntary urine leakage on effort or exertion, or during coughing [24] or exercise [24, 25]. Although its etiology is still an ongoing subject, it is mostly related to bladder neck hypermobility due to weakened or damaged pelvic floor muscles [26, 27], laxity of the fascia underlying the urethra, or damage of the pelvic ligaments [27–30]. Similarly, POP is common after injury to these support structures, which widens the *genital hiatus* and leads to organ prolapse, which may further stress or stretch ligaments. Hormonal changes are also related with weakened muscular and connective tissue support. A relation has been established between age and menopause, and degeneration of pelvic with estrogen receptors deficiency [31]. Moreover, progesterone is known to reduce muscular tonus of the ureters, bladder, and urethra because of its smooth muscle-relaxing and estrogen-antagonizing effects [32]. These features are typically seen in SUI and POP patients [27–30, 33, 34].

As the present results suggest, the bladder and uterus are the most affected by impaired ligaments. Despite the fact that the rectal portion of the pelvic floor seems to be the most movable (arrows on Figs. 3b and 4c), the puborectal muscle and the strong fascial involvement have a major role on maintaining rectal position. On the contrary, the urethra, the bladder neck, and the vagina get progressively compressed against the pelvic floor when the IAP is increased.

The FEM has been used by Marino et al. to study structural differences between lateral, trigone and anterior walls of the bladder, in correlation with the disposition of fibers of detrusor muscle and its thickness. When the simulation was performed in the absence of the PUL, the deflections of pelvic fascia modified the distributions of loads towards a centripetal orientation, which increases the stress over the perineal area and sphincter tract [35]. The author also confirmed the role of these ligaments between pubis and the cervix-urethra tract in dividing the global pressure load in the several components. Chen et al. confirmed the relevance of the *levator ani* in cystocele formation, since the decreased muscle resistance to counteract the stretch when the IAP is increased widens the *genital hiatus*. As a consequence, the vaginal wall is exposed to higher pressure, which resulted in larger cystocele size. Their model also helped to illustrate the role of apical support. With muscle impairment present and the anterior vaginal wall subjected to a differential loading, the tensile load has to be resisted by both apical and paravaginal connective tissue supports, as an 80 % impairment in apical support resulted in a 33 % larger cystocele size [16].

A model developed by Yip et al. [8] was employed to evaluate the impact of pelvic muscular defect on the vaginal apex support and bladder neck support, features which relates to SUI. Simulation showed that the compromise of muscular contributed to the descend of those structures, whcih is commonly seen in patients patients with SUI.

Our results are similar to the ones from Yip et al. [8] and Chen et al. [15, 16], regarding the fact that the middle and anterior compartments are more dependent on the support role of the pelvic ligaments.

5 Conclusion

Numerical simulation of damage on the pelvic ligaments lead to increased downward movement of the pelvic floor muscles and pelvic organs. These features are similar to what happens after trauma or when the age and hormonal effects weaken organ support. The results from this study are similar to the imaging studies that regularly evaluate organ prolapse or UI.

Acknowledgments The authors gratefully acknowledge to the funding by CNPq—from Brazil government and the project Pest-OE/EME/LA0022/2013 and also to the project "Biomechanics: contributions to the healthcare", reference NORTE-07-0124-FEDER-000035 co-financed by Programa Operacional Regional do Norte (ON.2—O Novo Norte), through the Fundo Europeu de Desenvolvimento Regional (FEDER).

References

1. Tasali, N., et al., MRI in stress urinary incontinence: endovaginal MRI with an intracavitary coil and dynamic pelvic MRI. Urol J, 2012. 9(1): p. 397-404.
2. Kim, J. K., et al., The urethra and its supporting structures in women with stress urinary incontinence: MR imaging using an endovaginal coil. AJR Am J Roentgenol, 2003. 180(4): p.1037-44.
3. Pregazzi, R., et al., Perineal ultrasound evaluation of urethral angle and bladder neck mobility in women with stress urinary incontinence. BJOG, 2002. 109(7): p. 821-7.
4. Ramanah, R., et al., Anatomy and histology of apical support: a literature review concerning cardinal and uterosacral ligaments. Int Urogynecol J, 2012. 23(11): 1483-94.

5. Wang, L., L. Y. Hanand, and H. L. Li, Etiological study of pelvic organ prolapse and stress urinary incontinence with collagen status and metabolism. Zhonghua Yi Xue Za Zhi, 2013. 93 (7): p. 500-3.
6. Baert AL, Kanuth M (2008) Imaging Pelvic Floor Disorders. 2nd Revised Edition. Springer ISBN 978-3-540-71966-3.
7. Law, Y. M. and J. R. Fielding, MRI of pelvic floor dysfunction: review. AJR Am J Roentgenol, 2008. 191(S6): p. 45-53.
8. Yip, C., et al., A biomechanical model to assess the contribution of pelvic musculature weakness to the development of stress urinary incontinence. Comput Methods Biomech Biomed Engin, 2014. 17(2): p. 163-76.
9. Parente, M. P., et al., Deformation of the pelvic floor muscles during a vaginal delivery. Int Urogynecol J Pelvic Floor Dysfunct, 2008. 19(1): p. 65-71.
10. Noakes, K. F., et al., Subject specific finite elasticity simulations of the pelvic floor. J Biomech, 2008. 41(14): p. 3060-5.
11. Saleme, C. S., et al., An approach on determining the displacements of the pelvic floor during voluntary contraction using numerical simulation and MRI. Comput Methods Biomech Biomed Engin, 2011. 14(4): p. 365-70.
12. Parente, M. P., et al., The influence of pelvic muscle activation during vaginal delivery. Obstet Gynecol, 2010. 115(4): p. 804-8.
13. Parente, M. P., et al., Computational modeling approach to study the effects of fetal head flexion during vaginal delivery. Am J Obstet Gynecol, 2010. 203(3): p. 217.e1-6.
14. Ashton-Miller, J. A., and J. O. L. DeLancey, On the biomechanics of vaginal birth and common sequelae. Annu Rev Biomed Eng, 2009. 11: p. 163-76.
15. Chen, L., et al., Interaction between Apical Supports and Levator Ani in Anterior Vaginal Support: Theoretical Analysis. Obstet Gynecol, 2006. 108(2): p. 324-32.
16. Chen, L., J. A., Ashton-Miller, and J. O. DeLancey, A 3-D Finite Element Model of Anterior Vaginal Wall Support to Evaluate Mechanisms Underlying Cystocele Formation. J Biomech, 2009. 42(10): p. 1371-7.
17. Patel U. Imaging and Urodynamics of the Lower Urinary Tract. Springer. 2010. © Springer-Verlag London Limited 2010. ISBN: 978-1-84882-835-3.
18. Rubod, C., et al., Biomechanical properties of human pelvic organs. Urology, 2012. 79(4): p. 968 e17–22.
19. Kirilova, M., et al., Experimental study of the mechanical properties of human abdominal fascia. Med Eng Phys, 2011. 33(1): p. 1-6.
20. Parente, M. P., et al., The influence of the material properties on the biomechanical behavior of the pelvic floor muscles during vaginal delivery. J Biomech, 2009. 42(9): p. 1301-6.
21. Lakenam, M. M., et al., Dynamic magnetic resonance imaging to quantify pelvic organ prolapse: reliability of assessment and correlation with clinical findings and pelvic floor symptoms. Int Urogynecol J, 2012. 23(11): p. 1547-54.
22. Tarhan, S., et al., The comparison of MRI findings with severity score of incontinence after pubovaginal sling surgery. Turk J Med Sci, 2010. 40 (4): p. 549-56.
23. Strohbehn, K., et al. Magnetic resonance imaging of the levator ani with anatomic correlation. Obstet Gyneco, 1996. 87(2): p. 277-85.
24. Abrams, P., et al., Reviewing the ICS 2002 terminology report: the ongoing debate. Neurourol Urodyn, 2009. 28(4): p. 287-90.
25. Kruger, J. A., H. P. Dietz, and B. A. Murphy, Pelvic floor function in elite nulliparous athletes. Ultrasound Obstet Gynecol, 2007. 30(1): p. 81-5.
26. Simeone, C., et al., Occurrence rates and predictors of lower urinary tract symptoms and incontinence in female athletes. Urologia, 77(2): p. 139-46.
27. Dietz, H. P., and J. M., Simpson, Levator trauma is associated with pelvic organ prolapse. BJOG, 2008. 15(8): p. 979-84.
28. Wu, Q., et al., Characteristics of pelvic diaphragm hiatus in pregnant women with stress urinary incontinence detected by transperineal three-dimensional ultrasound. Zhonghua Fu Chan Ke Za Zhi, 2010. 45(5): p. 326-30.

29. Siracusano, S., R., Mandras, and E. Belgrano, Physiopathology of the pelvic elements of support in stress urinary incontinence in women. Arch Ital Urol Androl, 1994. 66(S4): p. 151-3.
30. Wei, J. T., and J. O. L. DeLancey, Functional anatomy of the pelvic floor and lower urinary tract. Clin Obstet Gyneco, 2004. 47(1): p. 3-17.
31. Scheiner, D., et al., Aging-related changes of the female pelvic floor. Ther Umsch, 2010. 67 (1): p. 23-6.
32. Copas, P., et al., Estrogen, progesterone, and androgen receptor expression in levator ani muscle and fascia. J Womens Health Gend Based Med, 2001. 10(8): p. 785-95.
33. Zhu, L., J. H. Lang, and R. E. Feng, Study on estrogen receptor around levator ani muscle for female stress urinary incontinence. Zhonghua Fu Chan Ke Za Zhi, 2004. 39(10): p. 655-7.
34. Tinelli, A., et al., Age-related pelvic floor modifications and prolapse risk factors in postmenopausal women. Menopause, 2010. 17(1): p. 204-12.
35. Tinelli, A., et al., Age-related pelvic floor modifications and prolapse risk factors in postmenopausal women. Menopause, 2010. 17(1): p. 204-12.

Pelvic Floor Muscles Behavior in Practitioners of High and Low Impact Sports

Thuane Da Roza, Sofia Brandão, Teresa Mascarenhas, José Alberto Duarte and R.M. Natal Jorge

Abstract Physical activity has been promoted to all ages due to the benefits to health and as a tool to compensate for a sedentary lifestyle. Since the pelvic floor muscles have the function of keeping the sphincter functions and it were localized as a "floor" for the abdominal viscera. Maintain this muscles "healthy" is the great importance. It is known that some exercises can promote damage on the pelvic floor muscles. The impact of exercise on urinary incontinence has been previously considered, but not in a biomechanical perspective. Strengthening exercises performed through pelvic floor muscles contractions are the basis of physiotherapy treatment. The aim of this study was to verify whether practitioners of high-impact sports have differences in morphology and behavior of pelvic floor muscles when compared with low-impact activities practitioners. The results showed thickness differences at the level of midvagina between the swimmer and the trampolinist women. Additionally, differences in pubovisceral muscle behavior during maneuvers that increase intra-abdominal pressure were found. Further studies are required in this field to understand the impact of female training, and in what way its biomechanics related to urinary incontinence symptoms.

Keywords Pelvic floor muscles · Physical activity · Stress urinary incontinence · Intra-abdominal pressure

T.D. Roza (✉) · R.M. Natal Jorge
INEGI-Polo FEUP, Faculty of Engineering, University of Porto, Porto, Portugal
e-mail: thuaneroza@yahoo.com.br

R.M. Natal Jorge
e-mail: rnatal@fe.up.pt

S. Brandão
Department of Radiology, Centro Hospitalar de São João—EPE, Porto, Portugal

T. Mascarenhas
Department of Gynecology and Obstetrics, Centro Hospitalar de São João,
Faculty of Medicine, University of Porto, Porto, Portugal

T.D. Roza · J.A. Duarte
CIAFEL-Faculty of Sport, University of Porto, Research Centre in Physical Activity,
Health and Leisure, Porto, Portugal

© Springer International Publishing Switzerland 2015
J.M.R.S. Tavares and R.M. Natal Jorge (eds.), *Computational and Experimental Biomedical Sciences: Methods and Applications*, Lecture Notes in Computational Vision and Biomechanics 21, DOI 10.1007/978-3-319-15799-3_5

1 Introduction

The Pelvic floor muscles are a complex inter-related structure spatially arranged to maintain urinary continence and pelvic organs position inside the pelvic cavity. The pelvic floor diaphragm is a wide but thin muscular layer of tissue that forms the inferior border of the abdominopelvic cavity [1]. The deep pelvic floor is comprised of muscles which can be divided into pubococcygeus, ileococcygeuys, coccygeus and puborectalis muscles [1]. As there is some controversy about the nomenclature for the muscles of the pelvic floor, for the purposes of this study we adopted the terms defined by DeLancey [2], whereby "pubovisceral muscle" is used to represent both the muscles pubococcygeus and muscles puborectalis, as these two muscles cannot be easily differentiated when using ultrasound or Magnetic Resonance Imaging (MRI). Weakness or damage to these muscles can lead to pelvic floor dysfunction, including urinary incontinence (UI) [3] and pelvic organ prolapse [4, 5].

Stress UI (SUI) is the most common type of UI, affecting 6–33 % of the female population, with significant impact on their quality of life [6–8]. Currently, studies show a high rate of SUI in athletes, especially in the ones participating in sports that demand constant increase the intra-abdominal pressure (IAP) [9]. This situation can causes embarrassment and discomfort, depriving women of social conviviality abandonment of physical activities as well as it may affect sexual intercourse [10]. Gravitational forces of the abdominal content generate pelvic pressure, which is exacerbate by vigorous movements during sports practice. As SUI occurs when the IAP is greater than urethral pressure [11], it is expected that athletes of high-impact exercises have the higher frequency.

Structural defects of the neuromuscular and connective tissues supporting the bladder neck and urethra are implicated in the pathogenesis of SUI [12]. Until now, the knowledge published literature is limited regarding the identification of SUI in athletes, as the biomechanical behavior of the pelvic floor muscles remain unclear. The Finite Element Method, which may be based on MRI tridimensional morphology, allows to model the biomechanical behavior of the pelvic floor muscles. By modeling the muscles at rest and when active, it is possible to predict and evaluate the effects of vaginal birth or straining, as well as to test muscle ability to maintain urinary and fecal continence. Finally, it provide a good insight on the pelvic floor rehabilitation planning. As the IAP can be studied in a biomechanical perspective, the aim of this study was investigate the behavior and morphology of the pelvic floor muscles comparing two women who practice high-impact versus low-impact activities. For that propose pelvic MRI and the biomechanical analysis was performed using the finite element method.

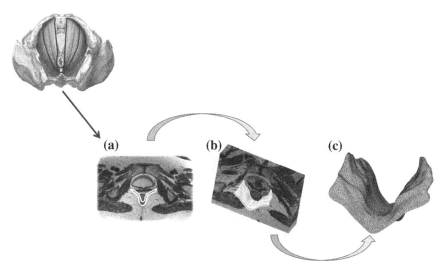

Fig. 1 Building the three-dimensional model with the finite element mesh

2 Method

Two asymptomatic sportswomen (trampoline and swimming athletes) without symptoms of UI or genital prolapse were included. Their age was 19 and 20 years, respectively. Trampoline was considered high-impact while swimming was assigned as low-impact. Both women performed clinical evaluation, and no pathological findings were described. Pelvic T2-weighted axial 3 mm images were acquired with the subjects in supine position using 3.0 tesla scanner.

Regarding the morphology, pubovisceral muscle thickness was measured at the levels of the midvagina and of the anal canal (right and left sides) and in the anorectal angle region. Finite element models of pubovisceral muscle of each woman were built from a set of twenty consecutive images. Inventor software (Inventor Professional 2010®) was used to manually draw the contour of the pubovisceral muscle (Fig. 1a) and to build the 3D models (Fig. 1b). Afterwards, these 3D solids were exported to ABAQUS software and the pubovisceral muscle meshes were generated (Fig. 1c) according to the methodology of Saleme et al. [13].

Some input conditions were established: the mesh consisted of tetrahedron solid elements type C3D4; the muscle was considered homogeneous and visco-hyper-elastic material, nodes were inserted in the coccyx to constrain the movement on the anteroposterior direction [14]; and boundary conditions were created on the left and right upper positions of pubovisceral muscle, where it inserts into the endopelvic fascia and internal obturator muscle (Fig. 2).

In order to simulate the IAP at rest, a distributed pressure of 60 cm H_2O was applied perpendicular to the ventral surface of the pubovisceral muscle.

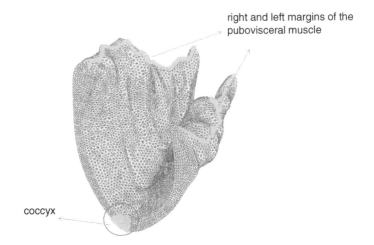

right and left margins of the
pubovisceral muscle

coccyx

Fig. 2 Boundary conditions on the *left* and *right upper* positions and in the coccyx region

Fig. 3 Displacement of
pubovisceral muscle in caudal
direction

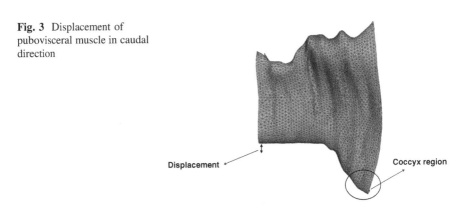

Displacement   Coccyx region

Afterwards, three additional IAP intensities were applied on the muscle: 100, 173 and 193 cm H_2O, corresponding to activities as up-stairs, cough and jump, respectively. The pubovisceral muscle displacement on the caudal direction was evaluated, Fig. 3.

3 Results

Regarding the morphologic aspects, thickness on the right and left sides (at level of anal canal) and in the anorectal angle region was similar. Figure 4 shows the location of each of these regions measurements (right and left sides at level of midvagina and anal canal; and in the anorectal angle region).

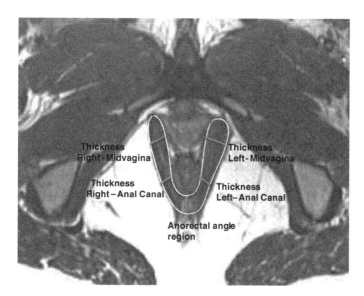

Fig. 4 Morphological measures on the axial static MR images. Pubovisceral muscle thickness measures: *left* and *right*—at the level of midvagina and at the level of anal canal; and in the anorectal angle region were taken

Table 1 Morphologic characteristics of pubovisceral muscle thickness in both women

	Midvagina (mm)		Anal canal (mm)		Anorectal region (mm)
	Left	Right	Left	Right	
Swimmer	0.33	0.35	0.43	0.44	0.51
Trampolinist	0.57	0.58	0.44	0.45	0.53

The differences were found midvagina with 0.35 and 0.33 mm for the swimmer and 0.58 and 0.57 mm for the trampolinist (right and left sides, respectively). The results from the static MR images measurements are displayed on Table 1.

Numerical simulation showed similar displacement of the pubovisceral muscle at rest for both women. When the IAP increased to 100 cm H_2O, the model of the trampolinist evidenced a displacement of 0.21 mm, slightly higher than that of the swimmer (0.19 mm). During simulation of cough, the displacement increased to 0.36 and 0.33 mm and during a jump to 0.48 and 0.39 mm for the trampolinist and for swimmer, respectively.

4 Discussion

The results of the present study showed a difference in the thickness of the mid-vagina and in the displacement of the pubovisceral muscle between the two athletes. Despite the similar thickness in anal canal and in the anorectal region of puboviscral muscle, the midvagina region was thicker in the trampolinist. In relation to the time and the practice of training no difference was found between the participants.

The mechanism of continence requires complex coordination of bladder, urethra, pelvic floor muscles and supporting ligaments. The pelvic floor muscles have the ability to resist to the downward movement through passive contraction that lifts the pelvic floor in an upward direction [15]. So far, there are two hypotheses for the pelvic floor muscles in athletes. The first states that athletes should have stronger muscles due to the continuous increases in IAP; the other suggests that athletes may have pelvic floor muscles stretched and damaged due to these stress over these muscles [16].

Kruger et al. [17] documenting the muscle morphology of the pelvic floor muscles in a group of nulliparous female athletes and comparing the findings with a similar group of age-matched nulliparous nonathletic women and showed that the cross-sectional area of these muscles was greater in the athlete women at level of canal anal. The results from the present study showed not differences at the level of canal anal which can be explained by the fact that both women performed exercise, so, probably both had an thickness increased at the level of anal canal. We found that the woman who practices high-impact sport shows an increase in muscle thickness at the level of midvagina, which could be due to recruitment of these muscles during the increase in IAP. As the pubovisceral muscle helps the sphincter urethrae muscle (the muscle that closes the urethra during micturition) to maintain the continence and that is localized at level of vagina, perhaps the pubovisceral muscle has strengthened at this level to keep the continence.

On the other hand, the trampolinist jumps induce greater forces affecting the pelvic floor muscles and connective tissue at every impact on the trampoline [9]. These jumps could cause slow increase in the mobility of the puboviscral muscle, not allowing them to hold the bladder neck and consequently leading to SUI. According to Jiang, direct damage to the pelvic floor, either the rupture of the pubocervical fascia or in the tendinous insertion of the endopelvic fascia, may occur when high-impact physical activities are practiced, and can be responsible for SUI complaints [18].

This study shows a greater displacement in pubovisceral muscle in the model built from MR images of the trampolinist when compared to the practitioner of low-impact exercise. This difference increases when simulating cough and is bigger when simulating a jump. It is possible that this displacement can increase with the years of training practice, and can lead to UI in the future. Therefore, the present work demonstrates that pubovisceral muscle have a greater thickness at level of midvagina when compared to the one of the swimmer and that the trampolinist had a greater pubovisceral muscle displacement while simulating the increase in IAP. Both morphological and functional differences may be consequences of exercise.

Importanlty, none of the young woman was diagnosed with UI or pelvic organ prolapse symptoms. Leakage of urine can also occur from the fatigue of the pelvic floor muscles, arising from repetitive muscular contraction during high impact exercises, although there is not enough evidence to sustain this hypothesis [19]. Additionally, the present numerical simulations were not able to predict muscle fatigue.

5 Conclusion

In conclusion, in this experimental study the practitioners of high-impact and low-impact sports showed different behavior of pubovisceral muscle during maneuvers that increase IAP. Furthermore, the region of midvagina region was thicker in trampolinist than in the swimmer. There were no major morphological differences in pubovisceral muscle between the two participants. A larger sample would be useful to confirm our findings. So, further studies are necessary in this area.

Acknowledgments The fist author gratefully acknowledge to the funding by CNPq-from Brazil government and the project Pest-OE/EME/LA0022/2013 and also to the project "Biomechanics: contributions to the healthcare", reference NORTE-07-0124-FEDER-000035 co-financed by Programa Operacional Regional do Norte (ON.2—O Novo Norte), through the Fundo Europeu de Desenvolvimento Regional (FEDER).

References

1. Raizada, V. and R.K. Mittal, Pelvic floor anatomy and applied physiology. Gastroenterol Clin North Am, 2008. 37(3): p. 493-509, vii.
2. DeLancey, J.O., The anatomy of the pelvic floor. Curr Opin Obstet Gynecol, 1994. 6(4): p. 313-6.
3. DeLancey, J.O., et al., Comparison of levator ani muscle defects and function in women with and without pelvic organ prolapse. Obstet Gynecol, 2007. 109(2 Pt 1): p. 295-302.
4. Shafik, A., Straining and its role in micturition. Urology, 2003. 62(1): p. 199-200; author reply 200-1.
5. Ashton-Miller, J.A. and J.O. DeLancey, Functional anatomy of the female pelvic floor. Ann N Y Acad Sci, 2007. 1101: p. 266-96.
6. Abrams, P., et al., The standardisation of terminology in lower urinary tract function: report from the standardisation sub-committee of the International Continence Society. Urology, 2003. 61(1): p. 37-49.
7. Minassian, V.A., H.P. Drutz, and A. Al-Badr, Urinary incontinence as a worldwide problem. Int J Gynaecol Obstet, 2003. 82(3): p. 327-38.
8. Hannestad, Y.S., et al., A community-based epidemiological survey of female urinary incontinence: the Norwegian EPINCONT study. Epidemiology of Incontinence in the County of Nord-Trondelag. J Clin Epidemiol, 2000. 53(11): p. 1150-7.
9. Eliasson, K., T. Larsson, and E. Mattsson, Prevalence of stress incontinence in nulliparous elite trampolinists. Scand J Med Sci Sports, 2002. 12(2): p. 106-10.
10. DeLancey, J.O., Structural support of the urethra as it relates to stress urinary incontinence: the hammock hypothesis. Am J Obstet Gynecol, 1994. 170(6): p. 1713-20; discussion 1720-3.
11. Haylen, B.T., et al., An International Urogynecological Association (IUGA)/International Continence Society (ICS) joint report on the terminology for female pelvic floor dysfunction. Int Urogynecol J, 2010. 21(1): p. 5-26.

12. Brostrom, S. and G. Lose, Pelvic floor muscle training in the prevention and treatment of urinary incontinence in women - what is the evidence? Acta Obstet Gynecol Scand, 2008. 87 (4): p. 384-402.
13. Saleme, C.S., et al., An approach on determining the displacements of the pelvic floor during voluntary contraction using numerical simulation and MRI. Comput Methods Biomech Biomed Engin, 2011. 14(4): p. 365-70.
14. Jing, D., J.A. Ashton-Miller, and J.O. DeLancey, A subject-specific anisotropic visco-hyperelastic finite element model of female pelvic floor stress and strain during the second stage of labor. J Biomech, 2012. 45(3): p. 455-60.
15. Bø, K., et al., Pelvic floor muscle exercise for the treatment of female stress urinary incontinence: II. Validity of vaginal pressure measurements of pelvic floor muscle strength and the necessity of supplementary methods for control of correct contraction. Neurourology and Urodynamics, 1990: p. 479 - 487.
16. Bø, K., Urinary incontinence, pelvic floor dysfunction, exercise and sport. Sports Med, 2004. 34(7): p. 451-64.
17. Kruger, J.A., B.A. Murphy, and S.W. Heap, Alterations in levator ani morphology in elite nulliparous athletes: a pilot study. Aust N Z J Obstet Gynaecol, 2005. 45(1): p. 42-7.
18. Jiang, K., et al., Exercise and urinary incontinence in women. Obstet Gynecol Surv, 2004. 59 (10): p. 717-21; quiz 745-6.
19. Ree, M.L., I. Nygaard, and K. Bo, Muscular fatigue in the pelvic floor muscles after strenuous physical activity. Acta Obstet Gynecol Scand, 2007. 86(7): p. 870-6.

Effects of a Pelvic Floor Muscle Training in Nulliparous Athletes with Urinary Incontinence: Biomechanical Models Protocol

M. Sousa, R. Viana, S. Viana, T. Da Roza, R. Azevedo, M. Araújo, C. Festas, T. Mascarenhas and R.M. Natal Jorge

Abstract Urinary Incontinence (UI) is a prevalent condition among active women, especially in young nulliparous athletes. However, up to now, only a few studies conducted pelvic floor muscles training (PFMT) in athletes with UI. So, the present study evaluated the effect of a comprehensive PFMT protocol on UI symptoms in young nulliparous athletes using biomechanical models. This was a experimental and longitudinal pre and post-test evaluations study with 9 young nulliparous athletes divided in 2 intervention groups: one group had supervision of a physiotherapist and another does not. The participants answered the questionnaires: CONTILIFE to investigate the quality of life, the Self-efficacy Scale of Broome to evaluate the capacity of pelvic floor muscles (PFM) contraction, the IPAQ-SF to quantify the physical activity level and socio-demographic characteristics, to characterize the sample. Additionally, they were clinically assessed by *Pad*-test to quantify urine loss and by the Oxford Grading Scale and Perineometry to evaluate the strength of PFM contraction. It was used the *T-test* for two independent samples and the *Manny-Whitney test* to compare the groups, as well as the *Spearman* Correlation to correlational analysis. The level of significance was p ≤ 0.05. Seven

M. Sousa (✉) · R. Viana · S. Viana · R. Azevedo · C. Festas
UFP—University of Fernando Pessoa, Porto, Portugal
e-mail: mbm.sousa@gmail.com

R. Viana · S. Viana
UFP—University of Fernando Pessoa; CHSJ—EPE, Porto, Portugal

T. Da Roza · R.M. Natal Jorge (✉)
INEGI—Polo FEUP, Faculty of Engineering, University of Porto, Porto, Portugal
e-mail: rnatal@fe.up.pt

M. Araújo
Department of Sport Gynecology, Escola Paulista de Medicina, Federal University of de São Paulo (EPM-UNIFESP), São Paulo, Brazil

T. Mascarenhas
Department of Obstetrics and Gynecology, CHSJ-EPE, Faculty of Medicine, University of Porto, Porto, Portugal

© Springer International Publishing Switzerland 2015
J.M.R.S. Tavares and R.M. Natal Jorge (eds.), *Computational and Experimental Biomedical Sciences: Methods and Applications*, Lecture Notes in Computational Vision and Biomechanics 21, DOI 10.1007/978-3-319-15799-3_6

athletes concluded the 8 weeks-protocol. The protocol shown to be effective in reduce the loss of urine. Further research is necessary to determine the specific PFMT protocol in women that perform exercise.

Keywords Urinary incontinence · Athletes · Pelvic floor muscle training · Biomechanical models

1 Introduction

Recent studies show high prevalence of UI in young nulliparous athletes [1, 2]. According with International Continence Society, UI is defined as "the complaint of any involuntary loss of urine" [1]. The authors suggest that stress UI is the type that mainly affects women who performed high-impact sports, such gymnastics, athletics and ball games [2–4]. These exercises may cause PFM disorders due a frequent increase in intra-abdominal pressure or by the reaction ground forces [4–6]. The loss of urine usually occurs during training, conditioning the concentration and performance of the athletes and can cause a barrier to sports and the quitting of the modalities, once it decreases the quality of life because of feelings such as discomfort, embarrassment and insecurity [2–4]. Since, the PFM is the principal component to maintain the urinary continence and the pelvic organs on the right position, is essential to strengthen these muscles and teach the correct contraction through PFMT which is a first line conservative treatment classified with the higher level of evidence—grade A [2, 7]. Therefore, the purpose of the present study was to evaluate the effect of a comprehensive PFMT protocol on UI symptoms in young nulliparous athletes using biomechanical models. We believe that the models can provide a better understanding and perception about the PFM localization and awareness improving UI. The goal of these biomechanical models was to reproduce PFM contraction to demonstrate how the pelvic floor behaves and function [8–23].

2 Method

This is a longitudinal study with pre and post-test evaluations divided in 3 steps. In the first step participants should answered the questionnaires to characterize the sample; on the second step participants should be evaluated to prove if they had urine leakage; and in the third step they should start the PFMT protocol.

The inclusion criteria were being nulliparous, with 18 years old or more, perform physical activity and wanted to participate in the study. For the second step the women need to be incontinent. Exclusion criteria were: pregnant, having had

Table 1 Inclusion and exclusion criteria

	Inclusion criteria	Exclusion criteria
Step 1	♀nulliparous; age ≥18 years; regular physical activity; consent to participate in the study	Pregnant; previous pelvic surgery; neurological problems; ongoing urinary tract infections; pelvic organ prolapse; inability to contract the PFM
Step 2	Urine leakage	

previous pelvic surgery, neurological problems, ongoing urinary tract infections, pelvic organ prolapse, or inability to contract the PFM (Table 1).

In the first step, the participants should answered the CONTILIFE to evaluate the quality of life; the Self-efficacy Scale of Broome to verify the capacity of contraction of PFM; and the socio-demographic questionnaires to characterize the sample. In the second step, executed in the Fernando Pessoa University, 9 participants performed the clinical examination and quantify their urine leakage by *Pad-test*; the PFM strength were evaluated by Oxford Grading Scale and by Perineometry. Additionaly, all athletes answered the International Physical Activity Questionnaire—Short Form (IPAQ-SF) to evaluate their activity level. In the total, 9 participants were incontinent and were divided in the intervention groups. The protocol had 8-weeks of the—third step.

The athletes were randomly divided into the two study groups. The first group (n=4) performed 8-weeks protocol with supervision of a physiotherapist and the other group (n=5) performed the same protocol at home without supervision. Both groups received a DVD instruction with the biomechanical models. At the end of the protocol, 2 women drop out the study. Therefore, 7 participants performed the revaluation.

The 3D models were built with CAD software (Inventor software) and simulated the contraction using ABAQUS software. The purpose of these models was to facilitate the women to see, through a video, the location, action and how perform a correct contraction of the PFM. Additionally, the DVD showed the exercises that should be performed. The PFMT protocol was divided in 4 phases: (1) stabilization, (2) strength, (3) power, and (4) contraction the PFM during sport activities and each one had duration of 2 weeks.

The female athletes were recruited in sports and affiliated clubs in Porto, Portugal and the study was approved by the Fernando Pessoa University Ethical Committee, Porto, Portugal.

Statistical analyses were performed using SPSS software (version 18.0). Descriptive analyses used the mean, standard deviations, maximum and minimum and absolute and relative frequencies. In inductive analyses were used the *T-test* for two independent samples and the *Manny-Whitney test* and in the correlational analysis the *Spearman* correlation was used. A p value of ≤0.05 was considered statistically significant.

3 Results

In the first step 50 participants answered to the questionnaires. However, out of 50 participants, one was excluded because did not answer to all questions in the questionnaire. The second and third steps were performed with a sample of 9 and 7 women, respectively (Table 2). The overall prevalence of UI was 74 % among the women. The age, BMI and age of menarche were characterized as we can see in Table 3.

All athletes of the supervised group registered improvements in quality of life (total score and score 28), in self-efficacy of the PFM contractions (scores A and B and total score), an increase of PFM strength by *Oxford Grading Scale* and Perineometry and a decrease in leakage of urine by *Pad-test*. The unsupervised group did not improve the score 28 of the CONTILIFE and the score B of the self-efficacy in the PFM contraction and did maintain the *Oxford Grading Scale* in grade 4 (Table 4). The PFM strength had a better improve in supervised group and the changes between groups can be observed in Figs. 2 and 3. Comparing pre and post-evaluation the *Pad-test* parameter was significant ($p = 0.05$)—Fig. 1.

Table 2 Schematization of the sample size in the different stages of the study

	Supervised group n	Unsupervised group n
Step 1	50	
Step 2	4	5
Step 3	4	3

Table 3 Sociodemographic characterization of the sample

	$n = 49$
Mean age (years)	21,78 ± 3, 6
Mean weight (kg)	62,39 ± 8,0
Mean BMI (kg/m^2)	22,40 ± 2,4
Mean age at menarche (years)	12,14 ± 1,5

Table 4 Pre and post–test evaluations in supervised group and in unsupervised group

	Supervised group		Unsupervised group	
	Pre-test ($n = 4$)	Post-test ($n = 4$)	Pre-test ($n = 5$)	Post-test ($n = 3$)
Mean CONTILIFE—total score	9,45 ± 1.0	9,79 ± 0.4	9,26 ± 1.2	9,45 ± 0.9
Mean CONTILIFE—score 28	1,50 ± 0.6	1,25 ± 0.5	1,30 ± 0.6	1,67 ± 1.2
Mean self-efficacy of broom—score A	46,25 ± 48.1	75,71 ± 17.9	61,90 ± 45.0	71,43 ± 25.1
Mean self-efficacy of broom—score B	69,45 ± 17.5	75,00 ± 12.5	71,48 ± 17.2	65,93 ± 25.7
Mean self-efficacy of broom—total score	57,85 ± 32.2	75,36 ± 15.0	66,69 ± 30.5	68,68 ± 25.2
Mean *pad-test*	1,34 ± 0.4	0,93 ± 0.3	1,08 ± 0.1	1,07 ± 0.2
Mean *Oxford scale*	3,50 ± 0.7	4,50 ± 0.7	4,00 ± 0.0	4,00 ± 0.0
Mean perineometry	34,61 ± 0.5	54,59 ± 11.2	41,23 ± 0.0	48,23 ± 0.0

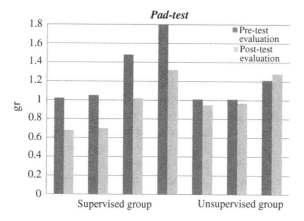

Fig. 1 Comparison between pre and post-test moments in *pad-test*

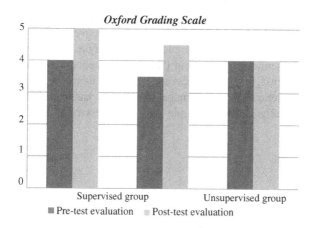

Fig. 2 Comparison between pre and post-test moments in *Oxford grading scale*

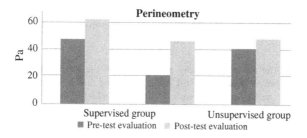

Fig. 3 Comparison between pre and post-test moments in perineometry

4 Discussion

Recent studies in the sports field and UI have shown a high prevalence of UI in nulliparous athletes, especially in those who perform high impact modalities [2–4]. This high prevalence was similar in the present study (74 %).

It was verified that the supervised group had better results than the unsupervised group. Urine leakage and PFM strength parameters has been associated with decrease in UI and with simultaneous increase of PFM strength, which can prevent the loss of urine [9, 10]. In fact, this study has registered improvements in urine leakage and in PFM strength, mainly in supervised group. Regarding the quality of life and self-efficacy in PFM contraction, the results obtained by the supervised group were tendentiously better when comparing to the other group. We suggest that this aspect may be related with a better reflection and reassessment of the UI that the supervisioned group was exposed. Studies have shown that the supervision is crucial for the correctly realization of PFMT protocols because can provide a greater awareness and understanding about this discipline, improve the perception and (re)assessment about the anatomy and exercises and the involvement is a motivation factor to increase the adherence and to recovery [3].

This study had some limitations such as the sample size due to the lack of information and openness to talk about UI, which can conditioned the adherence of athletes. We suggest further studies and more evidence, using biomechanical models and magnetic resonance image (MRI) to visualize and quantify PFM strength. Additionally, a larger sample will be necessary to confirm the present results.

5 Conclusion

The PFMT protocol seems to be effective in UI treatment in young nulliparous athletes. The supervised group demonstrated a significant improvement in *Pad-test* after 8-weeks protocol. The biomechanical models can be used as an alternative method to teach the women to contract their PFM. Additionally, biomechanical models can be used to a better understanding of physiological aspects of the pelvic floor by performing biomechanical simulations.

Acknowledgments The authors gratefully acknowledge to the funding by CNPq- from Brazil government and the project Pest-OE/EME/LA0022/2013 and also to the project "Biomechanics: contributions to the healthcare", reference NORTE-07-0124-FEDER-000035 co-financed by Programa Operacional Regional do Norte (ON.2—O Novo Norte), through the Fundo Europeu de Desenvolvimento Regional (FEDER).

References

1. Abrams P, et al, Fourth International Consultation on Incontinence Recommendations of the International Scientific Committee: Evaluation and treatment of urinary incontinence, pelvic organ prolapse, and fecal incontinence. Neurourol Urodyn, 2010. 29(1); p. 213–240.
2. Bo K, Berghmans B, Morkved S, & Van Kampen M, Evidence-Based PhysicalTherapy for the Pelvic Floor: Bridging Science and Clinical Practice. Elsevier Health Sciences, 2007.
3. Da Roza T, Araujo M, Viana R, Viana S, Jorge R, Bo K, & Mascarenhas T, Pelvic floor muscle training to improve urinary incontinence in young, nulliparous sport students: a pilot study. Int Urogynecol J, 2012. 23(8); p. 1069–1073.
4. Eliasson K, Larsson T, & Mattsson E, Prevalence of stress incontinence in nulliparous elite trampolinists. Scand J Med Sci Sports, 2002. 12(2); p. 106–110.
5. Fozzatti C, et al, Prevalence study of stress urinary incontinence in women who perform high-impact exercises. Int Urogynecol J, 2012.
6. Ree M, Nygaard I, & Bo K, Muscular fatigue in the pelvic floor muscles after strenuous physical activity. Acta Obstet Gynecol Scand, 2007. 86(7); p. 870–876.
7. Hay-Smith J, Herderschee R, Dumoulin C, & Herbison G, Comparisons of approaches to pelvic floor muscle training for urinary incontinence in women.[Meta-Analysis Review]. Cochrane Database Syst Rev (12), 2011.
8. Da Roza T, Araújo M, Mascarenhas T, Loureiro J, Parente M, & Natal Jorge R, Analysis of the contraction if the pubovisceral muscle based on a computational model. Portuguese Journal of Sport Sciences, 2011. 11 (2); p. 797–800.
9. Saleme C. et al, An approach on determining the displacements of the pelvic floor during voluntary contraction using numerical simulation and MRI. [Research Support, Non-U.S. Gov't]. Comput Methods Biomech Biomed Engin, 2011. 14(4); p. 365–370.
10. Parente M, Natal Jorge R, Mascarenhas T, Silva-Filho A, The influence of pelvic muscle activation during vaginal delivery: computational model. Obstetrics and Gynecology, 2010.115; p. 804–808.
11. D'Aulignac D, Martins J, Pires E, Mascarenhas T, Natal Jorge R, A Shell Finite Element Model of the Pelvic Floor Muscles. Computer Methods in Biomechanics and Biomedical Engineering, 2005. 8; p. 339–347.
12. Martins J, Pato M, Pires E, Natal Jorge R, Parente M, Mascarenhas T, Finite element studies of the deformation of the pelvic floor. Annals of the New York Academy of Sciences, 2007. 1101; p. 316–334.
13. Parente M, Natal Jorge R, Mascarenhas T, Fernandes A, Martins J, Deformation of the pelvic floor muscles during a vaginal delivery. International Urogynecology Journal, 2008. 19; p. 65–71.
14. Parente M, Natal Jorge R, Mascarenhas T, Fernandes A, Martins J, The influence of an occipito-posterior malposition on the biomechanical behavior of the pelvic floor. European Journal of Obstetrics, Gynecology & Reproductive Biology, 2009. 144S; p. S166-S169.
15. Parente M, Natal Jorge R, Mascarenhas T, Fernandes A, Martins J, The influence of the material properties on the biomechanical behavior of the pelvic floor during a vaginal delivery. Journal of Biomechanics, 2009. 42; p. 1301–1306.
16. Ma Z, Tavares J, Natal Jorge R, Mascarenhas T, A review of algorithms for medical image segmentation and their applications to the pelvic cavity., Computer Methods in Biomechanics and Biomedical Engineering, 2010. 13; p. 235–246.
17. Ma Z, Natal Jorge R, Tavares J, A shape guided C-V model to segment the levator ani muscle in axial magnetic resonance images. Medical Engineering Physics, 2010. 32; p. 766–774.
18. Parente M, Natal Jorge R, Mascarenhas T, Silva-Filho A, Computational modeling approach to study the effects of fetal head flexion during vaginal delivery. American Journal of Obstetrics and Gynecology, 2010. 203(217).

19. Ma Z, Natal Jorge R, Mascarenhas T, Tavares J, Novel approach to segment the inner and outer boundaries of the bladder wall in T2-weighted magnetic resonance images. Annals of Biomedical Engineering, 2011. 39; p. 2287–2297.
20. Martins P, Peña E, Natal Jorge R, Santos A, Santos L, Mascarenhas T, Calvo B, Mechanical characterization and constitutive modeling of the damage process in rectus sheath. Journal of the Mechanical Behavior of Biomedical Materials, 2012. 8; p. 111–122.
21. Ma Z, Natal Jorge R, Mascarenhas T, Tavares J, Segmentation of Female Pelvic Cavity in Axial T2-weighted MR Images towards the 3D Reconstruction. International Journal for Numerical Methods in Biomedical Engineering, 2012. 28; p. 714–726.
22. Ma Z, Natal Jorge R, Mascarenhas T, Tavares J, Segmentation of Female Pelvic Organs in Axial Magnetic Resonance Images using Coupled Geometric Deformable Models. Computers in Biology and Medicine, 2013. 43; p. 248–258.
23. Ma Z, Natal Jorge R, Mascarenhas T, Tavares J, A Level Set Based Algorithm to Reconstruct the Urinary Bladder from Multiple Views. Medical Engineering Physics, 2013. 35; p.1819–1824.

Biomechanical Study of the Cervical Spine

Tatiana Teixeira, Luísa Costa Sousa, R.M. Natal Jorge,
Marco Parente, João Maia Gonçalves and Rolando Freitas

Abstract The cervical spine is one of the most complex structures of the human skeleton. The knowledge of the cervical spine kinematics is a very important tool for many clinical applications such as diagnosis, treatment and surgical interventions and for the development of new spinal implants. The finite element method (FEM) is a well-known and widely used numerical method. In this study a three dimensional finite element (FE) model for the functional spine unit (FSU) C5-C6 was developed using computed tomography (CT) data. This model was used to study the internal stresses and strains of the intervertebral discs under static loading conditions of compression, extension, flexion, right lateral bending and left torsion. A hyperelastic constitutive model was used to describe the mechanical behavior of the nucleus pulposus. Maximum principal stresses in the disc were analyzed and higher values were found for the flexion movement. Maximum stresses in ligaments were observed for flexion and extension load cases.

Keywords Biomechanics · Finite element method · Cervical spine · Vertebrae C5/C6 · Intervertebral disc

T. Teixeira (✉)
Faculty of Engineering, University of Porto, Porto, Portugal
e-mail: tatiana.fsc.teixeira@gmail.com

L.C. Sousa · R.M. Natal Jorge · M. Parente
Department of Mechanical Engineering—Faculty of Engineering,
University of Porto, Porto, Portugal
e-mail: lcsousa@fe.up.pt

R.M. Natal Jorge
e-mail: rnatal@fe.up.pt

M. Parente
e-mail: mparente@fe.up.pt

J.M. Gonçalves · R. Freitas
Department of Spine Surgery, Orthopaedics Service—Centro Hospitalar de Vila
Nova de Gaia, Vila Nova de Gaia, Portugal
e-mail: maiagoncalves@gmail.com

1 Introduction

Spinal segments are subjected to repeated daily movements and loading by gravity and muscle forces. Taking into account the incidence of injuries in this region, which can result from trauma or degenerative diseases, it is sometimes necessary to resort to a surgical approach for maintaining the quality of life of the patient. The knowledge of the spinal kinematics is important into order to understand the load transfer through the intervertebral disc, the ligaments and the intervertebral joints. This knowledge facilitates diagnosis and treatment of instability, development and evaluation of spinal implants [1].

Any treatment of cervical spine injuries aims at returning to maximum functional ability with minimum of residual pain and residual deformity, decreasing of any neurological deficit and prevention of further disability. Furthermore, surgical treatment has some advantages like the immediate stability and the possibility for early mobilization. The use of computer models to study the biomechanical alterations of the cervical spine is a powerful tool to understand the mechanisms of injury. The finite element method is an excellent tool for studying the biomechanical behaviour of the cervical spine [2, 3] as it allows spine motion analysis for the purpose of planning surgical interventions.

In the past, several models were created, some of them consisting of a series of vertebrae (treated as rigid bodies) connected by ligaments and discs that are modeled as springs [4–6]; other detailed models in the representation of spinal geometries and materials, include the fiber-induced anisotropy to describe the behavior of the annulus fibrosus [7–9]. The first models could not accurately predict the mechanical behavior of the discs, and the last ones are limited by their dependence on model parameters that are difficult to determine. Recently more realistic models were used to study the behavior of healthy functional spine units [10–12], and to study surgical outcomes like anterior fusion and/or posterior fusion and spinal implants [13–16].

The main goal of this work was to demonstrate that a continuum model that considers a hyperelastic behavior of cervical nucleus pulposus is able to predict the stresses of the functional spine unit (FSU) C5-C6 and therefore foresee zones that are more likely to be damaged.

For this purpose a 3D finite element mechanical model of the C5-C6 FSU validated with experimental data was performed to investigate truly dynamic 3D motion data of the spine. First a FE model of the healthy C5-C6 FSU able to predict the relative movements of this pair of vertebrae under specific loads was created and validated considering flexion [3] and combined compression/flexion [13, 17, 18] load cases. Two types of material properties were used in order to find a combination of mechanical properties that allows obtaining accurate results. Then responses of the C5-C6 segment to static loads, such as axial compression, flexion, extension, lateral bending and torsion were calculated. This study was performed using the commercial code Abaqus Standard. The choice of this functional unit was due to the fact that these vertebrae are the most vulnerable to injury although they are still little studied [13].

2 Materials and Methods

The motion segment C5-C6 under consideration consists of two vertebral bodies, the intervertebral disc, spinal ligaments and facet joints. The intervertebral disc and ligaments contribute to the general flexibility of this spinal segment, having an important role in the spine kinematics. The finite element modeling of each component is described in the next sections.

2.1 Model Details

The construction of the C5-C6 FSU used in this study was established using CT scan data. The vertebra C5 has approximately 62.02 mm in width and 14.53 mm in height. The vertebra C6 has 59.54 mm in width and a height of 17.17 mm. The finite element mesh of the vertebrae was created using the commercial finite element package Abaqus. Vertebrae presented in Fig. 1 were modelled with four node tetrahedral elements C3D4.

After preparation of the vertebrae, the intervertebral disc was designed with its components, such as nucleus pulposus and annulus fibrosus bounded by two endplates [19, 20]. Due to its lower density, the intervertebral discs are not visible in a CT and disc geometry was defined using the lower surface of C5 and the upper surface of C6. Figure 2 shows the disc geometry with the two different regions, the inner nucleus pulposus and the peripheral annulus fibrosus. These two regions were created taking into account that the nucleus pulposus occupy between 30 and 50 % of the total area [21].

Aiming a refined mesh, a square was drawn in the centre of the nucleus pulposus in order to divide the intervertebral disc in four quadrants. The finite element mesh

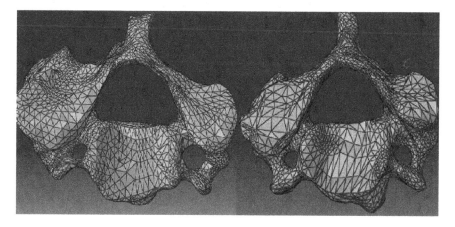

Fig. 1 Finite element mesh of vertebrae C5 and C6

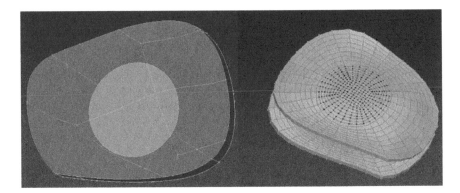

Fig. 2 Geometry and mesh of the intervertebral disc

was created with eight node hexahedral elements with a hybrid formulation C3D8H (Fig. 2). The definition of the endplates was performed considering the first and last layer elements and moving the nodes in order to decrease the thickness of the two plates (Fig. 2).

The annulus fibrosus is a viscous substance reinforced by a network of collagen fibres [22]. The arrangement of the elastic fibers plays a very important role in the overall mechanical properties of the annulus fibrosus [23]. The fibres present in the cervical spine are a set of eight layers making with each other an angle between 30° and 50° and having opposite directions from layer to layer [1, 10, 24]. Stiffness of fiber layers is higher at the outer side of disc, and decreased in center direction [25].

The fibres were modelled as tension-only truss elements, T3D2 [13] and embedded in the viscous matrix of the respective annulus layer. Figure 3a shows layer 1–2 of collagen fibres.

In order to model the intervertebral joints facet joints were created in the contact area of the two vertebrae (Fig. 3b). These facet joints were treated as a three-dimensional contact problem using surface-to-surface soft contact with exponential-pressure-over closure option available in ABAQUS.

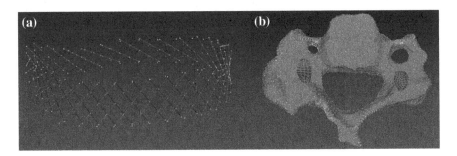

Fig. 3 a Layer 1–2 of collagen fibres; **b** facet joints

Finally the anterior longitudinal ligaments (ALL), the posterior longitudinal ligaments (PLL), the supraspinous ligament (SSL), the interspinous ligaments (ISL), the ligamentum flavum (LF) and the capsular ligaments (CL) were considered, and modeled with tension-only spring connector elements (truss elements T3D2), similar to the definition of the collagen fibres (Fig. 4). To simulate these ligaments, groups with different number of bars and equivalent sections were introduced between the anatomical insertion areas, as shown in Table 1.

2.2 Boundary and Loading Conditions

In FE modelling of spinal motion segments generally it is considered that the segment is supported rigidly along the inferior endplate of the lower vertebra, C6, and the loads are applied on the superior endplate of the upper vertebra. The loads can be applied as static or dynamic loads. Constant static loads or incrementally changing quasi-static loads are generally applied in cervical spine analyses.

In this study two types of static loading situations were used. The first type considers axial compression, pure flexion/extension, lateral bending and torsion types of cervical spine motion (Fig. 5). The second one is a combination of the pure flexion moments with a compression load. All the loads were applied in the superior surface of C5 through a reference node.

In numerical simulations of biomechanics, accuracy assessment can be obtained by experimental validation of numerical results. This enables to improve the agreement between the analytical and experimental data and consequently the quality and reliability of the FE model. The nucleus pulposus, mainly composed of water, was considered isotropic and almost incompressible. Two types of mechanical properties (Tables 2 and 3) were used in order to find the analytical results that best fit the experimental ones. In case 1 all the components where considered linear elastic and in case 2 a hyperelastic material was considered to characterize the behavior of the more gelatinous nucleus pulposus [5, 6].

The developed FE model was validated with previously published experimental results for two loading types: flexion [3], and a combination of flexion with a compressive force [13, 17, 18].

3 Results and Discussion

In first place the validation of the FE model was performed. Two analyses were performed considering two different loading types, flexion and a combination of the pure flexion with a compressive load. The accuracy of the developed model was validated by comparing output predictions with previously published experimental data. The results for flexion movement are shown in Fig. 6a and compared with the study of Wheeldon et al. [3]. The biggest differences (greater for properties case 1)

(a)

(b)

(c)

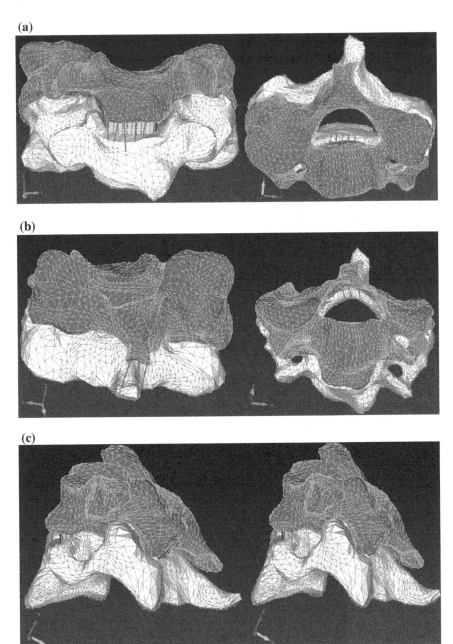

Fig. 4 Complete finite element model of the cervical spine: **a** ALL and PLL ligaments, **b** SSL and LF ligaments; **c** ISL and CL ligaments

Table 1 Ligaments definition

	Number of elements	Reference	Section area (mm^2)	Reference
ALL	5	[26]	12.1	[27]
PLL	5	[26]	14.7	[27]
ISL	4	[13]	13.4	[27]
LF	3	[26]	48.9	[27]
SSL	3	[13]	5.0	[17]
CL	6	[26]	46.6	[18]

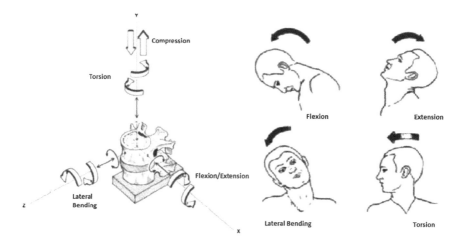

Fig. 5 Motions of the cervical spine: forces and movements of the mobile segment in three-dimensions [12, 13]

Table 2 Mechanical properties

Components	E (MPa)	ν	Reference
Vertebrae C5-C6	12,000	0.3	[13]
Annulus fibrosus	2.5	0.45	[13]
Fibres	500	0.3	[13]
LF	3.5	0.45	[13]
ALL	28	0.45	[13]
PLL	23	0.45	[13]
ISL	5	0.45	[13]
SSL	3	0.45	[26]
CL	5	0.45	[13]
Facet joints	5.5	0.4	[28]
End plates	300	0.3	[17]

Table 3 Mechanical properties of the nucleus pulposus

Components	Material	Reference
Case 1	Linear	[13]
	E = 0.1 MPa	
	v = 0.4999	
Case 2	Neo-Hookean	[10]
	C_1 = 0.16 MPa	
	D = 0.024 MPa^{-1}	

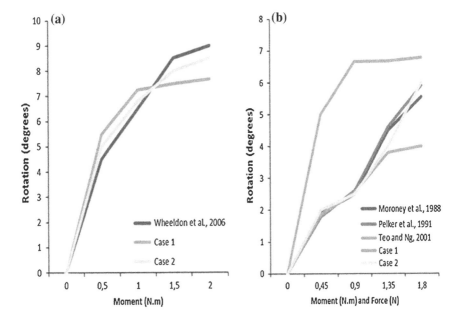

Fig. 6 Analitical versus experimental results: **a** flexion; **b** force/flexion

were obtained for the relative rotations coming from the highest moments. For the second load type, the predicted rotation, considering hyperelastic behavior for the nucleus pulposus, was in good agreement with the results in the literature.

The mechanical properties used in this work were chosen according to this study searching for accurate results. Hyperelastic material behavior assumed for the nucleus pulposus seems to be a realistic mechanical property and was adopted in the following analysis.

Figure 7 shows the displacement of the vertebral segment C5-C6 under a compression load. As expected, the displacement increased with higher loads, because the pressure applied on the vertebra C5 was higher, so this has tendency to slip on vertebra C6.

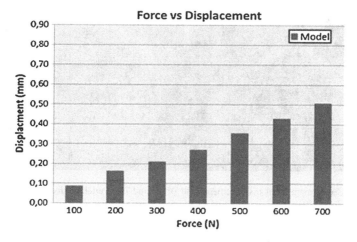

Fig. 7 Axial displacement of the vertebral segment C5-C6 under a compression load

Several movements were analyzed such as flexion, extension, lateral bending and torsion. For each load case displacements in direction z and the maximum principal stresses in the intervertebral disc were analyzed.

Considering load cases flexion and extension, moments of +2 and −2 nm were applied respectively. Output predictions for load case flexion, showed that a larger deformation of C5-C6 FSU was presented on the posterior zone, the apophysis (Fig. 8). Under extension, the opposite was verified on Fig. 9, and greater displacements occurred in the anterior zone.

Observing stress distribution on the disc the results were compression at the anterior zone and traction at the posterior zone, for the flexion load case. As expected, the opposite happened in the extension load case.

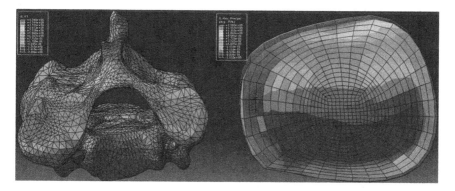

Fig. 8 C5-C6 segment axial displacement field (mm) and intervertebral disc stress distribution under flexion (MPa)

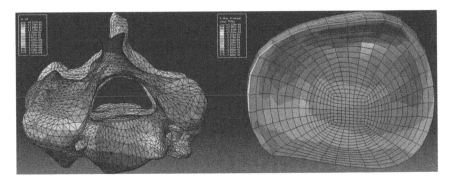

Fig. 9 C5-C6 segment axial displacement field (mm) and intervertebral disc stress distribution under extension (MPa)

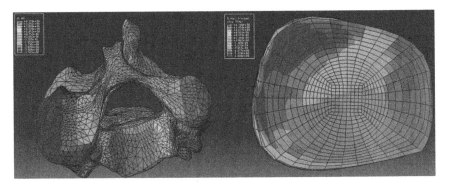

Fig. 10 C5-C6 segment axial displacement field (mm) and intervertebral disc stress distribution under lateral bending (MPa)

For right lateral bending load case a moment of 2 nm was applied. Figure 10 represents the displacement field of vertebral segment and stress distribution in intervertebral disc, under lateral bending. Output predictions were as expected, compression on the right side and traction on the left side.

Lastly, for left torsion load case a moment of 2 nm was applied. Figure 11 represents the displacement fields of vertebral segment and stress distribution in intervertebral disc. It can be seen that the right side of the intervertebral disc was under traction and the left side under compression.

Maximum values in ligament stress were observed for flexion and extension load cases. Flexion caused stretching of the interspinous, capsular, ligamentum flavum and posterior longitudinal ligaments and maximum value equal to 4.081 MPa, was observed in interspinous ligaments; extension yielded stretching of the anterior longitudinal ligament where maximum value is 3.279 MPa.

Although the current FEM model was based anatomically several limitations should be acknowledged. The definition of the vertebras was made considering

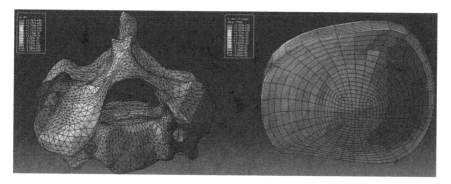

Fig. 11 C5-C6 segment axial displacement field (mm) and intervertebral disc stress distribution under *left* torsion (MPa)

them as rigid bodies. This simplification is not a relevant aspect in most of the cases since the stiffness of bones is much higher than the soft tissues. The work of Palomar et al. [10] compared two models, one considering and the other neglecting vertebrae deformation, and no significant differences were found in the stress patterns through the discs. A special effort was done to describe the intervertebral disc under a continuum model since this is an essential constituent of the intervertebral disc. The behavior of the highly reinforced annulus guided by the orientation of its collagen fibers is modeled by a elastic incompressible model while the nucleus pulposus that is mainly composed of water totally confined without fluid flow, is considered as an hiperelastic material. Weather this simplification is important or not it should be studied in a future work.

In this work the ligaments were represented using truss elements that only resisted tension. In order to obtain more accurate results the introduction of the real geometry of these elements like using solid elements would be necessary.

The obtained results with static load conditions allow the prediction of the most loaded parts of the discs related to the most susceptible zones of damage. Future analysis should be performed using dynamic load conditions aiming for example to mimic sudden car decelerations due to impacts, a common event responsible for cervical injuries.

Although the finite element model developed for this study is still not fully complete, as muscle forces and initial stresses of the ligaments were not considered it proved to be a useful tool for understanding the biomechanical behavior of the cervical spine.

4 Conclusions and Future Work

One purpose of this paper was to show the relevance of incorporating realistic constitutive models to accurately predict the internal stresses in the intervertebral disc of the C5-C6 segment under different loading scenarios. Finite element models present low costs and no risks to the biological tissue (bone), and they are able to provide data that are impossible to acquire in a cadaver body, such as strains and stresses on the disc. In summary, a three-dimensional cervical finite element model was validated with previously published experimental data and applied to obtain stresses in the intervertebral disc of a cervical unit under several spine movements. Obtained results allow the prediction of the most stressed parts of the discs corresponding to areas prone to damage.

This study was not exhaustive. The presented analysis can be considered as a first step in creating a complete model to study the evolution of different pathologies and concept implants, for example, the total disc replacement.

Acknowledgments The authors gratefully acknowledge the collaborative work of the medical team from Centro Hospitalar de Vila Nova de Gaia, a public hospital of Portugal.

References

1. V. Moramarco, A. P. Palomar, C. Pappalettere, and M. Doblare, "An accurate validation of a computational model of a human lumbosacral segment.," *Journal of Biomechanics*, vol. 43, pp. 334–342, 2010.
2. C. Calcavanti and J. L. Alves, "Understanding the role of the annulus fibrous in the biomechanics of the intervertebral disc," in *Proceeding of the 5th Portuguese Congress on Biomechanics*, 2013.
3. J. A. Wheeldon, F. A. Pintar, S. Knowles, and N. Yoganandan, "Experimental flexion/extension data corridors for validation of finite element models of the young, normal cervical spine.," *Journal of biomechanics*, vol. 39, pp. 375–380, Jan. 2006.
4. D. Stemper, N. Yoganandan, F. A. Pintar, and R. D. Rao, "Anterior longitudinal ligament injuries in whiplash may lead to cervical instability," *Medical Engineering & Physics*, vol. 28, pp. 515–524, 2006.
5. K. Brolin and P. Halldin, "Development of a finite element model of the upper cervical spine and a parameter study of ligament characteristics," *Spine*, vol. 29, pp. 376–385, 2004.
6. K. Brolin, P. Halldin, and I. Leijonhufvud, "The effect of muscle activation on neck response," *Traffic Injury Prevention*, vol. 6, pp. 67–76, 2005.
7. D. M. Elliott and L. . Setton, "A linear material model for fiberinduced anisotropy of the annulus fibrosus," *Journal of Biomechanical Engineering*, vol. 122, pp. 173–179, 2005.
8. S. M. Klish and J. C. Lotz, "Application of a fiber-reinforced continuum theory to multiple deformations of the annulus fibrosus," *Journal of Biomechanics*, vol. 32, pp. 1027–1036, 1999.
9. V. K. Goel, E. Y. Kim, T. H. Lim, and J. N. Weinstein, "An analytical investigation of the mechanics of spinal instrumentation," *Spine*, vol. 13, no. 1988, pp. 1003–1011.
10. A. P. Palomar, B. Calvo, and M. Doblare, "An accurate finite element model of the cervical spine under quasi-static loading," *Journal of Biomechanics*, vol. 41, pp. 523–531, 2008.
11. N. Bogduk and S. Mercer, "Biomechanics of the cervical spine . I : Normal kinematics," *Clinical Biomechanics*, vol. 15, pp. 633–648, 2000.
12. J. Wheeldon, B. D. Stemper, N. Yoganandan, and F. A. Pintar, "Validation of a finite element model of the young normal lower cervical spine.," *Annals of biomedical engineering*, vol. 36, pp. 1458–69, Sep. 2008.

13. F. Galbusera, A. Fantigrossi, M. T. Raimondi, M. Sassi, M. Fornari, and R. Assietti, "Biomechanics of the C5-C6 spinal unit before and after placement of a disc prosthesis," *Biomechan.Model Mechanobiol*, vol. 5, pp. 253–261, 2006.

14. A. Goel and V. Laheri, "Plate and Screw Fixation for Atlanto-Axial Subluxation," *Acta Neurochirurgia*, pp. 47–53, 1994.

15. M. D. Nabil Ebraheim, "Posterior Lateral Mass Screw Fixation : Anatomic and Radiographic Considerations," *The University of Pennsylvania Orthopaedic Journal*, vol. 12, pp. 66–72, 1999.

16. M. Aebi, "Surgical treatment of upper, middle and lower cervical injuries and non-unions by anterior procedures," *Eur Spine J.*, vol. 19, pp. 33–39, Mar. 2010.

17. A. Laville, S. Laporte, and W. Skalli, "Parametric and subject-specific finite element modelling of the lower cervical spine . Influence of geometrical parameters on the motion patterns," *Journal of Biomechanics*, vol. 42, pp. 1409–1415, 2009.

18. J. D. Clausen, V. K. Goel, V. C. Traynelis, and J. Scifert, "Uncinate Processes and Luschka Joints Influence the Biomechanics of the Cervical Spine : Quantification Using a Finite Element Model of the C5C6 Segment," *Journal of Orthopaedic Research*, vol. 15, pp. 342–347, 1997.

19. R. Seeley, T. Stephens, and P. Tate, *Anatomia e fisiologia*, 6ªEdição ed. Lusociência - EdiçõesTécnicas e Científicas, Lda, 2003.

20. K. L. Moore and A. F. Dalley, *Anatomia orientada para a clínica*, 4ª Edição. Lippincott Williams & Wilkins, 2006.

21. A. E. Castellvi, H. Huang, T. Vestgaarden, S. Saigal, D. H. Clabeaux, and D. Pienkowski, "Stress Reduction in Adjacent Level Discs via Dynamic Instrumentation: A Finite Element Analysis," *SAS Journal*, vol. 1, no. 2, pp. 74–81, Jun. 2007.

22. H. Gray, *Anatomy of the Human Body*, 20ªEdição ed. New York: Bartleby.com., 2000.

23. L. J. Smith and N. L. Fazzalari, "The elastic fibre network of the human lumbar anulus fibrosus: architecture, mechanical function and potential role in the progression of intervertebral disc degeneration," *Eur Spine J.*, pp. 18–439, 2009.

24. G. Denozière and D. N. Ku, "Biomechanical comparison between fusion of two vertebrae and implantation of an artificial intervertebral disc," *Journal of Biomechanics*, vol. 39, 2006.

25. Cheung, J. Tak-Man, M. Zhang, and D. Chow, "Biomechanical responses of the intervertebral joints to static and vibrational loading: a finite element study," *Clinical Biomechanics*, vol. 9, pp. 790–799, 2003.

26. N. Maurel, F. Lavaste, and W. Skalli, "A three-dimensional parameterized finite element model of the lower cervical spine . Study of the influence of the posterior articular facets," *Journal of Biomechanics*, vol. 30, no. 9, 1997.

27. N. Yoganandan, S. Kumaresan, and F. A. Pintar, "Biomechanics of the cervical spine Part 2. Cervical spine soft tissue responses and biomechanical modeling.," *Clinical biomechanics*, vol. 16, pp. 1–27, Jan. 2001.

28. M. Rodrigues, "Análise e projecto de estruturas para substituição do disco intervertebral.," Faculdade de Ciências e Tecnologia, 2012.

Injury Simulation of Anterior Cruciate Ligament Using Isogeometric Analysis

J.P.S. Ferreira, M.P.L. Parente and R.M. Natal Jorge

Abstract Many active sportsmen trend to get injured in knee ligaments. For that reason, singular researches on the deformations limits of Anterior Cruciate Ligament (ACL) which ensure the stability of knee have been made. Understanding in detail the running of the knee plays an important role in the design of orthotics and prosthetics, and may also modify surgical protocols. As a consequence, the injury risk will be minimized with the right knowledge of the knee functioning. The Isogeometric Analysis has the potential to facilitate the study of the most of bio-mechanical models, which are usually geometrically complex. In this work, we present the deformation of ACL at an injury position using the isogeometric approach (IGA), suggested by Cottrell (Isogeometric analysis toward integration of CAD and FEA. Wiley, Hoboken, 2009) and Hughes et al. (Comput Methods Appl Mech Eng 194:4135–4195, 2005). Also is emphasized the potential of IGA formulations in future of the Biomechanics.

Keywords Anterior cruciate ligament · ACL · Knee · Isogeometric analysis

1 Introduction

The Anterior Cruciate Ligament (ACL) connects from a posterio-lateral part of the femur to an anterio-medial part of the tibia. These attachments allow it to resist anterior translation of the tibia, in relation to the femur. More specifically, it is

J.P.S. Ferreira · M.P.L. Parente (✉) · R.M. Natal Jorge
Instituto de Engenharia Mecânica (IDMEC), Faculdade de Engenharia da
Universidade do Porto, Rua Dr. Roberto Frias, s/n, 4200-465 Porto, Portugal
e-mail: mparente@fe.up.pt

J.P.S. Ferreira
e-mail: em09029@fe.up.pt

R.M. Natal Jorge
e-mail: rnatal@fe.up.pt

© Springer International Publishing Switzerland 2015
J.M.R.S. Tavares and R.M. Natal Jorge (eds.), *Computational and Experimental Biomedical Sciences: Methods and Applications*, Lecture Notes in Computational Vision and Biomechanics 21, DOI 10.1007/978-3-319-15799-3_8

attached to the depression in front of the intercondyloid eminence of the tibia, being blended with the anterior extremity of the lateral meniscus. It passes up, backward, and laterally, and is fixed into the medial and back part of the lateral condyle of the femur [3]. The ACL tears appears upon a dislocation, tortion, or hyperextension of the knee. It is a very common injury in football, hockey, skiing, skating and basketball, due to the enormous amount of pressure, weight and number of impact solicitations, the knee must withstand [4].

The knee instability caused by high incidence of ACL injuries requires successful therapeutic solutions, otherwise leads to discomforting and painful situations. Thus, detailed knowledge of the ACL strain gradients during a injury situation helps in the design of orthotics and prosthetics, and may also modify surgical protocols. Several mechanical tests results shows that the ACL is able to withstand stretching up to 15 % in young adults [5]. It must be added that depending on the severity, the injuries can lead to complete rupture of the ligament or just the disruption of some ligament fibers, and in this second case, depending on the number of fibers broken the joint may become unstable or remain stable. Unstable joints can be surgically corrected and stable joints displacements, in the majority of cases, need to be controlled with a orthotic attached.

The combination of the physics involved by systems of partial differential equations and geometric description has promoted better and more efficient methods for solving mathematical problems numerically. This work was driven by the existing gap between Finite Element Analysis (FEA) and computer-aided design (CAD). Bridging these two tools it is even necessary to unify analysis and design fields. It would be of great advantage if there was interoperability between these two systems to facilitate computational analysis and engineering processes. That is the main goal of Isogeometric Analysis (IGA). In future, numerical computational simulations using IGA concept should provide accurate results and facilitating all the process.

Whereas CAD systems are characterized by exact (small gaps within predefined tolerances are allowed) descriptions of the inner and outer shells of the object and 3D models are sufficiently accurate for production purposes, in FEA the object is represented with a description of composed structures of finite elements, where there is a cruder representation of the shape of inner and outer hulls. In addition FEA needs compact geometric descriptions, where unnecessary detail is removed to focus the analysis on essential properties of the objects, namely, the simulation is performed only in the regions of interest to study the physical problem.

Right now, numerical simulation often involves using the Finite Element Method (FEM) where the geometry model, derived from CAD, usually will suffer a reparametrization of the CAD geometry by piecewise low order polynomials (mesh), generally applying linear Lagrange polynomials to approximate the geometry. This information transfer between models suitable for design (CAD) and analysis (FEM) is considered being a bottleneck in industry (industrial applications) of today, because it introduces significant approximation errors, or makes the simulations computational costly in FEM models with fine mesh, and entails a huge amount of man-hours to generate a suitable finite element mesh.

The IGA concept was introduced by Hughes et al. in [2] and was already applied in various engineering problems like: structural vibrations [6], linear and non-linear elasticity and plasticity [7], Reissner-Mindlin plates and shells [8, 9], and on other engineering problems 1. Their contribution to the biomechanics field seen bring some advantages like: The representation of trivariate models through splines allowed the representation of complex shapes without increased computational costs; Once the CAD geometry is build, further communication geometry is not necessary because mesh refinements can be made without geometry changes and; The development of global and local refinement techniques will allow improving the accuracy and efficiency of the method [10]. So, given the biomechanical models complexity, the IGA constitutes a very powerful tool.

However, since this is a recent method there are some challenges to overcome. Currently the CAD systems are programmed to define precisely the models geometry through surfaces but, in a general case, the FEM uses volume elements. The creation of a volumetric spline model from the surfaces of the CAD model suggests the study of local refinement techniques.

That said, this work seeks essentially to show the convergence of the method in a simplified elastostatic simulation of an common ACL injury event. In reality, the ACL has a anisotropic (bundles structure) viscoelastic behavior and is subject to fatigue and impact shocks. In this work ACL was considered with elastic and isotropic behavior and subjected to a static load. Also the geometry was created manually, leading to a simplified geometry of the ACL.

2 A Brief on Nurbs CAD Representation

2.1 Fundamental Concepts

In order to describe complex curves, surfaces or solids, parametric representations are used. NURBS parameterization is well suitable to describe the geometry of the model. A curve, surface, or solid can be described parametrically, respectively, as

$$\mathbf{C}(\xi) = (x(\xi), y(\xi), z(\xi)), \quad (\xi) \in [0, 1] \tag{1}$$

$$\mathbf{S}(\xi, \eta) = (x(\xi, \eta), y(\xi, \eta), z(\xi, \eta)), \quad (\xi, \eta) \in [0, 1] \times [0, 1] \tag{2}$$

$$\mathbf{G}(\xi, \eta, \zeta) = (x(\xi, \eta, \zeta), y(\xi, \eta, \zeta), z(\xi, \eta, \zeta)), \quad (\xi, \eta, \zeta) \in [0, 1] \times [0, 1] \times [0, 1] \tag{3}$$

The use of polynomials as a tool for computational modeling of geometric entities can approximate a large number of functions and these kind of functions are easily differentiated and integrated.

Several developments were made in order to develop well posed functions to describe complex geometries. First, Bernstein polynomials emerged [11]. Later, Bézier parameterization employing Bernstein polynomials allowed the parametric description of a curve, surface or solid. But, complex geometric entities cannot be represented using just one polynomial function to define the entire domain. It is then that emerges the idea to split the domain of the geometric entity (curve, surface or solid) into subdomains. Therefore, polynomials by parts have been employed to describe the geometric entities, where breakpoints are enforced up to some desired continuity order and are the end points for every subdomain. Note that these breakpoints are related to the knot vectors of the respective curve, surface or solid, in each direction. The B-spline and NURBS basis functions definitions contains this subdomain approach.

2.2 Knot Vector and Basis Function

The knot vector is a set of numerical values describing the knot coordinates in the parametric space, where non-decreasing sequence of parametric coordinates, $\xi_i \leq \xi_{i+1}$, $i = 1, \ldots n + p$. The ξ_i are called knots. Depending on the geometric topology, knot spans may represent points, lines or surfaces. After the knot coordinates are established, the knot spans knots spans are always surrounded by two consecutive knots, constituting the elementary entities for Isogeometric Analysis in the same manner as elements are basic entities for Finite Element Analysis (FEA).

If the the order of the polynomial basis functions is p, the parametric coordinates at the beginning and at the end of an open knot vector are repeated $p + 1$ times, and internal knots may be repeated p times. Open knot vectors are the most used by the geometric modeling packages. Each time a internal knot is repeated the continuity of the curve will decrease by one at respective control point. The basis functions are interpolatory at the end knots and in internal knots have multiplicity p (repeated p times). This is distinguish feature between knots and nodes in FEA (FEA elements are interpolatory).

The B-spline basis functions are defined by Cox-de-Boor recursion formula [11] for a given knot vector (Ξ, $\mathcal{H}$ and $\mathcal{Z}$) which are defined over the parametric space, the number of control points (n, m and l) and the polynomial degree (p, q and r) and over respective direction of the parametric space (ξ, η and ζ). So B-spline basis functions are defined as [11]

$$N_{i,p}(\xi) = \frac{\xi - \xi_i}{\xi_{i+p} - \xi_i} N_{i,p-1}(\xi) + \frac{\xi_{i+p+1} - \xi}{\xi_{i+p+1} - \xi_{i+1}} N_{i+1,p-1}(\xi) \tag{4}$$

over the knot vectors in respective directions

$$\Xi = \left\{ \xi_1, \ldots, \xi_{p+1}, \ldots, \xi_{n+1}, \ldots, \xi_{n+p+1} \right\}$$
$$\mathcal{H} = \left\{ \xi_1, \ldots, \eta_{q+1}, \ldots, \eta_{m+1}, \ldots, \eta_{m+q+1} \right\} \tag{5}$$
$$\mathcal{Z} = \left\{ \xi_1, \ldots, \zeta_{l+1}, \ldots, \zeta_{r+1}, \ldots, \zeta_{r+l+1} \right\}$$

starting with piecewise constants $(p = 0)$

$$N_{i,0}(\xi) = \begin{cases} 1, & \xi_i \leq t \leq \xi_{i+1} \\ 0, & otherwise \end{cases} \tag{6}$$

In addiction, B-spline geometries can be seen as a linear combination of B-spline basis functions presenting minimal support with respect to a given degree, continuity and domain partition.

2.3 NURBS Solid

For one-dimensional knot vector $\Xi = \left\{ \xi_1, \ldots, \xi_{n+p+1} \right\}$, a B-spline curve $\mathbf{C}_p(\xi)$ in $\mathbb{R}^3$ of order p is obtained by linear combination of the basis functions having as coefficients the coordinates of n control points $\mathbf{P}_i$. The mathematical expression is

$$\mathbf{C}_p(\xi) = \sum_{i=1}^{n} N_{i,p}(\xi) \mathbf{P}_i \tag{7}$$

A B-spline surface is constructed from a net of control points $\left\{ \mathbf{P}_{i,j} \right\}$ and from a two-dimensional knot set $\Xi \times \mathcal{H}$. The knot vector $\mathcal{H} = \left\{ \eta_1, \eta_2, \ldots, \eta_{m+q+1} \right\}$ of degree q have m control points or basis functions along the η direction. So, a tensor product B-spline surface is defined as

$$\mathbf{S}_{p,q}(\xi, \eta) = \sum_{i=1}^{n} \sum_{i=1}^{m} N_{i,p}(\xi) N_{j,p}(\eta) \mathbf{P}_{i,j} \tag{8}$$

In its turn, a tensor product B-spline solid are defined in analogous fashion. Given a control net $\left\{ \mathbf{P}_{i,j,k} \right\}$ and three-dimension knot set $\Xi \times \mathcal{H} \times \mathcal{Z}$, where $\mathcal{Z} = \left\{ \zeta_1, \zeta_2, \ldots, \zeta_{l+r+1} \right\}$ is a knot vector of degree r with l control points or basis functions along the ζ direction, is defined as

$$\mathbf{G}_{p,q,l}(\xi, \eta, \zeta) = \sum_{i=1}^{n} \sum_{j=1}^{m} \sum_{k=1}^{l} N_{i,p}(\xi) N_{j,q}(\eta) N_{k,r}(\zeta) \mathbf{P}_{i,j,k} \tag{9}$$

The rationalization of B-Splines involves a definition of a new basis functions, constructed from B-Spline basis functions. To define these rational basis functions is associated a weight w to a control point. So, a NURBS curve is defined by

$$\mathbf{C}_p(\xi) = \sum_{i=1}^{n} R_{i,p}(\xi) \cdot \mathbf{P}_i \tag{10}$$

where R_i^p is the NURBS basis functions for a curve and it's mathematical expression is

$$R_i^p(\xi) = \frac{N_{i,p}(\xi)w_i}{\sum_{i=1}^{n} N_{i,p}(\xi)w_i} \tag{11}$$

where w_i is the weight of control point $\mathbf{P}_i$.

Following the same reasoning, NURBS surfaces and solids are defined, respectively, by

$$\mathbf{S}_{p,q}(\xi,\eta) = \sum_{i=1}^{n} \sum_{j=1}^{m} R_{i,j}^{p,q}(\xi,\eta)\mathbf{P}_{i,j} \tag{12}$$

$$\mathbf{G}_{p,q,l}(\xi,\eta,\zeta) = \sum_{i=1}^{n} \sum_{j=1}^{m} \sum_{k=1}^{l} R_{i,j,k}^{p,q,r}(\xi,\eta,\zeta)\mathbf{P}_{i,j,k} \tag{13}$$

where rational basis functions are defined by the following equations

$$R_{i,j}^{p,q}(\xi) = \frac{N_{i,p}(\xi)N_{j,q}(\eta)w_{i,j}}{\sum_{i=1}^{n} \sum_{j=1}^{m} N_{i,p}(\xi)N_{j,q}(\eta)w_{i,j}} \tag{14}$$

$$R_{i,j,k}^{p,q,l}(\xi,\eta,\zeta) = \frac{N_{i,p}(\xi)N_{j,q}(\eta)N_{k,r}(\zeta)w_{i,j,k}}{\sum_{i=1}^{n} \sum_{j=1}^{m} \sum_{k=1}^{l} N_{i,p}(\xi)N_{j,q}(\eta)N_{k,r}(\zeta)w_{i,j,k}} \tag{15}$$

Additional information on NURBS may be found in [11]. As a comment to the previously equations, NURBS can be considered as a mapping from parametric space $\hat{\Omega}$ to physical space Ω. Now, remains the definition for the mapping from parametric space to the physical space.

3 An Isogeometric Formulation for Linear Elastostatic Models

Trivariate discretisations defined by Eq. 13 are not given in a explicitly way and usually some preprocessing is required before the application of the numerical solution. IGA and FEA are both isoparametric implementations of Galerkin's method, thus the code architectures are very similar [12].

3.1 Relevant Spaces

For the use of NURBS as a basis for analysis it is important to define the mappings and the spaces.

3.1.1 Index Space

The index space consists of a net of index knot points for all combinations of the NURBS patch, regardless of whether the knot is repeated or not. The index space is illustrative for analyzing the support of the basis functions, which can easily be read in this space, but are less apparent in the parametric space. Figure 1 shows a bivariate NURBS patch represented at the index space.

3.1.2 Parametric Space

Parametric space (the pre-image of the NURBS mapping) is formed by only the non-zero intervals between knot values forming the parametric space $\hat{\Omega} \subset \mathbb{R}^{d_p} \left(d_p = 1, 2, 3 \right)$ associated with a set of parametric coordinates $\boldsymbol{\xi} = (\xi, \eta, \zeta) = \left(\xi^1, \xi^2, \xi^3 \right)$.

Regarding the attention to Fig. 1, the region bounded by knot lines with non-zero area contains a set of unique knot values δ such that δ is the element domain. More formally, a set of n_s^i unique knot values δ^i in the parametric direction i such that

$$\delta^i = \left\{ \xi_1^i, \xi_2^i, \ldots, \xi_{n_s^i}^i \right\}, \quad \xi_j^i \neq \xi_j^i \tag{16}$$

represents the unique knot values for each parametric direction i. So, a generic element is defined in a multivariate case by

$$\hat{\Omega}^e = [\xi_i, \xi_{i+1}] \otimes [\eta_j, \eta_{j+1}] \otimes [\zeta_k, \zeta_{k+1}], \quad 1 \leq i, j, k \leq n_s^1, n_s^2, n_s^3 - 1 \tag{17}$$

Fig. 1 Bivariate NURBS
patch on index space
containing the parameter
space (*grey filled*)

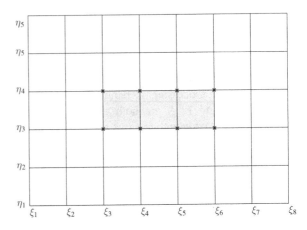

for the knots that are unique, that is, $\xi_i \in \delta^1$, $\eta_j \in \delta^2$, $\zeta_k \in \delta^3$, and n_s^i is the number of unique knots along parametric direction i. A possible numbering scheme for elements over a patch is

$$e = k\left(n_s^2 - 1\right)\left(n_s^1 - 1\right) + j\left(n_s^2 - 1\right) + i \tag{18}$$

3.1.3 Physical Space

The NURBS mapping transform coordinates in parameter space to the physical space $\Omega \subset \mathbb{R}^{d_p}$. For trivariate domains, a coordinate system $\boldsymbol{x} = (x, y, z) = (x^1, x^2.x^3)$ is associated for the physical space.

Note that neither the index knots in the index space nor the parameter space are directly linked with control points on the physical space.

3.1.4 Parent Space

The previous three spaces are inherent to NURBS but to perform the analysis routines it is required the definition of an additional space, the parent space $\tilde{\Omega}^e = [-1, 1]^{d_p}$. Parent space is used for numerical integration routines which are often defined over the interval $[-1, 1]$ and the respective coordinates are denoted as $\tilde{\boldsymbol{\xi}} = \left(\tilde{\xi}, \tilde{\eta}, \tilde{\zeta}\right) = \left(\tilde{\xi}^1, \tilde{\xi}^2.\tilde{\xi}^3\right)$.

3.2 Formulation

Accordingly to 13, the displacement field of a generalized linear elastostatic tri-variate model

$$\mathbf{u}(\xi) = \begin{bmatrix} u(\xi) \\ v(\xi) \\ w(\xi) \end{bmatrix} \tag{19}$$

is given by

$$\mathbf{u}(\xi) = \mathbf{R_a}(\xi)\mathbf{d_a} \tag{20}$$

where $\mathbf{d_a}$ contains the displacements over the N control points of the model.

Using the differential relation between strains and displacements, the strain field is defined as

$$\varepsilon(\xi) = \mathbf{LR}(\xi)\mathbf{d_a} \tag{21}$$

where differential operator $\mathbf{L}$ is defined as

$$\mathbf{L} = \begin{bmatrix} \frac{\partial}{\partial \xi} & 0 & 0 \\ 0 & \frac{\partial}{\partial \eta} & 0 \\ 0 & 0 & \frac{\partial}{\partial \zeta} \\ \frac{\partial}{\partial \xi} & \frac{\partial}{\partial \eta} & 0 \\ \frac{\partial}{\partial \zeta} & 0 & \frac{\partial}{\partial \xi} \\ 0 & \frac{\partial}{\partial \zeta} & \frac{\partial}{\partial \eta} \end{bmatrix} \tag{22}$$

Rewriting the equation above, the strain vector can be obtained by the following expression

$$\varepsilon(\xi) = \mathbf{B}(\xi)\mathbf{d}_a \tag{23}$$

Finally, the stress field is given by

$$\sigma = \mathbf{D}\varepsilon \tag{24}$$

where $\mathbf{D}$ is the elastic constitutive matrix.

$$\mathbf{D} = \frac{E}{(1+v)(1-2v)} \begin{bmatrix} 1-v & v & v & 0 & 0 & 0 \\ v & 1-v & v & 0 & 0 & 0 \\ v & v & 1-v & 0 & 0 & 0 \\ 0 & 0 & 0 & \frac{1-2v}{2} & 0 & 0 \\ 0 & 0 & 0 & 0 & \frac{1-2v}{2} & 0 \\ 0 & 0 & 0 & 0 & 0 & \frac{1-2v}{2} \end{bmatrix} \tag{25}$$

for a certain Young's Modulus E and Poisson's ratio v. Using the NURBS approximation, the stress field is can be rewritten as

$$\sigma = \mathbf{DB}(\xi)\mathbf{d_a} \tag{26}$$

Once the deformation matrix is already defined the stiffness matrix and load vector can be obtain establishing the element equilibrium. That is, for any virtual displacement of the element the work done by all the forces applied is zero (Virtual Work Principle). This principle leads to the follow equation:

$$\delta W_K + \delta W_P + \delta W_f = 0 \tag{27}$$

The first term is the work done by the inertial forces Once we have only static forces this term is zero.

$$W_K = 0 \tag{28}$$

The second term of Eq. 27 is related to the work done by the internal forces and is given by the following expression

$$W_P = \int_\Omega \sigma^T \varepsilon d\Omega \tag{29}$$

Applying virtual displacements to Eq. 29 and regarding the Eqs. 23 and 24, we obtain

$$\delta W_P = \int_\Omega \delta \mathbf{d_a}^T \mathbf{B}^T \mathbf{DB} \mathbf{d_a} d\Omega \tag{30}$$

The third term of Eq. 27 is the work done by external forces. In the case of the application of only surface forces $\mathbf{q}$ and volume forces $\mathbf{b}$ the work of external forces is given by

$$\delta W_f = -\int_S \delta \mathbf{d_a}^T \mathbf{R}^T \mathbf{q} dS - \int_\Omega \delta \mathbf{d_a}^T \mathbf{R}^T \mathbf{b} d\Omega \tag{31}$$

Returning to the Eq. 27, the principle of virtual work leads to the following equation

$$\int_\Omega \delta \mathbf{d_a}^T \mathbf{B}^T \mathbf{D} \mathbf{B} \mathbf{d_a} d\Omega - \int_S \delta \mathbf{d_a}^T \mathbf{R}^T \mathbf{q} dS - \int_\Omega \delta \mathbf{d_a}^T \mathbf{R}^T \mathbf{b} d\Omega = 0 \qquad (32)$$

The weak form derived from Eq. 32 can be expressed as the sum of integrals over which element for the entire domain.

$$\sum_{e=1}^{n_e} \left(\int_\Omega \delta \mathbf{d}_a^{e^T} \mathbf{B}^T \mathbf{D} \mathbf{B} \mathbf{d}_a^e d\Omega - \int_S \delta \mathbf{d}_a^{e^T} \mathbf{R}^T \mathbf{q} dS - \int_\Omega \delta \mathbf{d}_a^{e^T} \mathbf{R}^T \mathbf{b} d\Omega \right) = 0 \qquad (33)$$

which is valid for any virtual displacement. So, the last equation leads us to

$$\sum_{e=1}^{n_e} \left(\int_{\Omega_e} \hat{\mathbf{B}}^T \mathbf{D} \hat{\mathbf{B}} d\Omega_e \right) \mathbf{d_a}^e = \sum_{e=1}^{n_e} \left(\int_{S_e} \mathbf{R}^T \mathbf{q} dS_e + \int_{\Omega_e} \mathbf{R}^T \mathbf{b} d\Omega_e \right) \qquad (34)$$

Note that the displacements at the control points of the element $\mathbf{d}_a^e$ are restricted to the respective integration domain through Eqs. 20 and 34 leads to a system of linear algebraic equations where the unknowns are the displacements of control points of the model.

3.3 Discretization

For a given element e, using the isoparametric discrestization, the geometry is expressed as

$$x^e(\xi) = \sum_{a=1}^{n_{en}} R_a^e(\xi) \mathbf{P}_a^e \qquad (35)$$

where a is a local basis function index, $n_{en} = (p + 1)(r + 1)(s + 1)$ is the number of non-zero basis functions over the element e, $\mathbf{P}_{i,j,k}$ are the control points and $R_a^e(\bar{\varepsilon})$ is the NURBS basis function on parent domain associated with index a. The translation of a local basis function index to a global index is made by the connectivity array IEN [1] through

$$A = IEN(a, e) \qquad (36)$$

Global and local control points are therefore related through $\mathbf{P}_a^e = \mathbf{P}_{IEN(a,e)}$ with similar expressions for R_a^e.

So, the displacement field $\mathbf{u}(\mathbf{x})$ governed by our Partial Differential Equations (PDE) is discretized in a similar manner

$$\mathbf{u}^e\left(\tilde{\boldsymbol{\xi}}\right) = \sum_{a=1}^{n_{en}} R_a^e\left(\tilde{\boldsymbol{\xi}}\right)\mathbf{d}_a^e \tag{37}$$

where $\mathbf{d}_a^e$ are the control (nodal) variables.

The discretization process using NURBS introduces the concept of parametric space which is nonexistent in Finite Element simulations. As a consequence, we have an additional mapping in order to operate in parent element coordinates. Usually, there exist a mapping $\tilde{\phi}^e : \tilde{\Omega} \to \hat{\Omega}^e$ that relates parent space and parameter space and a mapping $\mathbf{S} : \hat{\Omega} \to \Omega$ which defines the relation between parameter and physical spaces. The composition $\mathbf{S} \circ \tilde{\phi}^e$ gives the mapping from parent to the physical domain $\mathbf{x}^e : \tilde{\Omega} \to \Omega^e$. Figure 2 shows the mappings defined previously.

Fig. 2 Representation of mappings thought from parent space to physical space

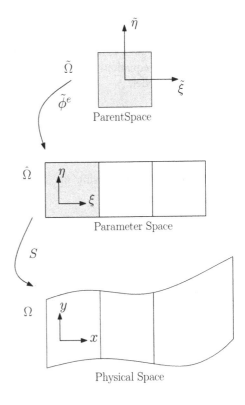

The relation between parent space and parameter space for an element is given by

$$\tilde{\phi}^e\left(\tilde{\xi}\right) = \begin{cases} \frac{1}{2}\left[(\xi_{i+1} - \xi_i)\tilde{\xi} + (\xi_{i+1} + \xi_i)\right] \\ \frac{1}{2}\left[(\eta_{i+1} - \eta_i)\tilde{\eta} + (\eta_{i+1} + \eta_i)\right] \\ \frac{1}{2}\left[(\zeta_{i+1} - \zeta_i)\tilde{\zeta} + (\zeta_{i+1} + \zeta_i)\right] \end{cases} \tag{38}$$

witch associated Jacobian determinant $\left|\mathbf{J}_{\tilde{\xi}}\right|$. In its turn the mapping from parameter space to physical space, given by Eq. 13 for a tridimensional case, leads to a Jacobian matrix (associated with respective Jacobian determinant $|\mathbf{J}_\xi|$) given by

$$\mathbf{J}_\xi = \begin{bmatrix} \frac{\partial x}{\partial \xi} & \frac{\partial x}{\partial \eta} & \frac{\partial x}{\partial \zeta} \\ \frac{\partial y}{\partial \eta} & \frac{\partial y}{\partial \eta} & \frac{\partial y}{\partial \zeta} \\ \frac{\partial z}{\partial \zeta} & \frac{\partial z}{\partial \eta} & \frac{\partial z}{\partial \zeta} \end{bmatrix} \tag{39}$$

obtained performing the following expression

$$\frac{\partial \mathbf{x}}{\partial \xi} = \sum_{a=1}^{n_{en}} \mathbf{P}_\mathbf{a}^\mathbf{e} \frac{\partial R_a^e(\xi)}{\partial \xi} \tag{40}$$

where n_{en} is the number of control points of the element.

Since the numerical integration is performed in the parent domain, the Jacobian determinant for the mapping $\mathbf{x}^e : \tilde{\Omega} \to \Omega^e$ is given by

$$|J| = \left|J_{\tilde{\xi}}\right| |J_\xi| \tag{41}$$

and the derivatives of basis functions in respect to the physical coordinates are calculated by

$$\left[\frac{\partial R_a{}^e}{\partial \mathbf{x}}\right] = \left[\frac{\partial R_a{}^e}{\partial \xi}\right] \mathbf{J}_\xi^{-1} \tag{42}$$

Finally, with the mappings previously defined it is possible to integrate a function $f : \Omega \to \mathbb{R}$ over the physical domain using the parent domain in the following way

$$\int_\Omega f(x)d\Omega = \sum_{e=1}^{n_{el}} \int_{\tilde{\Omega}} f\left(\tilde{\xi}\right)|J|d\tilde{\Omega} \tag{43}$$

In this work, the typical Gaussian quadrature procedure was used. It should be emphasized that Gaussian quadrature is not optimal for IGA [12]. Optimal integration procedures have been studied in [13, 14].

4 Numerical Results

Based on [1, 3] a suitable physical net of control points $\mathbf{P}_{i,j,k}$ and respective weights $w_{i,j,k}$ and a proper choice of the knot vectors in each direction, that is the NURBS trivariate patch $\Xi \times \mathcal{H} \times \mathcal{Z}$ the simplified ACL geometry was created.

The ACL anatomy was checked in [8], using average sizes for an adult. Thus, the geometry of the ACL was approximated by a cylinder with a radius of 11 mm and a length of 38 mm, where the ends have a gradually increasing radius to emphasize the connections to the femur and the tibia. The obtained geometry is shown in Fig. 3.

Studies in [4] shows a viscoelastic behavior in the longitudinal direction of the ligament. For young adults, the average unidirectional tensile test results are present in Fig. 4. Observing Fig. 4, for a certain range of deformations, the ACL has an approximate elastic behavior with Young's modulus 0.8 GPa. The Poisson's ratio was arbitrated value was equal to 0.33.

As an attempt to match the injury position, the ligament was placed in a approximate position in order to make compatible to the situation of the most common injury position. That is, leg 10° bent, interior rotation of 15° with foot constraint.

Therefore, it can be stated in an approximate way, that the ACL-femur connection is fixed and the ACL-tibia connection is subjected to a static load consisting of a transverse tensile stress and a torsional moment. This situation is shown in Fig. 5. However, the equivalence situation for the application of this loads was made by imposing prescribed displacements (Dirichlet boundary conditions) on control points of ACL-tibia connection to approximate the injury position.

Fig. 3 ACL approximated geometry

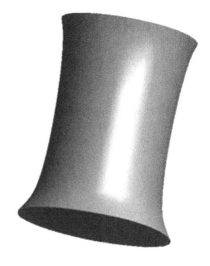

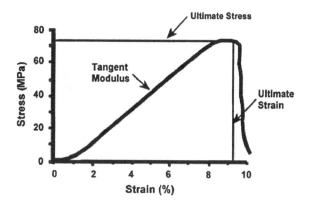

Fig. 4 Stress-strain curve from ACL longitudinal tensile tests [4]

The establishment of the ACL stiffness matrix was made using Gaussian quadrature, which varied in the number of Gaussian points for each knot span. Figures 6 and 7 shows the obtained results and displacement field, respectively.

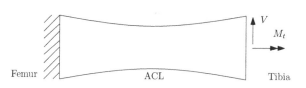

Fig. 5 Approximate boundary conditions of the ACL injury

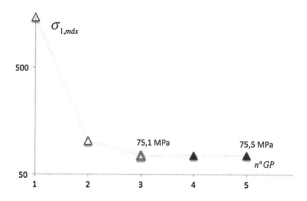

Fig. 6 Maximum Von Mises stress as a function of the number o gauss points per knot span

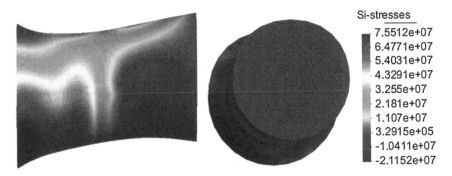

Si-stresses
7.5512e+07
6.4771e+07
5.4031e+07
4.3291e+07
3.255e+07
2.181e+07
1.107e+07
3.2915e+05
-1.0411e+07
-2.1152e+07

Fig. 7 ACL displacement field using 5 gauss points per knot span

5 Conclusions

The design of the model was subjected to simplifications: geometric, relative to material characterization, and on the prescribed displacements. In fact, the ACL deformed position is complex and difficult to represent and we only can represent the real ACL demeanor including in the model the around the ACL structures and obtaining realistic geometries.

The linear elastostatic IGA model using NURBS converged to a maximum Von Mises stress to approximately 75 MPa using 3 Gauss points per knot span in each parametric direction.

In the future, obtaining trivariate spline models directly from a CAD software will allow the analysis of biomechanical complex models in a friendly way. To reach a more realistic model it is necessary include anisotropy, viscoelasticity, fatigue and impact loads, differentiate areas with distinct mechanical behavior (distinguish bundles and matrix), and study the influence of model refinement on the final results.

Acknowledgments The authors truly acknowledge the funding provided by Ministério da Ciência, Tecnologia e Ensino Superior Fundação para a Ciência e a Tecnologia (Portugal), under grant SFRH/BPD/75072/2010, and by FEDER/FSE, under grant PTDC/EMETME/098050/2008.

References

1. J Cottrell. *Isogeometric analysis toward integration of CAD and FEA*. Wiley, Chichester, West Sussex, U.K. Hoboken, NJ, 2009.
2. T.J.R. Hughes, J.A. Cottrell, and Y. Bazilevs. Isogeometric analysis: Cad, finite elements, nurbs, exact geometry and mesh refinement. *Computer Methods in Applied Mechanics and Engineering*, 194(39 – 41):4135 – 4195, 2005.
3. Gerard J. Tortora and Bryan H. Derrickson. *Principles of Anatomy and Physiology, 12th Edition*. Wiley, 2008.

4. FREDDIE H. FU, CHRISTOPHER D. HARNER, DARREN L. JOHNSON, MARK D. MILLER, and SAVIO L.-Y. WOO. Biomechanics of knee ligaments basic concepts and clinical application. *The Journal of Bone & Joint Surgery*, 75(11):1716–1727, 1993.
5. Savio L.-Y. Woo, Steven D. Abramowitch, Robert Kilger, and Rui Liang. Biomechanics of knee ligaments: injury, healing, and repair. *Journal of Biomechanics*, 39(1):1 – 20, 2006.
6. J.A. Cottrell, A. Reali, Y. Bazilevs, and T.J.R. Hughes. Isogeometric analysis of structural vibrations. *Computer Methods in Applied Mechanics and Engineering*, 195(41–43): 5257 – 5296, 2006. John H. Argyris Memorial Issue. Part {II}.
7. T. Elguedj, Y. Bazilevs, V.M. Calo, and T.J.R. Hughes. and projection methods for nearly incompressible linear and non-linear elasticity and plasticity using higher-order {NURBS} elements. *Computer Methods in Applied Mechanics and Engineering*, 197(33–40): 2732 – 2762, 2008.
8. Chien H. Thai, H. Nguyen-Xuan, N. Nguyen-Thanh, T-H. Le, T. Nguyen-Thoi, and T. Rabczuk. Static, free vibration, and buckling analysis of laminated composite reissnermindlin plates using nurbs-based isogeometric approach. *International Journal for Numerical Methods in Engineering*, 91(6):571–603, 2012.
9. D.J. Benson, Y. Bazilevs, M.C. Hsu, and T.J.R. Hughes. Isogeometric shell analysis: The reissnermindlin shell. *Computer Methods in Applied Mechanics and Engineering*, 199 (5–8):276 – 289, 2010. Computational Geometry and Analysis.
10. J.A. Cottrell, T.J.R. Hughes, and A. Reali. Studies of refinement and continuity in isogeometric structural analysis. *Computer Methods in Applied Mechanics and Engineering*, 196(41–44):4160 – 4183, 2007.
11. Les Piegl. *The NURBS book*. Springer, Berlin New York, 1997.
12. V. Phu Nguyen, S. P. A. Bordas, and T. Rabczuk. Isogeometric analysis: an overview and computer implementation aspects. *ArXiv e-prints*, May 2012.
13. T.J.R. Hughes, A. Reali, and G. Sangalli. Efficient quadrature for nurbs-based isogeometric analysis. *Computer Methods in Applied Mechanics and Engineering*, 199(5–8):301 – 313, 2010. Computational Geometry and Analysis.
14. F. Auricchio, F. Calabr, T.J.R. Hughes, A. Reali, and G. Sangalli. A simple algorithm for obtaining nearly optimal quadrature rules for nurbs-based isogeometric analysis. *Computer Methods in Applied Mechanics and Engineering*, 249–252(0):15 – 27, 2012. Higher Order Finite Element and Isogeometric Methods.

Influence of Flexing Load Position on the Loading of Cruciate Ligaments at the Knee—A Graphics-Based Analysis

A. Imran

Abstract Injuries of the cruciate ligaments of the knee, particularly the anterior cruciate ligament (ACL), is a common problem in young athletes. Therefore, identification of high-risk factors that lead to injury of the knee ligaments is required to avoid loading or protecting the ligaments from injury or during rehabilitation. In the present study, mechanics of the knee was analyzed for the influence of external flexing load positions on loading of the cruciate ligaments in the sagittal plane during 0° to 120° flexion. Experimental data was taken from literature. Mechanical equilibrium of the tibia was considered due to four types of forces, namely, a force in the patellar tendon, a ligament force, a tibio-femoral joint contact force, and an external flexing load applied distally on the tibia. The analysis suggests that during the muscle exercise at the knee, loading of the cruciate ligaments depends on flexion angle as well as on the position of external load on the tibia. Far distal placements of flexing loads on the tibia can stretch the ACL significantly at low flexion angles. The PCL is stretched during mid-to-high flexion range for all positions of the external flexing loads on the tibia. However, during the mid-flexion range, the effects of placement are modest. Therefore, rehabilitation exercises requiring protection of the ligaments need to pay attention to the position of external flexing load on the tibia as well as flexion angle at which the exercise is performed.

Keywords Ligament injuries · ACL rehabilitation · Ligament mechanics

A. Imran (✉)
Ajman University of Science & Technology, P. O. Box 346, Ajman, UAE.
e-mail: ai_imran@yahoo.com; ajac.ai_imran@ajman.ac.ae

© Springer International Publishing Switzerland 2015   123
J.M.R.S. Tavares and R.M. Natal Jorge (eds.), *Computational and Experimental
Biomedical Sciences: Methods and Applications*, Lecture Notes in Computational
Vision and Biomechanics 21, DOI 10.1007/978-3-319-15799-3_9

1 Introduction

Injuries of the cruciate ligaments of the knee, particularly the anterior cruciate ligament (ACL), is a common problem in young athletes. Studies suggest that the ACL injured patients are at a high risk of developing osteoarthritis 10–15 years after injury, irrespective of treatment [1, 10]. Therefore, identification of high-risk factors that lead to injury of the knee ligaments is required to avoid loading or protecting the ligaments from injury or during rehabilitation. Previous studies have identified positions of the external loads on the tibia that have the potential of loading either the anterior or the posterior cruciate ligament (ACL or PCL) [5, 11]. In the present study, mechanics of the knee was analyzed for the influence of flexing load positions on loading of the cruciate ligaments in the sagittal plane during 0° to 120° flexion. The analysis is based on considerations of mechanical equilibrium of the joint with external loads balanced by forces and moments developed in the internal structures like, tendons and ligaments as well as bone-to-bone joint contact force.

2 The Knee in the Sagittal Plane

Figure 1a gives a simplified representation of the knee in the sagittal plane with main load bearing structures as the two cruciate ligaments, muscle tendons and the bones. Straight lines were used to show the net forces in the respective tendons or ligaments. Other soft tissues, like articular cartilage or the menisci were not taken into consideration. Also, the collateral ligaments were not included in the analysis as they are shown to have minimal contributions in the sagittal plane [6, 7].

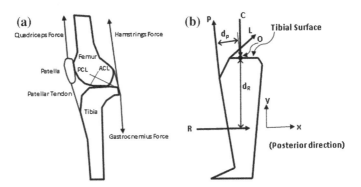

Fig. 1 Major load-bearing structures of the knee in the sagittal plane. **a** Outlines of the femoral and tibial bones and the patella are shown. *Straight lines* represent the net forces in the ligaments and muscle tendons. **b** Equilibrium of the lower leg during simulated quadriceps muscle exercise. External flexing load (R) is balanced by internal forces P, C and L. ('L' represents either the ACL or the PCL forces)

3 Equilibrium of the Joint During a Simulated Quadriceps Contraction

Figure 1b shows the lower leg in equilibrium during a simulated quadriceps muscle contraction which resists flexion due to an externally applied load on the leg. There are four types of forces involved, namely an external load, muscle force transmitted to the tibia through patellar tendon, a ligament force and a joint contact force. Each of these forces is described below.

3.1 External Load (R)

The external flexing load (R) acts on the tibia parallel to the tibial surface and a known distance below the joint line in the posterior direction. In practice, the external loads on the leg may arise due to gravity, ground reaction or other sources during activity like a reaction force when a player hits a ball with his leg.

3.2 Muscle Force

A force in the patellar tendon (P) due to a pull exerted by the quadriceps muscle contraction and transmitted to the tibia via the quadriceps tendon, patella and the patellar tendon. The force P has an extending effect at the joint and can also translate the lower bone or tibia relative to the upper bone or femur. The orientation of P changes with flexion, directed more anteriorly near extension and more posteriorly in high flexion. The orientation of P is also influenced by the tibial translation, for example, an anterior translation of the tibia would decrease the anterior component of P near extension or increase the posterior component of P in high flexion.

3.3 Ligament Force (L)

The ligaments (ACL or PCL) exert forces on the tibia when stretched due to relative translation or distraction of the two bones. An anterior translation of the tibia relative to the femur stretches the ACL, while a posterior translation stretches the PCL. The angle of ACL with the tibial articular surface decreases with increasing flexion [3] or with increasing anterior translation of tibia [5]. The angle of PCL with the posterior direction first decreases from low-to-mid flexion range and then increases from mid-to-high flexion range [3]. A posterior translation of tibia results in reduced inclination of the PCL with tibial articular surface.

3.4 Joint Contact Force (C)

A compressive contact force (C) exists between the femoral and tibial bones at the joint. As the healthy joints are known to have nearly zero friction [9], the contact force acts normal to the surfaces at their contact. Also, in normal healthy joints, articular surfaces and menisci (not considered for this analysis) help in reducing stresses by increasing the area of contact [2].

3.5 Kinematics

At full extension or 0° flexion, the long axes of the tibial and femoral bones are parallel. With flexion, the angle between the two axes increases to a maximum of about 140°. Any change in the flexion angle results in changed orientations and/or locations of the internal joint forces.

3.6 Conditions of Equilibrium

Equation (1) gives the condition for equilibrium of moment; Eqs. (2) and (3) give the conditions for equilibrium of forces in the anterior-posterior and proximal-distal directions, respectively.

With reference to Fig. 1, the flexing moment generated by R about the knee is balanced mainly by an extending moment provided by P due to a pull from the quadriceps muscles transmitted to the tibia through patella. As the patellar tendon is located much closer to the joint center of rotation than the external loads, the moment arm available to P is normally much smaller than that available to R. As a consequence, the force P is much bigger than R, as given by Eq. (1).

Forces parallel to the tibial articular surface have translational effect. Any unbalanced horizontal force in Fig. 1b would translate the tibia relative to the femur. As a consequence, the ligaments would stretch and resist the translation with a force (L). When excessive, such translations have the potential of overstretching the ligament fibers, possibly resulting in injury to the involved ligament.

Forces perpendicular to the tibial surface either push the bones into each other or distract them. The joint contact force (C) resists interpenetration of the bones while ligamentous structures resist distraction of the bones.

$$P * d_P + R * d_R = 0 \tag{1}$$

$$P * \cos(\phi_P) + R * \cos(\phi_R) + L * \cos(\phi_L) = 0 \tag{2}$$

$$P * \sin(\phi_P) + L * \sin(\phi_L) + C * \sin(\phi_C) = 0 \tag{3}$$

where,

R, P, L and C are the forces as defined earlier in this section.

ϕ is the angle with the positive x-axis for a force given by its respective subscript.

'd' is the moment arm from the tibio-femoral contact point (point O in Fig. 1b) for a force given by its respective subscript.

By definition, $\phi_R = 0°$.

4 Factors that Influence the Loading of Cruciate Ligaments

During a simulated quadriceps exercise, the effects of position of external flexing load on tibia and the orientation of patellar tendon are analyzed below in terms of their influence on the loading of cruciate ligaments. The situations that would load or unload each of the cruciate ligaments are described below and also illustrated in Figs. 2 and 3.

4.1 Proximal—Distal Position of the External Flexing Load

Distal placement of flexing load on the tibia results in an increased moment arm available to R, thus, flexing moment about the joint center of rotation is also increased. The balancing effect in the form of an extending moment is provided

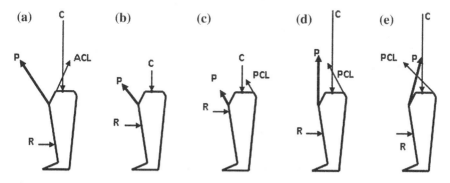

Fig. 2 Diagrammatic representation of the factors that influence the loading of cruciate ligaments at the knee. The *lines* showing the respective forces in each illustration are in proportion to their magnitudes as calculated using Eqs. (1–3). **a** Anterior component of P is greater than R, the joint equilibrium requires a force in the ACL. **b** Anterior component of P equals to R, the joint equilibrium does not require any ligament force. **c** Anterior component of P is smaller than R, the joint equilibrium requires a force in the PCL. **d** P is perpendicular to the tibial surface, the joint equilibrium requires a force in the PCL. **e** P is directed posteriorly, the joint equilibrium requires a force in the PCL

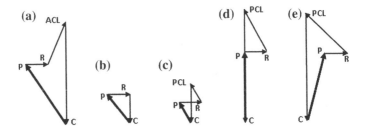

Fig. 3 Equilibrium of forces acting on the lower leg shown graphically corresponding to the five different situations illustrated in Fig. 2. ACL force is required in (**a**), while PCL force is required in (**c**–**e**). No ligament force is required in (**b**)

mainly by quadriceps muscle force through the patellar tendon. However, in comparison to the external load, the patellar tendon force is located closer to the joint center with a much smaller moment arm. As a consequence, the force P required for equilibrium of moment is much larger than the force R. As given by Eq. (1), the force ratio, P/R is inversely proportional to the ratio of their moment arms, d_R/d_P.

4.2 Orientation of the Patellar Tendon

The patellar tendon, therefore, the force P is shown to have an anterior direction in the flexion range from 0° to nearly 70°, and posterior direction for higher flexion angles [4, 8].

A force in the ACL would be required if P has an anterior component that is greater than R, as illustrated in Fig. 2a. A force in the PCL would be required if P has an anterior component that is smaller than R, or if P is not directed anteriorly, as illustrated in Fig. 2c–e. No ligament force would be required if the anterior component of P exactly balances the posterior R (Fig. 2b).

Figure 3 graphically shows the equilibrium of forces at the knee for five different situations leading to loading or unloading of the cruciate ligaments during quadriceps exercise. The force estimates follow Eqs. 1–3.

4.3 Shear Force on the Tibia

Shear force (T) on the tibia is defined here as the sum of the components of P and R that are parallel to the tibial surface. Using Eq. (2) without the ligament force, the equation for T is as given by Eq. 4.

$$T = P * \cos(\phi_P) + R * \cos(\phi_R) \tag{4}$$

where, the meaning of the symbols is same as defined earlier.

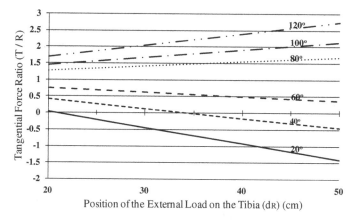

Fig. 4 Tangential force ratio (T/R) plotted against increasing values of the moment arm d_R for different flexion angles of the knee. Negative is anterior

As explained in the sections above, for balancing the shear force, a negative value of T would require a force in the ACL and a positive value of T would require a force in the PCL. Using Eq. (1), the ratio P/R can be calculated in terms of moment arms of the respective forces. Further, utilizing experimental measurements from Herzog and Read [3] for moment arms and orientations of the patellar tendon during flexion, the values of T are calculated per unit of R for known positions and orientations of the external load. Figure 4 shows the force ratio T/R plotted for increasing values of 'd_R' while $\phi_R = 0°$. The ratios are plotted for flexion angle = 20, 40, 60, 80, 100 and 120°. The following important observations can be made from the plot:

- At 20° flexion, the T/R ratio is negative, requiring ACL force, for $d_R > 20.5$ cm.
- At 40° flexion, the T/R ratio is negative, requiring ACL force, for $d_R > 34$ cm.
- At all other flexion positions shown, the T/R ratio is positive, requiring a force in the PCL.
- For all flexion positions, the magnitude of shear force increases with increasing values of d_R.
- At low as well as at high flexion angles, the force ratio increases relatively sharply as the distance d_R increases. In the mid-flexion range, the increase in the shear force due to an increase in d_R is relatively modest.

5 Conclusions

Based on the model results, analysis suggests that during the muscle exercise at the knee, loading of the cruciate ligaments depends on flexion angle as well as on the position of external load on the tibia.

Far distal placements of flexing loads on the tibia can stretch the ACL significantly at low flexion angles. The PCL is stretched during mid-to-high flexion range for all positions of the external flexing loads on tibia. However, during the mid-flexion range, such effects of variation in placement are relatively modest.

Therefore, rehabilitation exercises requiring protection of the ligaments need to pay attention to the position of external flexing load on the tibia as well as the flexion angle at which the exercise is performed.

References

1. Gillquist J and Messner K (1999) Anterior cruciate ligament reconstruction and the long-term incidence of gonarthrosis. Sports Med. 27: 143–56.
2. Goodfellow J and O'Connor J (1978) The mechanics of the knee and prosthesis design. J Bone Jt Surg. Br. 60(B): 358–369.
3. Herzog W and Read LJ (1993) Lines of action and moment arms of the major force-carrying structures crossing the human knee joint. J Anatomy 182: 213–230.
4. Imran A, Huss R, Holstein H and O'Connor J (2000) The variation in the orientations and moment arms of the knee extensor and flexor muscle tendons with increasing muscle force: a mathematical analysis. J Engineering in Medicine 214(H): 277–286.
5. Imran A and O'Connor J (1998) Control of knee stability after ACL injury or repair: interaction between hamstrings contraction and tibial translation. Clin Biomech. 13(3): 153–62.
6. Masouros SD, Bull A and Amis (2010) Biomechanics of the knee joint. Orthopaedics and Trauma. 24(2): 84–91.
7. Mommersteeg T, Blankevoort L, Huiskes R, Kooloos J and Kauer J (1996) Characterization of the mechanical behavior of human knee ligaments: a numerical-experimental approach. J Biomechanics 29(2): 151–160.
8. O'Connor J, Shercliff T, Biden E and Goodfellow J (1989) The geometry of the knee in the sagittal plane. J Engineering in Medicine 203 (H4): 223–233.
9. Unsworth A, Dowson D and Wright V (1975) Some new evidence on human joint lubrication. Ann. Rheum. Dis. 34: 277–285.
10. von Porat A, Roos EM and Roos H (2004) High prevalence of osteoarthritis 14 years after an anterior cruciate ligament tear in male soccer players: a study of radiographic and patient relevant outcomes. Ann Rheum Dis. 63: 269–73.
11. Zavatsky AB and O'Connor J (1993) Ligament forces at the knee during isometric quadriceps contractions. J Engineering in Medicine 207(H1): 7–18.

Modelling and Simulation in Orthopedic Biomechanics—Applications and Limitations

A. Imran

Abstract Modelling and simulation in orthopedic biomechanics involves the use of computational methods to study mechanics of load-bearing structures of the human musculoskeletal system. Such joints as the hip, knee, ankle, elbow and shoulder provide us mobility with stability during various activities. Changes in the internal configurations of a joint due to an abnormality, injury or surgical intervention, can affect the ability of a person to perform common activities. The internal structures, like ligaments, tendons and bones are not readily amenable to direct observation or measurement. Also, certain effects are difficult to analyze using experiment, for example, the influence of surgical techniques on the resulting joint mechanics. Modeling and simulation using computational methods, therefore, provides an opportunity to gain insight into the behavior of the joints and to predict effects due to a variety of internal joint configurations which are otherwise difficult, cost prohibitive, unethical or impossible to implement using the available experimental techniques. However, sensitivity analysis, relevant validation and an understanding of limitations is important in order to have practical significance. This paper discusses various approaches, applications and limitations of computational methods used to study the mechanics of human joints.

Keywords Joint biomechanics · Computational biomechanics · Ligament mechanics

1 Introduction

Modelling and simulation in orthopedic biomechanics involves the use of computational methods to study mechanics of load-bearing structures of the human musculoskeletal system. This paper discusses various approaches, applications and

A. Imran (✉)
Ajman University of Science and Technology, P. O. Box 346, Ajman, UAE
e-mail: ai_imran@yahoo.com; ajac.ai_imran@ajman.ac.ae

© Springer International Publishing Switzerland 2015
J.M.R.S. Tavares and R.M. Natal Jorge (eds.), *Computational and Experimental Biomedical Sciences: Methods and Applications*, Lecture Notes in Computational Vision and Biomechanics 21, DOI 10.1007/978-3-319-15799-3_10

131

limitations of such methods used to study the joints, such as the hip, knee, ankle, elbow and shoulder. These joints provide us mobility with stability during various activities. Changes in the internal configurations of a joint due to an abnormality, injury or surgical intervention, can affect the ability of a person to perform common activities. The internal structures, like ligaments, tendons and bones are not readily amenable to direct observation or measurement. Also, certain effects are difficult to analyze using experiment, for example, the influence of surgical techniques on the resulting joint mechanics. Modeling and simulation using computational methods, therefore, provides an opportunity to study mechanics of the joints with a variety of internal changes. Validation of outcomes, however, has been a challenging task for the investigators.

2 Modelling and Simulation—Various Approaches

In developing a model, anatomical data and material properties of load bearing structures of the joint are required as input parameters. The joint mechanics during specific activities is simulated using theoretical or empirical approach [2–9]. The outcomes are normally validated either directly with specially designed experiments, or indirectly with relevant experimental or simulation studies from literature. Validated models can then be used, for example, to explain clinical observations or mechanisms of injury as well as to predict outcomes corresponding to different joint conditions. As an example, in a mathematical study of the knee joint with an artificial prosthesis, Imran [2] analyzed the surgical effects of component placement on resulting joint laxity during a simulated clinical test. The results agreed with common clinical observations and explained that how small errors in component placement could cause significant changes in the joint laxity. However, the analysis was limited to two dimensions only.

2.1 An Example of Application

In this example, a model of the knee is used in the sagittal plane to study the effects of relative movements of bones on forces in the internal structures of the joint. It will be shown that relatively small variations in positions of the internal structures of the joint have the potential to influence the resulting estimates of internal forces significantly.

Figure 1a illustrates the anatomy of knee joint in the sagittal plane, showing outlines for the femoral and tibial bones as well as the patella. The net muscle forces through their respective tendons are shown by straight lines. Two ligaments, the anterior and posterior cruciate ligaments (ACL and PCL, respectively) are also shown by straight lines. Other soft tissues, like articular cartilage or the menisci were not taken into consideration.

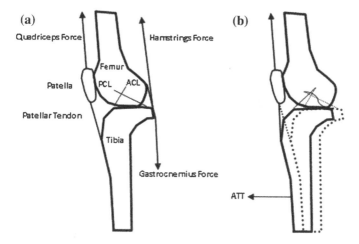

Fig. 1 Major load-bearing structures of the knee in the sagittal plane. **a** Outlines of the femoral and tibial bones and the patella are shown. *Straight lines* represent the net forces in the ligaments and muscle tendons. **b** The effects of anterior translation of tibia relative to the femur (ATT). The patellar tendon is shown to have re-oriented while the ligaments either re-orient and stretch or become slack, as illustrated. Also, the contact position between the bones has shifted posteriorly. Hamstrings and gastrocnemius muscle forces are not shown for the sake of clarity

Figure 1b illustrates the effects of translation of the lower bone anterior to the upper bone. As a result of the translation the orientations of the tendon and ligament forces are altered as well as the location of contact between the bones is changed. Further, the moment arms available to the forces may also change.

Figure 2 illustrates a simulated muscle exercise in which a posteriorly directed flexing load (R) acts on the tibia, shown here parallel to the tibial surface. The joint equilibrium is provided by a force in the patellar tendon (P), a joint contact force acting between the two bones (C) and a ligament force (L) (either ACL or PCL as shown in Fig. 1a, b). Moment arms are shown by the letter M with a subscript corresponding to the respective force.

In this example, the rotational effect of R about the point O is balanced by the rotational effect of P. The rotational effects due to L were ignored. Since P is located much closer to the point O, the force P must be much larger than the force R. Further, an unbalanced tangential force (T) parallel to the tibial surface can translate the tibia relative to the femur and stretch either the ACL or the PCL as explained below.

When P has an anterior component greater than R, the tibia would translate anterior to the femur, thus, stretching the ACL. Similarly, when P has a component smaller than R, the tibia would translate posterior to the femur, thus, stretching the PCL. If the anterior–posterior component of P exactly balances R, no ligament force would be required.

Figure 3 shows the tangential force T plotted as a ratio of R over the flexion range 0°–120°. The values are compared for the joint in the neutral state and after

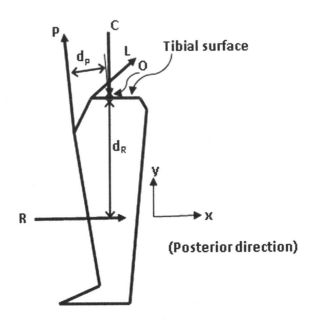

Fig. 2 Equilibrium of the lower leg during a simulated muscle exercise. External flexing load (R) is balanced by internal forces P, C and L

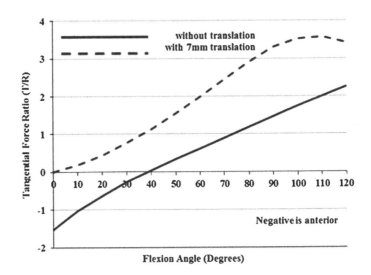

Fig. 3 Tangential force ratio (T/R) plotted during flexion with and without tibial translation

7 mm translation of the tibia anterior to the femur. For these calculations, ana-tomical parameters as well as orientations and moment arms of patellar tendon were taken from experimental measurements on cadaver knees [1, 8]. Without tibial

translation, the T/R ratio was negative for nearly 0°–40° flexion and positive thereafter. With 7 mm translation the ratio was altered significantly and became positive for all flexion positions of the joint. This effect may explain a possible compensatory mechanism in the form of large tibial translations observed in the knees with ACL–deficiency [4].

3 Limitations of Modelling and Simulation

Literature shows large variations in input parameters as well as in force and motion data obtained from in vivo or in vitro experimental studies. Even in some investigations outcomes are found to be contradictory to other similar studies or to general observations. Such variations or contradictions have been found to arise due to individual differences in the living subjects or cadaver specimens as well as due to the applied experimental set-up and measuring techniques. Therefore, the models and simulations of the joints are limited in their applicability and interpretation of results. An understanding of such limitations is important for this exercise to be of practical relevance.

3.1 Parameter Sensitivity

In general, the simulation outcomes are found to be more sensitive to certain input parameters than others. For example, in a theoretical study of the anterior cruciate ligament, Toutoungi et al. [9] found that variations in certain anatomical parameters of the model changed the ligament force by 130 % while altering the mechanical parameters produced smaller differences in force of less than 15 %. In another theoretical study of the knee mechanics, Imran et al. [3] found relatively small differences between incompressible and compressible contact conditions for a simulated test. A sensitivity analysis is, therefore, needed in order to understand the behavior of the model and the nature of errors, particularly while utilizing the model for individualized or for predictive applications.

4 Conclusions

In conclusion, computational models and simulations of the human mobile joints provide an opportunity to gain insight into the behavior of the joints and to predict effects due to a variety of internal joint configurations which are otherwise difficult, cost prohibitive, unethical or impossible to implement using the available experimental techniques. However, sensitivity analysis, relevant validation and an understanding of limitations is important in order to have practical significance.

References

1. Herzog W and Read LJ (1993) Lines of action and moment arms of the major force-carrying structures crossing the human knee joint J Anatomy 182: 213–230.
2. Imran A (2010) Unicompartmental knee arthroplasty (UKA) – effects of component placement on joint mechanics studied with a mathematical model. IFMBE Proc (Springer) 31: 616–619.
3. Imran A, Huss R, Holstein H and O'Connor J (2000) The variation of orientations and moment arms of the knee extensor and flexor muscle tendons with increasing muscle force. J Engineering in Medicine 214(H): 277–286.
4. Imran A and O'Connor J (1998) Control of knee stability after ACL injury or repair: interaction between hamstrings contraction and tibial translation. Clin Biomech. 13(3): 153–62.
5. Lewis C, Sahrmann S and Moran D (2010) Effect of hip angle on anterior hip joint force during gait. Gait & Posture 32(4): 603–607.
6. Morrow M, Kaufman K and An KN (2010) Shoulder model validation and joint contact forces during wheelchair activities. J Biomechanics 43(13): 2487–2492.
7. Nikooyan A, Veeger H, Chadwick E, Praagman M and van der Helm FCT (2011) Development of a comprehensive musculoskeletal model of the shoulder and elbow. Med Biol Eng Comput. 49: 1425–1435.
8. O'Connor J, Shercliff T, Biden E and Goodfellow J (1989) The geometry of the knee in the sagittal plane. J Engineering in Medicine 203 (H4): 223–233.
9. Toutoungi D, Zavatsky A and O'Connor J (1997) Parameter sensitivity of a mathematical model of the anterior cruciate ligament. J Engineering in Medicine 211(H): 235–246.

One-Dimensional Modelling of the Coronary Circulation. Application to Noninvasive Quantification of Fractional Flow Reserve (FFR)

Etienne Boileau and Perumal Nithiarasu

Abstract In guiding intervention in patients with coronary artery disease (CAD), measurements of fractional flow reserve (FFR) usually complement the anatomic information. With the development of noninvasive imaging and computational-based technologies to interpret clinical data, new approaches have emerged to quantify CAD severity. In parallel with three-dimensional models, models combining lumped and one-dimensional segments have been proposed as a tool to investigate myocardium-vessel interactions. Although they have been used extensively to provide a better understanding of the dynamics of the coronary circulation, they may face a number of limitations, when used as predictive tools. We present herein an example of an open-loop model to estimate FFR values, using an 'average' description of the human coronary geometry.

1 Introduction

Coronary circulation supplies blood to the heart muscle, or myocardium, for its own metabolic needs. Myocardial oxygen supply depends on the oxygen content of the blood, and is subject to variations in blood flow. In coronary arteries, oxygen extraction is as much as three times higher than in the rest of the body. As supply closely matches any changes in demand, coronary blood flow adapts to meet oxygen consumption, and to prevent tissue hypoxia and functional impairment of the cardiac muscle [1]. Myocardial perfusion depends on the aortic pressure, or the cardiac output, i.e. the volume of blood being pumped by the heart, and also on the vascular resistance of the coronary bed. Since blood pressure is subject to the baroreflex and maintained within a limited range under normal conditions, flow through the

E. Boileau (✉) · P. Nithiarasu
Computational Bioengineering and Rheology, Swansea University, Swansea SA2 8PP, UK
e-mail: e.boileau@swansea.ac.uk

P. Nithiarasu
e-mail: P.Nithiarasu@swansea.ac.uk

© Springer International Publishing Switzerland 2015
J.M.R.S. Tavares and R.M. Natal Jorge (eds.), *Computational and Experimental Biomedical Sciences: Methods and Applications*, Lecture Notes in Computational Vision and Biomechanics 21, DOI 10.1007/978-3-319-15799-3_11

coronary vascular tree depends largely on its resistance. Changes in arteriolar vessel calibre thus constitutes a primary determinant of vascular resistance. The capacity of the coronary vascular bed to supply blood to the myocardium in excess of the normal resting conditions is referred to as coronary flow reserve (CFR) [2].

1.1 Coronary and Fractional Flow Reserve

A reduction in CFR is usually accompanied by inadequate perfusion in some part of the myocardium. In the presence of coronary artery disease (CAD), with occluded and stenotic vessels, insufficient blood supply (ischaemia) will often result in chest pain, or angina, and myocardial infarction. Anatomical indices, such as diameter of a stenosis, serve to quantify CAD severity, but identifying coronary stenoses responsible for ischaemia can be challenging. Lesions of intermediate severity are difficult to assess, and their functional significance cannot be predicted by coronary angiography alone [3, 4]. In guiding intervention in patients with CAD, intracoronary physiologic measurements of CFR or myocardial fractional flow reserve (FFR) complement the anatomic information [5]. Since noninvasive imaging provide little or no physiologic information, this combined evaluation of CAD can have a significant impact on clinical-decision making for coronary revascularization, potentially improving event-free survival [6, 7].

FFR is performed invasively in the catheterization laboratory and represents the fraction of the normal maximal coronary blood flow that is achieved in the presence of a stenotic artery. Under hyperaemic conditions, coronary resistance will be minimal, and flow can be assumed to be proportional to pressure. If, in addition, venous pressure is neglected, FFR is calculated as the ratio of the mean hyperaemic distal pressure (measured with the pressure wire) to the mean arterial or aortic pressure (measured simultaneously with the coronary catheter). There is some debate on the reliability of pressure-derived CFR, as compared with flow- or velocity-derived CFR (typically measured with a Doppler guide wire or transthoracic Doppler echocardiography) [8, 9]. At present, however, FFR is the gold standard for evaluating the functional severity of coronary stenoses [10, 11]. It is certainly one of the most simple and reliable indices to assess the haemodynamic significance of coronary lesions, and to determine if a stenosis can be responsible for myocardial ischaemia [12]. But due to its invasive nature, FFR can be associated with medical complications, such as coronary dissections, and is not entirely suitable for the follow-up of medically treated stenoses.

1.2 Diagnosis of Coronary Artery Disease

Better strategies for risk stratification and noninvasive testing are needed to increase the diagnostic yield of cardiac catheterization. This has been evidenced, amongst others, in a study performed in the United-States, where a relatively small proportion of obstructive CAD was found at elective catheterization [13]. But coronary computed tomography (CTA)-guided diagnosis demonstrates an unreliable relationship to lesion-specific ischæmia, and numerous studies have shown that visual and quantitative coronary angiography (high-definition multidetector CTA, single-photon emission CT or other modalities) does not always predict the functional relevance of coronary stenoses, nor does it correlates well with the functional assessment of FFR [3, 14–16]. Anatomical indices may seem insufficient to quantify CAD severity, as the impact of a stenosis will also depend on the location, its length and other physiological factors, all of which can affect its hæmodynamic significance. These findings emphasize the need for additional physiologic measures in patient selection for invasive angiography and coronary revascularization. To avoid procedural shortcomings, it would be useful to develop a noninvasive predictive model of FFR, only based on clinical measurements and information that can be obtained from CTA-based approaches. Much progress has been made over the last few years regarding diagnostic tools and computational-based model interpretation of clinical data [17].

1.3 Computational Modelling: Towards Translational Medicine

Estimation of FFR from CTA data (FFR_{CTA}) has emerged as a noninvasive method for identifying ischæmia-causing stenosis in patients with suspected or known CAD (see [18], for instance). The technique relies on the use of CTA images and computational fluid dynamics (CFD) for the prediction of coronary hæmodynamics. HeartFlow Inc. recently funded a multi-centre diagnostic performance study, aiming to determine if this novel approach could improve the per-patient diagnostic accuracy. The latest trial, the DeFACTO study, was designed to evaluate the accuracy of the HeartFlow FFR_{CTA} approach, as compared with the standard FFR, on a targeted population of patients referred for a clinically-indicated non-emergent invasive coronary angiography [19]. Although the study did not attain the pre-specified level of per-patient diagnostic accuracy, enhanced diagnostic accuracy was generally achieved, compared with CTA alone [20, 21]. These results support a potential role for FFR_{CTA} in identifying individuals with ischæmic stenoses. Its increased discriminatory ability, when used in conjunction with anatomic CTA, may give clinicians enough additional information in deciding whether a patient should be referred for invasive angiography.

The diagnostic performance of FFR_{CTA} relies on the accurate calculation of coronary pressure from acquired CTA scans, using CFD, and requires the construction of a realistic physiological model. Computation of FFR_{CTA} has been performed so far in a number of studies using three-dimensional (3D) models of the coronary tree and ventricular myocardium [18–20, 22]. The patient anatomy is modelled from a mid-diastolic time point, extracted from semi-automated segmented data. Since flow and pressure are unknown a priori, the 3D model requires the coupling of lumped parameter models of the microcirculation. These models need to be tuned so that both the cardiac output and the mean aortic pressure are 'matched with' the clinical data. This process required approximately 6 h per case [20]. While this approach is being extensively advertised, others have tried to develop one-dimensional (1D) or lumped (0D) models, with the additional advantage of providing accurate time-dependent information at lower costs [23–28]. These models have also been used to provide a better understanding of the dynamics of the coronary circulation, and to explain the underlying mechanisms of myocardium-vessel interactions.

1.4 Coronary Geometry and Myocardium-Vessel Interactions

Coronary circulation normally originates in two ostia, or openings, in the aortic sinus, just above the aortic valve. The left main coronary artery (LMCA) branches into the left anterior descending artery (LAD) and the the circumflex artery (LCx). The LAD runs along the anterior longitudinal sulcus, or interventricular groove, towards the apex of the heart, while the LCx follows the coronary sulcus to the left. Left coronary circulation supplies both the lateral and anterior walls of the left ventricle, and part of the anterior interventricular septum. The right coronary artery (RCA) supplies the right ventricle and, in a great majority of human hearts, the posterior wall of the left ventricle and part of the interventricular septum, via the posterior descending artery (PD) [29]. Coronary circulation is then referred to as 'right dominant'.

All main arteries traverse the surface of the heart, the epicardium, and divide into epicardial vessels. Crossing the under surface of the heart, intramuscular arteries penetrate the myocardium to form subendocardial vessels. Since the left ventricular intramural pressure is greater, the interaction between muscle contraction and coronary vessels is different on each side of the heart, particularly in the subendocardial layers [30].

1.4.1 Intramyocardial Pressure and Systolic Flow Impediment

Differences in epi- and subendocardial circulation are important, and this distinction is useful to explain coronary hæmodynamics, as discussed below. Although perfusion pressure is greatest in systole, coronary flow is predominantly diastolic. An explanation for this phenomenon is found in the concept of intramyocardial pressure (IMP), which is fundamental in modelling the coronary circulation. An increase in IMP leads to a temporary reduction in blood volume delivered to the myocardium, and causes impediment of arterial inflow and augmentation of venous outflow during systole. As a consequence, reduction in vessel diameter further increases the resistance to flow. Systolic flow impediment (SFI) is prominently observed in the left arteries, whereas the RCA is exposed to more uniform time-varied resistances throughout the cardiac cycle [31].

Models and Mechanisms of Myocardium-Vessel Interactions

There has been much controversy concerning the origin and the precise mechanisms by which IMP affect coronary circulation. Different mathematical models were used to reproduce the effect of SFI, and describe the nature and distribution of IMP, the manner by which it affects coronary flow, and the relation between resistance and compliance of the tree. A relatively simple description is given by the 'vascular waterfall' mechanism, proposed by Downey and Kirk [32], where a reduction in flow is explained by an increase in resistance from the collapse of the vascular bed. This would occur when IMP exceeds the actual intravascular pressure, and would also restrain the venous outflow during systole, which has not yet been observed [33]. By introducing capacitance, differences in systolic and diastolic flow are related to intramyocardial volume variations [34], providing a 'pump effect', where filled vessels are discharged through the low-pressure venous side during diastole [35]. This concept has been used extensively, and extended to account for variations in resistance and compliance [36–40]. In both the waterfall and the intramyocardial pump model, IMP is proportional or equal to the ventricular pressure, and increase towards the endocardium. Other mechanisms of myocardium-vessel interactions and modelling approaches can be summarized as follows (see also [41, 42]):

1. Ventricular elastance. This approach was proposed by Krams et al. [43–45]. A number of studies have shown that SFI still occur when cavity pressure is kept constant [43, 46]. By employing a time-varying elastance model, changes in vascular volume and cavity pressure are generated by variations in myocardial stiffness. Contractility causes impediment of arterial inflow and increase of systolic venous outflow. This concept does however not explain the differences in epi- and subendocardial flow [47]. Other studies also suggest that rather than contributing to SFI, systolic stiffening shields subendocardial vessels from the effect of ventricular pressure, and tends to resist vessel expansion caused by changes in intravascular pressure [48, 49].
2. Cavity-induced extracellular pressure (CEP). This is the mechanism originating from both the intramyocardial pump and the vascular waterfall model. Extravascular pressure is proportional to left cavity pressure, giving rise to a linear IMP distribution, with respect to transmural position, or myocardial depth. Modelling and in vivo studies support this hypothesis [30, 33].
3. Shortening-induced intracellular pressure (SIP). This mechanism is based on the hypothesis that contractile shortening leads to radial thickening of the cardiac myocyte, and an increase in intracellular pressure transmitted to the vessel, thus contributing to IMP [50]. See Algranati et al. for a comprehensive assessment of myocardial-vessel interaction mechanisms [49].

With the increase in complexity, however, parameter sensitivity analysis becomes difficult, especially if one has no access to experimental data. It is nevertheless possible to reproduce some of the main features of coronary hæmodynamics with 1D-0D models [23, 24]. From the clinical point of view, this might not be so important, and the interest may lie in getting additional information, that is difficult to obtain from traditional diagnostic tools. In this case, it might be sufficient to have a very simple model of the coronary circulation, such as the one presented below.

2 One-Dimensional Models of the Coronary Circulation

One-dimensional modelling of the systemic circulation has been carried out extensively, for gaining a better understanding of pressure-flow propagation, and can provide useful information at a reasonable computational cost (see [51–58] for instance, and references therein). Predictions from 1D models exhibit many of the features of the systemic and coronary arteries of both normal and diseased physiologic and geometric data. Changes resulting from diseases such as aortic valve stenosis or coronary atherosclerosis have been quantified and compared with experimental observations in the published literature. Although a large number of modelling approaches are followed, the major interest lies in evaluating the applicability of such models in the clinical decision-making process. Application of 1D models to the coronary circulation in this context is relatively new.

2.1 Governing Equations

Assuming a flat velocity profile, the relation between velocity (u), cross-sectional area (A) and pressure (p) is described by the following system:

$$\frac{\partial \mathbf{U}}{\partial t} + \frac{\partial \mathbf{F}}{\partial x} = \mathbf{S}$$

$$\mathbf{U} = \begin{bmatrix} A \\ u \end{bmatrix} \quad \mathbf{F} = \begin{bmatrix} Au \\ \frac{u^2}{2} + \frac{p}{\rho} \end{bmatrix} \quad \mathbf{S} = \begin{bmatrix} 0 \\ f \end{bmatrix} \tag{1}$$

where ρ is the blood density and f is a loss term related to viscous friction, that also depends on the chosen velocity profile. The system is closed by a constitutive relation of the form [35]:

$$p - p_{ext} = \frac{2\rho c_o^2}{b} \left[\left(\frac{A}{A_0} \right)^{\frac{b}{2}} - 1 \right] + p_0 \tag{2}$$

where $p - p_{ext}$ is the transmural pressure, A_0 is the cross-sectional area at zero transmural pressure and c_0 is the wave speed at the reference pressure p_0. A commonly-used expression is obtained when $b = 1$, which is then equivalent to assuming a thin, homogeneous Hookean wall material (see [52, 55] for instance).

The value of b can otherwise be determined empirically, or approximated with an estimated collapse pressure (pressure for which $A = 0$) [59].

To impose the appropriate boundary conditions, and couple 1D segments to instances of the 0D model, the governing equations are expressed in terms of the forward w_+ and backward w_- characteristic variables:

$$w_\pm = u \pm \int_{A_0}^{A} \frac{c'}{A'} \, dA' \quad c' = c(A') \tag{3}$$

which are obtained after diagonalizing the quasi-linear form of Eq. (1). At boundaries, the primitive variables are recovered by adding or subtracting the two equations in (3). In the present work, the 1D equations are solved using a finite element method, ensuring continuity of total pressure at vessel junctions. The interested reader is referred to the extensive literature on the subject for a detailed presentation [55].

2.2 Coronary Model

There exists wide variations in coronary anatomy, which makes an exact geometrical description impractical. From the modelling point of view, it seems sufficient to identify the principal vessels and their functional layout, allowing an average representation of the coronary circulation. If needed, specific anatomical information can be added to personalize the model. While all of the major arteries are incorporated, only a small number of side branches are included (c.f. Sect. 1.4). Length, diameter and wall thickness are derived from anatomical measurements [60–66], and are given in Table 1. A graphical representation of the model is shown in Fig. 1. The diagonal artery (D) arises at or near the bifurcation of the LMCA, but due to anatomical variability it is sometimes included as a bifurcation in the LAD. The choice made here is arbitrary. The LCx is divided into three segments, by the obtuse marginal (OM) and its subendocardial terminal segment. Branches of the LAD include two septal perforator (S1-S2). The RCA is divided into two segments by the acute marginal branches (AM) and PD.

2.2.1 Coupling 1D Segments and Lumped Elements

Representation of the downstream circulation and hæmodynamic effects beyond 1D segments are simulated using a combination of linear taper, to account for multiple wave reflections, and lumped parameter or 0D models. Several instances of the latter are then coupled to the 1D formulation using a time-domain algorithm. At the 0D-1D interface, the problem is expressed in terms of the characteristic variables, and the solution is achieved as described in [67].

Table 1 Vessel length (l), wall thickness (h) and reference proximal diameter (d_0) of the 1D segments in the coronary model

Vessel	l (cm)	h (cm)	d_0 (cm)	Taper
LMCA	0.5	0.12	0.45	
LAD1	2.3	0.09	0.37	0.05
LAD2	1.2	0.087	0.29	0.21
LAD3	1.2	0.05	0.2	0.3
S1	1.7	0.04	0.14	0.29
S2	1.5	0.03	0.11	0.18
LCx1	1.7	0.09	0.34	
LCx2	0.9	0.08	0.28	0.39
D	2.4	0.06	0.21	0.43
OM	2.7	0.06	0.21	0.45
RCA1	3.0	0.11	0.4	0.05
RCA2	1.2	0.10	0.35	0.09
AM1	1.9	0.07	0.25	
AM2	1.9	0.06	0.21	
PD	2.7	0.06	0.22	0.36

The degree of tapering, or reduction in diameter, is expressed in terms of d_0. Names correspond to those of Fig. 1. Terminal arteries of the LAD, LCx and RCA also connect to 0D vascular beds

Fig. 1 Geometrical representation of the 1D coronary model

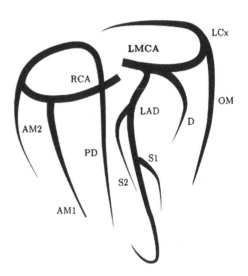

Coronary Lumped Model

The present model is comparable to models presented earlier by Mynard [58] and Mynard et al. [28], and is based on prior lumped models proposed by Beyar and Sideman [68], Bruinsma et al. [69] and Spaan et al. [40]. It consists of several 'terminals', as depicted in Fig. 2, each connecting to terminal arteries of the LAD, LCx and RCA. A terminal is divided into two layers $l = epi, endo$, representing the epi- and subendocardial circulation, and each layer consists of two compartments, characterized by arterial C^a and venous C^v compliances, initially set to 0.013 and 0.25 ml mmHg^{-1} 100 g^{-1}, respectively, with a subendocardial-to-subepicardial ratio ~ 1 [40, 69]. Compliance values are then distributed according to the inverse cube of the radius, for each coupled 1D segment, and then equally to each layer. The total resistance is similarly divided into arterial R^a, capillary R^c and venous R^v components.

All resistances are volume (V)-dependent, and the capillary resistance is shared by both compartments, i.e. it depends simultaneously on the volume of the arterial and venous compartments. According to Poiseuille, and if only the radius vary with volume, $R \propto V^{-2}$. By expanding to first order, an expression is obtained for the update of the resistances:

$$R_l = R_l(V_l)_{t=n} + \left.\frac{dR_l(V_l)}{dV_l}\right|_{t=n} \left(V_l - V_{l,t=n}\right) \tag{4}$$

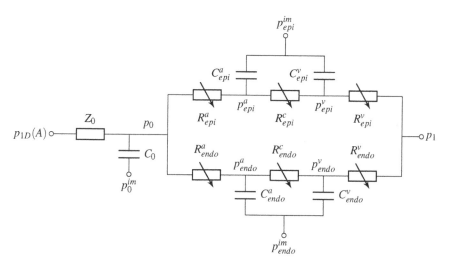

Fig. 2 One instance of a 0D terminal model of the coronary bed. $p_{1D}(A)$ is the area-dependent pressure at the terminal 1D segment, and $Z_0 = \rho c/A$ the characteristic impedance. The terminal consists of an epi- and subendocardial layer, each characterised by arterial C^a and venous C^v compliances, arterial R^a, capillary R^c and venous R^v volume-dependent resistances and time-varying intramyocardial pressures p^{im}. Flow across each resistance is expressed in terms of pressure variations p_0, p_a and p_v, as explained in the text

where values are taken at time step $t = n$, with compartment volume given by:

$$V_l = V_{l,t=n} + \int_0^t C_l \frac{d}{dt'} \left(p_l - p_l^{im} \right) \ dt' \tag{5}$$

for each layer $l = epi, endo$, and for both arterial a and venous v compartments. The middle or capillary resistance is calculated by adding contributions of $R_l^{c_1}$ and $R_l^{c_2}$, according to:

$$R_l^{c_1} = \theta R_l^c \qquad R_l^{c_2} = (1 - \theta) R_l^c \tag{6}$$

where $\theta = 3/4$ is a proportion of the capillary resistance assigned to the arterial and venous compartments, respectively. The layer-dependent IMP p^{im} expressed in Eq. (5) is applied to the vascular compliances of each compartment, as described below. Compartment volumes are specified based on estimates of coronary compliance distribution, and assuming that venous volume initially equals twice the arterial volume [36]. Flow q across the resistances is expressed in terms of pressure variations:

$$q_l^a - q_l^c = C_l^a \frac{d}{dt} \left(p_l^a - p_l^{im} \right) \qquad q_l^c - q_l^v = C_l^v \frac{d}{dt} \left(p_l^v - p_l^{im} \right) \tag{7}$$

The numerical solution of the 0D pressures is also advanced in time explicitly via a first-order discretisation of Eq. (7), for each instance of the model (Fig. 2), and for each layer $l = epi, endo$. Since only the arterial system is represented, the venous pressure p_1 is assumed to be constant, with a value of 5 mmHg. Once the pressures are calculated, the flows are updated, with the total inflow equal to the sum of arterial flows through the epi- and subendocardial layers:

$$q_l^a = \frac{p_0 - p_l^a}{R_l^a} \qquad q_l^c = \frac{p_l^a - p_l^v}{R_l^c} \qquad q_l^v = \frac{p_l^v - p_1}{R_l^v} \tag{8}$$

Coupling to the 1D domain is achieved partly via a characteristic impedance $Z_0 = \rho c / A$, and ensuring that the upwind state satisfies the relation dictated by the 0D model. The 1D area is then determined by solving:

$$Au = \frac{p_{1D}(A) - p_0}{Z_0} \tag{9}$$

where the velocity u is expressed in terms of the characteristic variables using Eq. (3), and extrapolating the forward characteristic between discrete time steps. By rearranging Eq. (2), it is possible to express the 1D pressure in terms of area, and to solve for A using Newton's method.

A time-varying IMP p^{im} is applied to the vascular compliances of each compartment, but only in the form of CEP, with $1/3$ of left ventricular pressure to the epicardial layer, and the remaining $2/3$ to the subendocardial layer. Extravascular pressure is also applied to the arterial compliance C_0, with p_0^{im} varying according to the prescribed IMP. For the right coronary vessels, the effect of IMP is uniformly reduced by a factor of $1/5$. Septal 1D segments are also subject to extravascular pressures, by imposing $p_{ext} = p_{endo}^{im}$ through Eq. (2).

In summary, for each terminal 1D segments and for each layer $l = epi, endo$, the new pressures are updated using Eq. (7), given the flows Eq. (8) at the previous discrete time step. The new volumes are then calculated using Eq. (5), and the resistances are updated according to Eq. (4). The primitive variables A and u are finally obtained by solving Eq. (9), using Eqs. (2) and (3).

2.2.2 Open-Loop with Ventricular Pressure

The open-loop model relies on the use of a pressure-source ventricle, prescribed in the form of a time-varying pressure input [55, 57]. Inlet boundary conditions are then imposed by prescribing the incoming characteristic variables, using Eqs. (3) and (2). The aortic valve is modelled using a varying index of valve state, where the rates of opening and closure are function of the pressure difference across the valve, and the state of the valve (open, closed, opening or closing) [59]. Flow through the valve is calculated using the Bernoulli equation. All valve parameters are taken from Mynard et al. [59].

It is known that, although the three-element windkessel can produce realistic aortic pressures and flows, it often does with parameters values that differ from the vascular properties. The comparative advantage of adding an inertial term in parallel with the characteristic impedance, as proposed by Stergiopulos et al. [70], is nevertheless arguable. In practice, the inertance may be difficult to estimate, and while pulsatility and inertia may be important in larger arteries, flow is dominated by viscosity in smaller vessels.

Instead of coupling one arterial segment directly to a terminal windkessel, we found that better results are obtained by adding an 'arterio-venous bed' compartment. The systemic circulation is thus replaced with two 1D segments, coupled together through a lumped compartment, and terminated with the usual peripheral three-element windkessel model, as shown in Fig. 3. Physiologically, the last element can be interpreted as a venous load, while the middle compartment accounts for the arterial compliance and resistance. In fact, microvascular compliance is not accounted for in the middle compartment. All resistances and compliances are based on values used in previous systemic arterial models (see [51, 59] for instance), and are given along with geometrical information in Table 2. For the middle compartment, the discrete equations are similar to the ones presented in Sect. 2.2.1, and the solution of the three-element windkessel is standard. Coupling to the 1D segments is achieved in the same manner as described previously in Sect. 2.2.1.

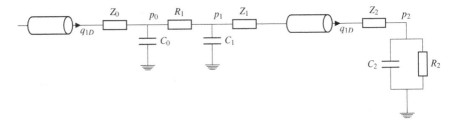

Fig. 3 Representation of the open-loop model. Segment information is given in Table 2. At the inlet (LVOT), a time-varying pressure is applied, with a model aortic valve. The aortic root (AR) divides into left and right coronary arteries, as represented in Fig. 1 and Table 1, and into the first segment (SEG1). A lumped compartment connecting 1D segments (SEG1 and SEG2, represented by '*transmission lines*'), stands for the systemic arterial compliance and resistance, and is characterised by characteristic impedances Z_0, Z_1, resistance R_1 and compliances C_0, C_1. The open-loop is terminated with a standard three-element windkessel (Z_2, R_2, C_2). Lumped pressures are p_0, p_1 and p_2, and q_{1D} are the flows at the 1D-0D interfaces, c.f. Eq. (9)

Table 2 Vessel length (l), wall thickness (h) and reference proximal diameter (d_0) of the 1D segments in the open-loop model

Vessel	l (cm)	h (cm)	d_0 (cm)	R_1	R_2	C_0	C_1	C_2
				(mmHg s ml^{-1})		(ml mmHg^{-1})		
LVOT	1.0	0.168	2.49					
AR	1.7	0.168	2.49					
SEG1	10.0	0.163	2.94	0.9		1.0		
SEG2	10.0	0.163	2.88		6.0		11.0	0.2

Only the aortic root (AR) increases in diameter by 30 % of its proximal value. Values of the resistances and compliances are assumed constant, and based on values used in previous models. Names correspond to those of Fig. 3. *LVOT* left ventricular outflow tract, *SEG* segment

Figure 4 compares the predicted values at the aortic root (AR), just after the aortic valve, with the ones obtained by other investigators using a complete arterial network. Baseline computed values of mean arterial pressure of 91 mmHg, pulse pressure of 44 mmHg and cardiac output of 6 l min^{-1} are within the normal range, for a heart rate of 75 bpm. The numerical solution, obtained within a few seconds, contains all the expected features of the aortic waveforms. If one is interested in coronary hæmodynamics, this may present additional benefits. Although the simplifications made here can be regarded as a limitation, they are rather seen as an advantage, in view of the intended application.

While the open-loop model is convenient, it does not allow a complete investigation of ventricular dynamics, and limits further development of a more complete coronary model. As previously described, the interactions between the myocardium and its vasculature affect coronary flow, and this could not be given full consideration with the open-loop pressure-source model. As a result, some features of coronary hæmodynamics cannot be reproduced. A more comprehensive model, such as the time-varying elastance model, may offer additional advantages, when included in a closed-loop, albeit at the expense of increasing the complexity.

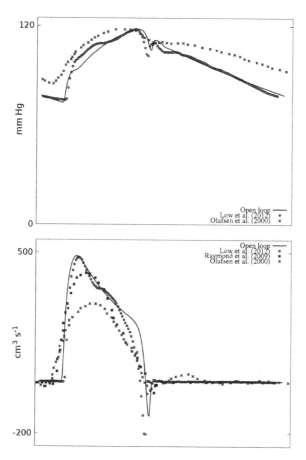

Fig. 4 Waveform of aortic pressure and flow. *Solid lines* represent the predicted pressure-flow waveform using the open-loop model. Other waveforms are taken from Olufsen et al. [71], Raymond et al. (aortic arch) [72], and Low et al. (ascending aorta) [57]

2.2.3 Estimation of FFR Using 1D Models

The open-loop model is used to estimate FFR in the proximal LAD (LAD1). By changing a limited number of parameters, values were obtained that match experimental observations described in the literature. The stenosis was modelled axisymmetrically at the mid-length of the segment. A subset of the data presented in [73] was used to validate the efficacy of the open-loop model in calculating FFR values. Since only pressure and diameters were given, the length of the stenosis had to be adjusted in each case to obtain the values shown in Table 3. By matching the given mean arterial pressure (MAP), values of mean post stenotic pressure (MPSP) and FFR were obtained that are close to the experimental data. As the actual values of pressure were obtained under hyperæmic conditions, the effect of adenosine does

Table 3 Intracoronary pressure measurement and FFR values obtained by Baumgart et al. and computed values, indicated by an asterisk

Lesion	Diam. stenosis (%)	MAP (mmHg)	MPSP (mmHg)	FFR	MAP* (mmHg)	MPSP* (mmHg)	FFR*
1	77.6	98	48	0.49	97.8	48.2	0.49
2	68.4	99	52	0.53	100.0	52.3	0.53
5	61.3	90	63	0.70	90.5	63.6	0.70
8	60.0	85	66	0.78	84.8	65.7	0.78
13	47.1	70	58	0.83	70.7	59.3	0.84
19	53.1	95	90	0.95	94.9	88.8	0.94

Six cases of stenosis in the LAD have been selected for comparison. For the simulation, the stenosis was placed in the LAD1. The lesion number refers to the individual data presented in [73]. *MAP* mean arterial pressure. *MPSP* mean post stenotic pressure

not need to be explicitly modelled. Nevertheless, change from baseline to hyperæmia was accounted for by a decrease in the initial values of the arteriolar resistances in Fig. 2. As no specific data was available, this was done arbitrarily, but uniformly. This did not seem to affect substantially the results, as compared to varying the geometrical description of the stenosis. Values of the resistances during the cardiac cycle were neither affected by the upstream stenosis, suggesting that 'normal values' of downstream parameters could also be used for stenotic cases, providing that the source pressure is properly adjusted. As a consequence, we assumed that only changes in the axisymmetric geometry and input pressure would affect the computed results. It is however well-known that flow and resistive losses depend on factors that cannot be directly modelled using a 1D approach, and that are not taken into account in the present description of the stenosis. As an example, other investigators have included 'stenosis elements' in their model [26, 74], based on earlier work by Young [75]. The use of a single shaped-stenosis model, without any relation to account for losses, or to take into account the hæmodynamics of irregular stenoses, is obviously a limitation of the model.

A complete sensitivity analysis of the model parameters may be helpful in understanding the relationship between instances of the 0D model and the response of the 1D coronary model, especially with a view to include patient-specific information. Although the results show that this approach is capable of achieving accurate estimates of FFR, substantial work needs to be done to make the model applicable to a variety of cases, in the manner of a 'blackbox'.

3 Summary, Limitations and Future Directions

With the development of noninvasive imaging and computational-based technologies to interpret clinical data, it now becomes possible to envisage a different approach in estimating hæmodynamic parameters, and thereby quantifying CAD severity. Estimation of FFR from CTA data has thus emerged as a novel method for identifying ischæmia-causing stenosis in patients with CAD. Although an approach based on 1D-0D models may present some major advantages, it also faces a number of important limitations. In the present work, the assumptions concerning the pressure-area relationship do not reflect the viscoelastic properties of the vessel wall. Similarly, the form of the assumed radial velocity profile is not accurate, and does not take into account phasic changes that may have a non-negligible impact. In addition, losses due to viscous and flow separation effects have been ignored, whereas they are expected to be important when investigating CAD. But 3D models are also associated with inherent and similar limitations, as briefly described in Sect. 1.3.

The open-loop model presented in Sect. 2.2.2 is convenient and can provide a solution within seconds. When combined with the coronary model, and by appropriately matching input pressure and stenosis geometry, it yields estimates of FFR that are close to measured values of intracoronary pressures. It is not known, however, if the computed values correspond to the true anatomical data, and what is the actual performance and precision of the method. Future work will address these limitations, with a view to include patient-specific CTA data and other physiologic information. As mentioned previously, the open-loop model does not allow a detailed representation of myocardium-vessel interactions, and various other possibilities are currently being investigated to include some of the mechanisms mentioned in Sect. 1.4.1. Due to its rapidity and ease of use, such an approach may seem very promising.

References

1. Guyton AC, Hall JE, (eds) Textbook of Medical Physiology, 9th Edn. Philadelphia: WB Saunders, 1996.
2. Spaan JAE Coronary Blood Flow. Kluwer Academic Publishers, Dordrecht, The Netherlands, 1991.
3. Tonino PAL, de Bruyne B, Pijls NHJ et al for the FAME study investigators (2009) Fractional flow reserve versus angiography for guiding percutaneous coronary intervention. N Engl J Med 360:213–24.
4. Pijls NHJ, Fearon WF, Tonino PAL et al (2010) Fractional flow reserve versus angiography for guiding percutaneous coronary intervention in patients with multivessel coronary artery disease: 2-year follow-up of the FAME study. J Am Coll Cardiol 56:177–84.
5. Pijls NHJ, de Bruyne B, Peels K et al (1996) Measurements of fractional flow reserve to assess the functional severity of coronary artery stenoses. N Engl J Med 334:1703–1708.
6. Bech GJW, de Bruyne B, Pijls NHJ et al (2001) Fractional flow reserve to determine the appropriateness of angioplasty in moderate coronary stenosis. A randomized trial. Circ 103:2928–2934.
7. Pijls NHJ, van Schaardenburgh P, Manoharan G et al (2007) Percutaneous coronary intervention of functionally nonsignificant stenosis: 5-year follow up of the DEFER study. J Am Coll Cardiol 49:2105–2111.
8. Akasaka T, Yamamuro A, Kamiyama N et al (2003) Assessment of coronary flow reserve by coronary pressure measurement comparison with flow- or velocity-derived coronary flow reserve. J Am Coll Cardiol 41:1554–1560.

9. MacCarthy P, Berger A, Manoharan G et al (2005) Pressure-derived measurement of coronary flow reserve. J Am Coll Cardiol 45:216–220.

10. Kern MJ, Lerman A, Bech J-W et al (2006) Physiological assessment of coronary artery disease in the cardiac catheterization laboratory: a scientific statement from the American Heart Association Committee on Diagnostic and Interventional Cardiac Catheterization, Council on Clinical Cardiology. Circ 114:1321–1341.

11. Kern MJ, Samady H (2010) Current concepts of integrated coronary physiology in the catheterization laboratory. J Am Coll Cardiol 55:173–185.

12. Bishop AH, Samady H (2004) Fractional flow reserve: Critical review of an important physiologic adjunct to angiography. Am Heart J 147:792–802.

13. Patel MR, Peterson ED, Dai D et al (2010) Low diagnostic yield of elective coronary angiography. N Eng J Med 362:886–895.

14. Hacker M, Jakobs T, Hack N et al (2007) Sixty-four slice spiral CT angiography does not predict the functional relevance of coronary artery stenoses in patients with stable angina. Eur J Nucl Med Mol Imaging 34:4–10.

15. Meijboom WB, van Mieghem CAG, van Pelt N et al (2008) Comprehensive assessment of coronary artery stenoses. Computed tomography coronary angiography versus conventional coronary angiography and correlation with fractional flow reserve in patients with stable angina. J Am Coll Cardiol 52:636–643.

16. Melikian N, De Bondt P, Tonino PAL. Fractional flow reserve and myocardial perfusion imaging in patients with angiographic multivessel coronary artery disease. J Am Coll Cardiol Intv 3:307–314.

17. Zhang J-M, Zhong L, Su B et al (2014) Perspective on CFD studies of coronary artery disease lesions and hemodynamics: A review. Int J Numer Meth Biomed Engng, doi: 10.1002/cnm. 2625.

18. Koo BK, Erglis A, Doh JH et al (2011) Diagnosis of ischemia-causing coronary stenoses by noninvasive fractional flow reserve computed from coronary computed tomographic angiograms. Results from the prospective Mmlticenter DISCOVER-FLOW (Diagnosis of Ischemia-Causing Stenoses Obtained Via Noninvasive Fractional Flow Reserve) study J Am Coll Cardiol 58:1989–1997.

19. Min JK, Berman DS, Budoff MJ et al (2011) Rationale and design of the DeFACTO (Determination of Fractional Flow Reserve by Anatomic Computed Tomographic Angiography) study J Cardiovasc Comput Tomogr 5:301–309.

20. Min JK, Leipsic J, Pencina MJ et al (2012) Diagnostic accuracy of fractional flow reserve from anatomic CT angiography JAMA 308:1237–1265.

21. Nakazato R, Park H-B, Berman DS et al (2013) Non-invasive fractional flow reserve derived from CT angiography (FFRCT) for coronary lesions of intermediate stenosis severity: results from the DeFACTO study. Circ Cardiovasc Imaging, online September 30.

22. Taylor CA, Fonte TA, Min JK (2013) Computational fluid dynamics applied to cardiac computed tomography for noninvasive quantification of fractional flow reserve. Scientific basis. J Am Coll Cardiol 61:2233–2241.

23. Geven MCF, Boht VN, Aarnoudse WH et al (2004) A physiologically representative in vitro model of the coronary circulation. Physiol Meas 25:891–904.

24. Boveendeerd PHM, Borsje P, Arts T, van de Vosse FN (2006) Dependence of intramyocardial pressure and coronary flow on ventricular loading and contractility: A model study. Annals Biomed Eng, doi: 10.1007/s10439-006-9189-2.

25. Huo Y, Kassab GS (2007) A hybrid one-dimensional/Womersley model of pulsatile blood flow in the entire coronary arterial tree. Am J Physiol Heart Circ Physiol 292:2623–2633.

26. van der Horst A, Boogaard FL, vant Veer M et al (2013) Towards patient-specific modeling of coronary hemodynamics in healthy and diseased state. Comput Math Methods Med, http://dx. doi.org/10.1155/2013/393792.

27. Huo Y, Svendsen M, Choy JS et al (2012) A validated predictive model of coronary fractional flow reserve. J R Soc Interface 9:1325–1338.

28. Mynard JP, Penny DJ, Smolich JJ (2013) Validation of a multi-scale model of the coronary circulation in adult sheep and newborn lambs. Conf Proc IEEE Eng Med Biol Soc 3857–60.

29. Valentin F, Wayne AW, O'Rourke RA et al (eds) Hurst's The Heart, 11th Edn. McGraw-Hill, 2004.

30. Heineman FW, Grayson J (1985) Transmural distribution of intramyocardial pressure measured by micropipette technique. Am J Physiol Heart Circ Physiol 249:1216–1223.

31. Heller LI, Silver KH, Villegas BJ et al (1994) Blood flow velocity in the right coronary artery: assessment before and after angioplasty. J Am Coll Cardiol 24:1012–1017.

32. Downey JM, Kirk ES (1975) Inhibition of coronary blood flow by a vascular waterfall mechanism. Circ Res 36:753–760.

33. Hoffman JI, Spaan JA (1990) Pressure-flow relations in coronary circulation. Physiol Rev 70:331–390.

34. Spaan JAE, Breuls NPW, Laird JD (1981) Diastolic–systolic coronary flow differences are caused by intramyocardial pump action in the anesthetised dog. Circ Res 49:584–593.

35. Smith NP, Pullan AJ, Hunter PJ (2001) An anatomically based model of transient coronary blood flow in the heart. SIAM J Appl Math 62:990–1018.

36. Spaan JAE (1985) Coronary diastolic pressure-flow relation and zero flow pressure explained on the basis of intramyocardial compliance. Circ Res 56:293–309.

37. Arts T, Reneman RS (1985) Interaction between intramyocardial pressure and myocardial circulation. J Biomech Eng 107:51–56.

38. Kresh JY, Fox M, Brockman SK, Noordergraaf A (1990) Model-based analysis of transmural vessel impedance and myocardial circulation dynamics. Am J Physiol Heart Circ Physiol 258:262–H276.

39. Zinemanas D, Beyar R, Sideman S (1994) Relating mechanics, blood flow and mass transport in the cardiac muscle. Int J Heat Mass Transf 37:191–205.

40. Spaan JAE, Cornelissen AJM, Chan C et al (2000) Dynamics of flow, resistance, and intramural vascular volume in canine coronary circulation. Am J Physiol Heart Circ Physiol 278:383–403.

41. Beyar R, Manor D, Zinemans D, Sideman S (1993) Concepts and controversies in modelling the coronary circulation. In: Maruyama Y, Kajiya F, Hoffman JIE and Spaan JAE (eds) Recent Advances in Coronary Circulation, Springer Japan, Tokyo.

42. Westerhof N, Boer C, Lamberts RR, Sipkema P (2006) Cross-talk between cardiac muscle and coronary vasculature. Physiol Rev 86:1263–1308.

43. Krams R, Sipkema P, Westerhof N (1989) Varying elastance concept may explain coronary systolic flow impediment. Am J Physiol 257:1471–1479.

44. Krams R, Sipkema P, Zegers J, Westerhof N (1989) Contractility is the main determinant of coronary systolic flow impediment. Am J Physiol Heart Circ Physiol 257:1936–1944.

45. Krams R, van Haelst ACTA, Sipkema P, Westerhof N (1989) Can coronary systolic-diastolic flow differences be predicted by left ventricular pressure or time-varying intramyocardial elastance? Basic Res Cardiol 84:149–159.

46. Baan J Jr, Steendijk JP, Mikuniya A, Baan J (1996) Systolic coronary flow reduction in the canine heart in situ: Effects of left ventricular pressure and elastance. Basic Res cardiol 91:468–478.

47. Goto M, Flynn AE, Doucette JW et al (1991) Cardiac contraction affects deep myocardial vessels predominantly. Am J Physiol 261:1417–1429.

48. Spaan JAE (1995) Mechanical determinants of myocardial perfusion. Basic Res Cardiol 90:89–102.

49. Algranati D, Kassab GS, Lanir Y (2010) Mechanisms of myocardium–coronary vessel interaction Am J Physiol Heart Circ Physiol 298:861–873.

50. Rabbany SY, Funai JT, Noordergraaf A (1994) Pressure generation in a contracting myocyte. Heart Vessels 9:169–174.

51. Stergiopulos N, Young DF, Rogge TR (1992) Computer simulation of arterial flow with applications to arterial and aortic stenoses. J Biomech 25:1477–1488.

52. Sherwin SJ, Franke V, Peiro J, Parker K (2003) One-dimensional modelling of a vascular network in space-time variables. J eng Math 47:217–250.
53. Formaggia L, Lamponi D, Quarteroni A (2003) One-dimensional models for blood flow in arteries. J Eng Math 47:251–276.
54. Alastruey J (2006) Numerical modelling of pulse wave propagation in the cardiovascular system: Development, validation and clinical applications. PhD Thesis, Imperial College, London.
55. Mynard JP, Nithiarasu P (2008) A one dimensional arterial blood flow model incorporating ventricular pressure, aortic valve and regional coronary flow using the locally conservative Galerkin (LCG) method. Commun Numer Meth En 24:367–417.
56. Reymond P, Merenda F, Perren et al (2009) Validation of a one-dimensional model of the systemic arterial tree. Am J Physiol Heart Circ Physiol 297:208–222.
57. Low K, van Loon R, Sazonov I et al (2012) An improved baseline model for a human arterial network to study the impact of aneurysms on pressure-flow waveforms. Int J Numer Meth Biomed Engng 28:1224–1246.
58. Mynard, JP (2011) Computer modelling and wave intensity analysis of perinatal cardiovascular function and dysfunction. PhD Thesis, Murdoch Childrens Research Institute, The University of Melbourne.
59. Mynard JP, Davidson MR, Penny DJ, Smolich JJ (2012) A simple, versatile valve model for use in lumped parameter and one-dimensional cardiovascular models. Int J Numer Meth Biomed Engng 28:626–641.
60. Dodge Jr JT, Brown BG, Bolson EL and Dodge HT (1988) Intrathoracic spatial location of specified coronary segments on the normal human heart. Applications in quantitative arteriography, assessment of regional risk and contraction, and anatomic display. Circ 78:1167–1180.
61. Douglas PS, Fiolkoski J, Berko B and Reichek N (1988) Echocardiographic visualization of coronary artery anatomy in the adult. J Am Coll Cardiol 11:565–571.
62. Dodge Jr JT, Brown BG, Bolson EL and Dodge HT (1992) Lumen diameter of normal human coronary arteries. Influence of age, sex, anatomic variation, and left ventricular hypertrophy or dilation. Circ 86:232–246.
63. Pennell DJ, Keegan J, Firmin DN, Gatehouse PD et al (1993) Magnetic resonance imaging of coronary arteries: technique and preliminary results. Br Heart J 70:315–326.
64. Seiler C, Kirkeeide RL and Gould KL (1993) Measurement from arteriograms of regional myocardial bed size distal to any point in the coronary vascular tree for assessing anatomic area at risk. J Am Coll Cardiol 21:783–797.
65. Holzapfel GA, Sommer G, Gasser CT and Regitnig P (2005) Determination of layer-specific mechanical properties of human coronary arteries with nonatherosclerotic intimal thickening and related constitutive modeling. Am J Physiol Heart Circ Physiol 289:2048–2058.
66. Tops LF, Wood DA, Delgado V, Schuijf JD et al (2008) Noninvasive Evaluation of the Aortic Root With Multislice Computed Tomography Implications for Transcatheter Aortic Valve Replacement. J Am Coll Cardiol 1:321–330.
67. Alastruey J, Parker KH, Peiro J, Sherwin S (2008) Lumped parameter outflow models for 1D blood flow simulations: effect on pulse waves and parameter estimation. CiCP 4:317–336.
68. Beyar R, Sideman S (1987) Time-dependent coronary blood flow distribution in left ventricular wall. Am J Physiol Heart Circ Physiol 252:417–433.
69. Bruinsma P, Arts T, Dankelman J, Spaan JAE (1988) Model of the coronary circulation based on pressure dependence of coronary resistance and compliance. Basic Res Cardiol 83:510–524.
70. Stergiopulos N, Westerhof BE, Westerhol N (1999) Total arterial inertance as the fourth element of the windkessel model. Am J Physiol Heart Circ Physiol 45:81–88.
71. Olufsen MS, Peskin CS, Kim WY et al (2000) Numerical Simulation and Experimental Validation of Blood Flow in Arteries with Structured-Tree Outflow Conditions. Annals Biomed Eng 28:1281–1299.
72. Reymond P, Merenda F, Perren F et al (2009) Validation of a one-dimensional model of the systemic arterial tree. Am J Physiol Heart Circ Physiol 297:208–H222.

73. Baumgart D, Haude M, Goerge G, Ge J et al (1998) Improved assessment of coronary stenosis severity using the relative flow velocity reserve. Circ 98:40–46.
74. Stergiopulos N, Spriridon M, Pythoud F, Meister JJ (1996) On the wave transmission and reflection properties of stenoses. J Biomech 29:31–38.
75. Young DF (1973) Flow characteristics in models of arterial stenoses. Unsteady flow. Biomech 6:547–559.

Prediction of Carotid Hemodynamic Descriptors Based on Ultrasound Data and a Neural Network Model

Catarina F. Castro, Carlos Conceição António and Luísa Costa Sousa

Abstract The goal of this study was to analyse the hemodynamics in the carotid bifurcation and to evaluate its dependence on bifurcation geometry and presence of internal carotid artery (ICA) stenosis. Based on patient-specific ultrasound data, an optimal artificial neural network (ANN) model was developed searching data dimensional reduction. ANN estimated pulsatile conditions were used as boundary conditions along different points of the common carotid artery (CCA) and ICA for fluid dynamic simulations. Toward faster patient-specific hemodynamic and stenosis interpretation, ANN estimated blood flow descriptors were calculated and analysed.

1 Introduction

Each artery in the human body has a unique flow profile by which it may be identified, but this unique profile can be also modified by the presence of diseases. Doppler ultrasound acquisition can give reliable information on certain hemodynamic changes by screening both systolic and diastolic blood flow velocities of the carotid arteries [1, 2]. An efficient imaging and accurate analysis of these disturbed flow fields can help in diagnosing arterial disease at an early stage and contribute to our understanding of cardiovascular disease development and progression. However, Doppler images are not always able to portray the true flow behaviour, especially for complex vessel geometries and non-axial flow patterns such as vortex formations [3]. Simulation of arterial blood dynamics has received substantial attention owing to its flow prediction abilities and to the enormous motivation for obtaining insight into the consequences of surgery on the pathophysiology of arterial disease, e.g. hypertension, atherosclerosis, and aneurysm formation [4–6].

Artificial neural network (ANN) models are an extraordinarily flexible tool for nonlinear modelling and their capability to classify patterns under variability and

C.F. Castro (✉) · C.C. António · L.C. Sousa
Faculdade de Engenharia da Universidade do Porto, Porto, Portugal
e-mail: ccastro@fe.up.pt

© Springer International Publishing Switzerland 2015
J.M.R.S. Tavares and R.M. Natal Jorge (eds.), *Computational and Experimental Biomedical Sciences: Methods and Applications*, Lecture Notes in Computational Vision and Biomechanics 21, DOI 10.1007/978-3-319-15799-3_12

differentiation of assorted pathological data has been proven [7, 8]. Based on the four most commonly used duplex ultrasound velocity measurements, peak systolic velocity and end-diastolic velocity in the internal carotid artery (ICA) and common carotid artery (CCA), neural network algorithms were able to predict the degree of ICA stenosis with reasonable accuracy [9]. Decisions on individual bifurcation geometry alterations could benefit from hemodynamic descriptors correlating with markers of abnormal bifurcation geometry. Sophisticated patient-specific fluid dynamic three-dimensional simulations present prohibit cost times. Implementing virtual computational hemodynamic platforms for clinical use to determine the severity of a stenosis and give guidance for surgical decision making has been an ongoing project [8–11]. Artificial intelligence techniques, such as ANN could be used to search for descriptors used by the overseeing physician to enrich and complement the anatomical information for more in-depth evaluation of stenosis in reasonable time duration.

The purpose of this study was to evaluate the possible use of ANN predictions of hemodynamic descriptors based on daily clinical ultrasound carotid examinations to establish a feasible and efficient framework to assess atherosclerosis disease. The basic idea of this approach was to construct patient-specific ANN model from input Doppler data and subsequently predict descriptive outputs of interest [10, 11]. In this paper, a time efficient ANN model is proposed for prediction of hemodynamic indicators processing image data. A carotid artery bifurcation with a moderately high ICA stenosis was reconstructed from ultrasound B-mode images. Arterial flow patterns were predicted with an optimal ANN learning from Doppler data acquired at specific vessel locations. ANN predictions were also used as inlet and outlet boundary conditions for simulating stenosis induced flow patterns obtained using a finite element code with a structured mesh and a Newtonian viscosity model [12–14]. Pre-stenosis and post-stenosis flow behaviours were examined.

2 Carotid Hemodynamic Simulations

Computational fluid dynamics has been used extensively for several decades and proven itself as a reliable approach to predict complex fluid flow phenomena [6]. Numerical simulation methodology for carotid disease is increasingly sophisticated exploring complex geometries, fluid-structure interaction and time-dependent pulsatile solutions. Finite-element methods have been widely used because of their ability to handle complex geometries and have shown to accurately capture cycle-to-cycle variations in unsteady flow [15]. Models are typically constructed from magnetic resonance imaging, computed tomography or ultrasound data, including detailed anatomy with multiple vessel bifurcations and outlets. Patient-specific boundary conditions for simulations are often derived from magnetic resonance imaging or Doppler measurements of flow.

Blood flow is governed by the incompressible Navier-Stokes equations for conservation of mass and momentum. 3D computational fluid dynamics simulations were performed to analyse blood flow patterns at carotid bifurcation highlighting disturbed flow patterns due to alterations in arterial geometry and identifying regions susceptible to atherosclerotic pathogenesis and pathophysiology [16, 17]. Hemodynamic simulations can augment imaging methods, systematically predicting surgical outcomes and device performance at little or no risk to the patient and on a patient-specific basis [18].

Carotid arteries are easily accessible with ultrasound and due to their susceptibility to atherosclerosis and the complexity of the local flow field model construction and simulation have been an ongoing project. Based on ultrasound and PW-Doppler data, Fig. 1 shows the typical steps for model construction and simulation for a patient-specific model of the carotid arteries in a patient with detectable carotid stenosis [12, 13].

Ideally, numerical simulations ought to be carried out in a very fast way, to rapidly provide a quantitative output/response on each new patient-specific geometrical configuration. Assuming that realistic geometry definition of bifurcation is time consuming, methodologies for evaluation of output related to blood flows based on deformation of a reference configuration have been suggestively presented [19]. A different approach has been presented by Swillens et al. [3] suggesting a simulation environment for improving and developing imaging algorithms. The development of flow-related ultrasound algorithms coupled with a computed flow field with an ultrasound model offers flexible control of flow and ultrasound imaging parameters for complex flow fields existing in carotid arteries [20]. Realistic prediction of blood behaviour, visualization and diagnosis to elucidate internal zones that are unreachable in bi-dimensional images, is associated to a large computational

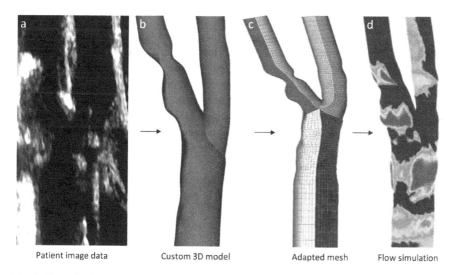

Patient image data   Custom 3D model   Adapted mesh   Flow simulation

Fig. 1 Steps in the process of patient-specific modelling for a patient with detectable carotid stenosis: **a** Grey-scale imaging data, **b** patient-specific model with common, external and internal arteries, **c** adapted mesh, and **d** contours of time average wall shear stress from simulation results

cost. The total time cost for a complete 3D computational hemodynamic modelling of each single carotid bifurcation can take from one up to several days. The two most time consuming jobs are 3D geometry reconstruction and fluid dynamics simulation. The first involves image segmentation and structured meshing that are very user-intensive as the shape varies among individuals due to different branch curvatures and stenosis severity and the second one due to the need for accurate results by solving the linearized equations in an incremental iterative manner, requiring repetitive solution of a large system of equations [21]. To simplify the decision job, when the time costs become important or even critical for the treating physician in practice, research on new methodologies toward realistic predictions in a quick time-frame have been addressed [22–24]. The advances in artificial neuron network (ANN) technologies allow the identification of the most relevant parameters and increase the possibility of correctly interpreting the results.

3 ANN Developments

Correction and registration methods of image acquisition devices have received much attention to improve the quality and eliminate most of the error sources of model input data. 3D models based on ultrasound images still have inherent errors associated with the process of thresholding the region of interest or variable distortion introduced by the boundary conditions. Due to the importance of accuracy in models used for medical applications, several methods have been developed for reducing the complexity of the problem.

An artificial neuron network (ANN) is a computational model based on the structure and functions of biological neural networks. Learning from input and output information that flows through the network, ANNs are considered fairly simple mathematical models managing to enhance existing data analysis technologies. ANNs have been successfully used in a variety of medical applications [2, 7, 10]. Until now, there has been no study on combining neural network predictions for minimizing simulation errors associated with boundary conditions of 3D hemodynamic models based on Doppler ultrasonography image data, identifying characteristics of the flow that were not apparent from the original PW Doppler velocity envelope. The fuzzy appearance of the Doppler signals sometimes makes physicians suspicious about the existence of artery diseases and causes false diagnosis. The goal of this work gets around this problem using ANN to assist the physician to make the final judgment in confidence.

3.1 The ANN Architecture

The developed ANN has three layers that are interconnected. As shown in Fig. 2, the first layer consists of input neurons, the input variables to the problem. Those

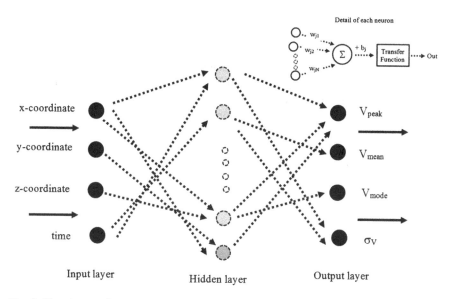

Fig. 2 Neural network topology for carotid artery PW velocity data

neurons send data on to a hidden layer of N neurons, which in turn sends the output neurons to the third layer representing the dependent variables (what is being modelled). The linkages between input and hidden nodes and between hidden and output nodes are denoted by synapses. Input weights (linking the input layer to the first hidden layer) and hidden layer biases need to be adjusted in all learning algorithms of feed forward neural networks and thus there exists the dependency between different layers of parameters (weights and biases). Each neuron j in the hidden or output layer ($k = 1$ or 2) sums its input signals x_i after multiplying them by the strengths of the respective connection weights w_{ij} and then computes its output y_i as function

$$y_j = f_k\left(\sum w_{ij}x_i + b_j\right) \tag{1}$$

where f_k is the activation function and b_j is the bias. The activation functions, the weights of the synapses and the bias applied on the neurons at the hidden and output layers are to be controlled during the supervised learning process.

In real applications, the neural networks are trained in finite training set. In this work, the input data vector is defined by a set of position and time values of Doppler measurements on the carotid artery bifurcation. The corresponding output data vector contains the blood flow velocity parameters (maximum, mean, mode and standard deviation) measured from the Doppler ultrasound signal at the corresponding time and sample volume. The optimal ANN minimizes an error $E(N, w, b, f)$ defined as the sum of the squared differences between the desired and actual values of the neurons of the output layer, being N the number of nodes in the hidden layer and w, b, f the matrixes containing respectively the weights, bias and activation functions of each particular ANN.

A hybrid method for configuring the optimal neural network is proposed using the hierarchy process methodology. An iterative process based on a developed genetic algorithm (GA) optimizes the topology of the ANN, that is, number of nodes of the hidden layer, and the training procedure, allowed variations for the weights and bias and choice of activation functions. The Levenberg-Marquardt (LM) algorithm is one of the most efficient learning algorithms used to tune weights and bias of individual ANN topologies [25]. The GA iterates over populations of chromosomes. In the addressed problem, each chromosome encodes a particular ANN configuration and the GA searches the highest fitness value calculated as

$$FIT = 1/[E(N, w, b, f) + 1] \tag{2}$$

3.2 Encoding ANN Topology

Genetic algorithms (GAs) are based on Darwinian evolutionary principles and can be used to implement efficient search strategies for optimal ANN configurations and training procedure. The implemented GA starts with N randomly created chromosomes. Each chromosome, consisting of genes of binary numbers, represents a specific architecture. As shown in Fig. 3, the chromosome is divided in four parts. The first part represents the number N of hidden neurons; the second part corresponds to the initial weight range; the third part corresponds to the initial bias range and the fourth part corresponds to the activation function selection. Two of the most commonly used functions were considered: the linear transfer function and the sigmoidal function. Each ANN topology encoded by a chromosome is then trained using the LM algorithm given input and output patterns. The fitness function of the chromosome is calculated using the validation set.

The fitness function is a function of the mean-square error in the validation set of the corresponding ANN configuration. Once the fitness functions of the initial

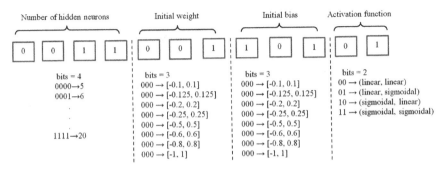

Fig. 3 Encoding hidden neurons, initial weights, initial bias and activation functions

population of chromosomes are estimated, the population is updated by using three genetic operators: selection, crossover and mutation supported by an elitist strategy that always preserves a core of best individuals of the population. Selection operator chooses the population part that will be transferred into the next generation after the fitness ranking of the actual population. An elitist strategy where only the best chromosomes from the actual population will pass into the next population was adopted. With this methodology the increase of the fitness of the future populations will be guaranteed [26]. Crossover operator transforms two chromosomes (parents) into a new chromosome (offspring) having genes from both progenitors. After the fitness ranking of the population, the two progenitors are selected: one belongs to the population part with best fitness (elite) and the second one is selected from the inferior fitness group. The offspring genetic material is obtained using a modification of the Parameterized Uniform Crossover, a multipoint combination technique applied to the binary string of the selected chromosomes. To avoid the rising of local minima a chromosome set group which genes are generated in a random way is introduced into the population. This operation is called mutation being quite different from classic techniques where a reduced number of genes are changed. Furthermore, the Implicit Mutation can affect all genes of the chromosome and guarantees the diversity of the population in each generation. The genetic search convergence is established based on the relative change of the fitness function.

3.3 The ANN Optimized via GA

The analysis of the clinician of the Doppler flow velocity is based on manual identification of some important points, such as the systolic and diastolic peaks. When the lumen of the vessel is narrow, the sample volume catches effectively the whole velocity profile and looking at the wave envelope means looking to the highest velocities reached by the blood flow. On the other hand, the Doppler spectrum of velocities can also be read as a histogram that varies over time. At one specific time of the cardiac cycle, the grey intensities represent the number of red blood cells moving at that specific velocity in the sample volume and, thus, a density of points. From this, the idea of the extraction of statistical indexes at fixed time arises and using those indexes could be a method to represent carotid hemodynamics.

Aiming to obtain a good representation of the carotid artery blood flow behaviour, sample volumes at specific locations were considered in the collection of clinical Doppler data in the common (CCA), internal (ICA) and external carotid (ECA) arteries. Collected data and statistical indexes will be used as input/output patterns in ANN learning procedure.

As previously stated, ANN learning procedure may be regarded as an optimization problem. Each pattern, consisting of an input and output vector, was normalized to avoid numerical error propagation during the ANN learning process. Firstly, an initial population was assigned by randomly generating the number of neurons, the activation function selection and allowed variations for weights and bias. Then, every individual of the population represents a particular ANN. Each network was trained with Levenberg-Marquardt back propagation. During supervised training, the input and target data were randomly divided into training, test, and validation data sets. The network was trained on the training set until its performance began to decrease on the validation data, which signals that generalization was peaked with minimal mean squared error. The test data provided a completely independent test of network generalization.

GA optimization algorithm will iterate over a population of ANN networks, each one with an assigned mean squared error. With a fixed population of 15 individuals and an elite group defined by the fittest 5 individuals, the evolutionary process will evolve through the previously specified genetic operators. At every generation a set of 3 randomly generated individuals will be inserted into the population through implicit mutation to guarantee the diversity. The details of the GA used to obtain the optimal configuration of ANN were described by Conceição António [26].

4 Pulsatile Hemodynamic Results

The efficacy of computational models to predict whether or not a medical intervention will be successful often depends on subtle factors operating at the level of unique individuals. The present study examines the detailed flow field within a subject-specific carotid bifurcation with a stenosis. Pulsatile hemodynamics is presented for one patient, female, age 84, with local degree of stenosis (ECST) 70 % and peak systolic velocity at ICA up to 160.0 cm/s measured during Doppler data acquisition.

Examination of the extra-cranial carotid system was performed using a commercial colour ultrasound scanner (model Vivid-e ultrasound system from GE Healthcare, Milwaukee, WI, USA) and a linear array probe (model 8L-RS from GE Healthcare) at the Neurosonology Unit of the Department of Neurology of Hospital São João in Portugal. A C-mode image was acquired along the longitudinal plane to delineate the carotid environment. To allow the correct reconstruction of the carotid bifurcation luminal surface, B-mode longitudinal images were also acquired and complemented with B-mode images of the carotid vessels and bifurcation along the transverse plane registered at end-diastole to control the physiologic variations of the vessel diameter along the cardiac cycle. DICOM files were imported into MATLAB framework and the B-mode images were segmented to produce smooth lumen and plaque contours by using an image segmentation MATLAB algorithm [28, 29]. Aiming at obtaining a good representation of the carotid artery hemodynamic behaviour, sample volume PW Doppler was recorded at five different locations of the carotid bifurcation, as pointed at Fig. 4.

The first objective of this section was to present a bi-dimensional numerical simulation system for the study of arterial blood flow under pulsatile conditions using the ANN with optimal configuration. Locations and PW Doppler records

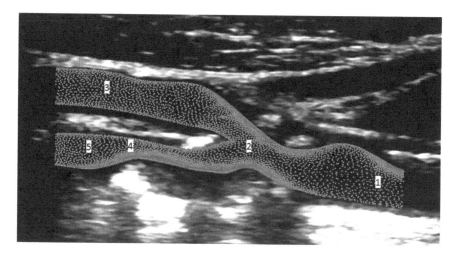

Fig. 4 Volume discretization of the region of interest for hemodynamic simulation superposed on an acquired longitudinal B-mode image and locations of PW Doppler velocity records: *1* Distal CCA; *2* Bifurcation; *3* Distal ECA; *4* Stenotic ICA; *5* Distal ICA

were used as input/output patterns in the ANN learning procedure described previously. The optimal ANN assigned a hidden layer of ten nodes and a sigmoid transfer function for the hidden layer and a linear transfer function for the output layer. To validate the proposed surrogate model, the performance of the optimal ANN is illustrated in Fig. 5 by comparing ANN centreline velocity outputs with the correspondent data targets at distal CCA and distal ICA. The ANN velocities were simulated at the exact same locations as in the ultrasound image. Agreement between ANN predictions and Doppler data is observed at the three important phases of the cardiac cycle: systolic acceleration, systolic deceleration, and diastole.

The developed innovative algorithm found an ANN surrogate model capable of data dimensional reduction and axial velocity analysis. Based on output predictions

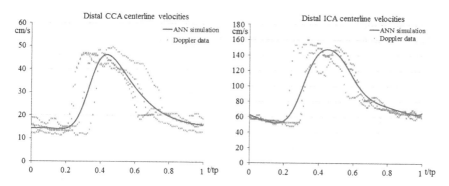

Fig. 5 Distal CCA (*left*) and distal ICA (*right*) velocity waveforms: Doppler acquisition and ANN derived input used for hemodynamic simulation

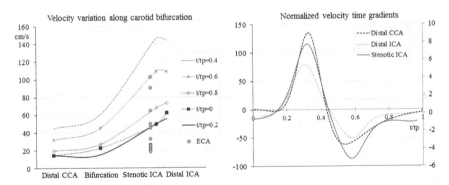

Fig. 6 Velocity analysis: Velocity variation along carotid bifurcation at specific cardiac cycle instants (*left*) and normalized velocity time gradients at specific locations (*right*). The secondary vertical axis on the right displays the stenotic ICA values

of the optimal ANN model, Fig. 6 displays the temporal variation of the flow: velocity variation along carotid bifurcation at specific cardiac cycle instants (left) and normalized velocity time gradients at specific locations (right). Blood velocity at distal CCA presents values from around 20–40 cm/s with a mean flow velocity of approximately 30 cm/s, which are within physiologic levels [30, 31]. These low values are typical in the common carotid artery suggesting no plaque at the beginning of the ICA that is to say at the level of the bifurcation [32, 33]. On the other hand, values up to 150 cm/s were found at distal ICA stenosis enforcing the classification of a moderate to high degree of ICA stenosis. A hemodynamically significant stenosis is assumed when peak systolic flow velocities reaches values greater than 120 cm/s, while an intermediate or high grade stenosis is assumed for values higher than 180 cm/s. For comparison, the distal ECA velocity values assigned by the optimal ANN model go from a low 20 cm/s at diastole to around 100 cm/s at systole, as reported in Fig. 6.

Time gradient velocity considerations can also be deduced from the output predictions of the optimal ANN model. The flow analysis at the bifurcation site is to be avoided since vortex formation in the bifurcation is not readily available from only axial velocity information. Due to the closeness to the bifurcation, blood flow is more turbulent and, in some cases, it is already divided into two flows, heading towards ICA and ECA. Also it has been shown that it is easier to detect the presence of a plaque downstream in the ICA using data 2 cm before the bifurcation than 5 mm before the bifurcation [34]. Figure 6 presents the normalized time velocity gradients at three specific sites, before and after flow division. Time velocity gradients have been normalized using the average values along the cardiac cycle. A common behaviour is observed at the three sites: high gradient values along systole and negative values after systolic peak. High gradients were observed not only in post-stenotic region, but also at CCA.

Doppler ultrasound is useful in screening certain hemodynamic alterations in arteries [35]. The ANN output values found for this analysed stenotic bifurcation can be compared with ANN results presented by António et al. [14] for a non-stenotic bifurcation. The envelope velocity found at distal CCA presents a very similar behaviour as well as similar values (Fig. 5). On the contrary, the velocity values found in this work for the stenotic ICA triple the values found around the same bulb region of the stenosis free bifurcation. In ICA stenotic cases, the bulb region is narrowed by the atherosclerotic plaque formation and there is much more streamlined flow, with reduced or disappeared areas of weakly turbulent flow. The variation of the velocity field along the longitudinal axis of the carotid bifurcation, as reported in Fig. 6, exhibits high gradient values even at the bulb region. This behavior is opposite to the one found for the normal bifurcation where stagnation areas were found at the carotid bulb [14].

The second goal of this section is to introduce ANN outputs as boundary conditions for 3D carotid flow simulations. Using the previous ultrasound data, a 3D model of the lumen and wall boundaries was reconstructed from B-mode ultrasound images. The fluid domains were meshed to create finite-volume hexahedral elements. Blood motion in vessels is highly directional and the use of computational meshes with well-organized elements along the main flow direction assures faster convergence and more accurate numerical solutions [30, 31]. Small meshes were generated near the bifurcation walls to enhance local resolution while keeping the total number of elements within reasonable bounds. Computational fluid dynamics simulations were performed in a similar manner as described previously [27]. The smallest grid size was 0.1 mm in the vicinity of the vessel wall. The number of elements in the model ranged from approximately 50 thousand to 70 thousand, which was confirmed to be adequate to calculate the velocity and wall shear stress (WSS). Approximately doubled grid densities showed 5 % differences in velocity and WSS confirming grid independence [13]. Blood was modelled as a Newtonian fluid with an attenuation of 1060 kg/m^3 and a viscosity of 0.0035 kg/m/s. A rigid-wall no-slip boundary condition was implemented at the vessel walls. Pulsatile flow simulations were performed with a developed solver, the accuracy of which had been validated previously [12, 13, 27]. For the inlet and outlet flow boundary conditions, Womersley profiles based on velocity waveforms built with the optimal ANN were considered (Fig. 5). The width of the time-step for calculation was set at 0.005 s [27]. Calculations were performed for 3 cardiac cycles, and the result of the last cycle was used for analysis.

Flow is weakly turbulent inside the ICA during the systolic phase and laminar during diastole while it remains laminar within the CCA and ECA throughout the cardiac cycle. This elevated disturbance in the decelerating phase was also observed by Long et al. [33]. Figure 7 reports simulated velocity and wall shear stress (WSS) results. As expected, due to the increased extent of stenosis, stronger blood jets formed at the portion of narrowing, and more prominent eddy flows and slow back flows were found at ICA stenosis. During systolic peak, high spatial velocity gradients were detected due to the sharp unevenness of ICA wall, with reduced or disappeared areas of weakly turbulent flow. The jet flow exiting the stenosis and impinging on the inner distal ICA wall is characteristic of flow in moderate to severe stenosis. Regions of elevated WSS were predicted at the portion of stenosis

Fig. 7 Carotid bifurcation systolic values: **a** Velocity field, and **b** *front* and *back* view of WSS contours

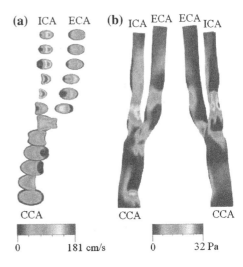

and in the path of the downstream jet. Instantaneous WSS values within the ICA were relatively high during systole (25–32 Pa) compared to that in a healthy carotid [32, 36]. Stagnation zones were detected at distal CCA and distal ICA away from the stenotic area. At these same areas, low WSS were predicted locating slowly turbulent flows. On the contrary, at ICA stenosis, areas of low WSS were reduced or even disappeared. Localized region of WSS > 10 Pa occurred close to the outer wall of ECA and around bifurcation. Low WSS contiguous patches were observed in CCA and ECA. Similar simulated hemodynamic results were obtained by Sousa et al. [36] using the same code but Womersley inlet and outlet flow profiles based on Doppler acquired data without the ANN approached model.

5 Conclusions and Future Work

The purpose of this work was to analyse flow patterns and hemodynamic distribution in stenotic carotid bifurcation in vivo based on ultrasound clinical acquisitions. Treating ultrasound and Doppler data is a difficult task due to its high variability. In fact, not only the morphology of the carotid bifurcation and type or location of the stenosis plaque are a source of variability, but also the acquisition procedure is highly sensitive leading to distorted or dirty images. Keeping all these factors in mind, the characteristics of blood flow in a stenotic carotid artery were extracted with the aim of developing a patient-specific ANN based simulator capable of detecting abnormal flow features. Concluding, the presented ANN approach can simulate flow patterns and calculate hemodynamic variables in stenotic carotid bifurcations as well as normal ones. It provides a new method to investigate the relationship of vascular geometry and flow condition with atherosclerotic pathological changes.

The presented analysis is not exhaustive. This research intends to illustrate new tools available for blood behaviour investigation and to stimulate future developments. It would be useful to repeat the analysis on a large sample of patients with different degrees of stenosis. New and continuing advances in ultrasound technology and the application of model simulations will provide more tools for assessment of carotid disease.

Acknowledgments This work was partially done in the scope of project PTDC/SAU-BEB/ 102547/2008, "Blood flow simulation in arterial networks towards application at hospital", financially supported by *FCT—Fundação para a Ciência e a Tecnologia* from Portugal. The authors acknowledge the support and dedication of the clinical group at Unidade de Neurossonologia do Serviço de Neurologia do Hospital de S. João, Porto, Portugal.

References

1. Grant E.G., Benson C.B., Moneta G.L., Alexandrov A.V., Baker J.D., Bluth E.I., et al.: Carotid artery stenosis: gray-scale and Doppler US diagnosis–Society of Radiologists in Ultrasound Consensus Conference. Radiology 229, 340–346 (2003)
2. Eckstein H.H., Winter R., Eichbaum M., Klemm K., Schumacher H., Dörfler A., et al.: Grading of internal carotid artery stenosis: Validation of Doppler/duplex ultrasound criteria and angiography against endarterectomy specimen. Eur J Vasc Endovasc Surg. 21, 301–310 (2001)
3. Swillens A., Løvstakken L., Kips J., Torp H., Segers P.: Ultrasound simulation of complex flow velocity fields based on computational fluid dynamics. IEEE Trans Ultrason Ferroelectr Freq Control 56(3), 546–556 (2009)
4. Lee S.E., Lee S.W., Fischer P.F., Bassiouny H.S., Loth F.: Direct numerical simulation of transitional flow in a stenosed carotid bifurcation. J Biomech. 41(11), 2551–2561 (2008)
5. Markl M., Wegent F., Zech T., Bauer S., Strecker C., Schumacher M., Weiller C., Hennig J., Harloff A.: In vivo wall shear stress distribution in the carotid artery: effect of bifurcation geometry, internal carotid artery stenosis, and recanalization therapy. Circulation Cardiovascular Imaging, 3, 647–655 (2010)
6. Marsden A.L.: Optimization in Cardiovascular Modeling. Annu. Rev. Fluid Mech. 46, 519–546 (2014)
7. Übeyli E.D., Güler I.: Improving medical diagnostic accuracy of ultrasound Doppler signals by combining neural network models. Comput. Biol. Med. 35(6), 533–554 (2005)
8. Güler I., Übeyli E.D.: A recurrent neural network classifier for Doppler ultrasound blood flow signals. Pattern Recognition Letters 27(13), 1560–1571 (2006)
9. Mofidi R., Brabazon A., Powell T., Hurson C., Sheehan S., Mehigan D., MacErlaine D., Keaveny T.V.: Assessment of degree of internal carotid artery stenosis based on duplex velocity measurements using an artificial neural network. British Journal of Surgery 88 (4), 600 (2001)
10. Mougiakakou S.G., Golemati S., Gousias I., Nicolaides A.N., Nikita K.S.: Computer-aided diagnosis of carotid atherosclerosis based on ultrasound image statistics, laws' texture and neural networks, Ultrasound in Med. & Biol. 33 (1), 26–36 (2007)
11. Dirgenali F., Kara S.: Recognition of early phase of atherosclerosis using principles component analysis and artificial neural networks from carotid artery Doppler signals. Expert Systems with Applications 31 643–651(2006)
12. Sousa L.C., Castro C.F., António C.A.C., Chaves R. Blood flow simulation and vascular reconstruction. J Biomech. 45, 2549–2555 (2012)
13. Sousa L.C., Castro C.F., Antonio C.A.C. Blood flow simulation and applications. Technologies for Medical Sciences: Lecture Notes in Computational Vision and Biomechanics, 67–86 (2012)

14. António C.C., Castro C.F., Sousa L.C., Chaves R.: Predictions of blood flow variations based on artificial neural network and doppler signal. ICEM15 - 15th International Conference on Experimental Mechanics, 1089–1090 (2012)
15. Kaazempur-Mofrad M.R., Isasi A.G., Younis H.F., Chan R.C., Hinton D.P., Sukhova G., LaMuraglia G.M., Lee R.T., Kamm R.D.: Characterization of the Atherosclerotic Carotid Bifurcation Using MRI, Finite Element Modeling and Histology. Annals of Biomedical Engineering 32(7), 932–946 (2004)
16. Tang D., Teng Z., Canton G., Yang C., Ferguson M., Huang X., Zheng J., Woodard P.K., Yuan C.: Sites of rupture in human atherosclerotic carotid plaques are associated with high structural stresses: an in vivo MRI-based 3D fluid-structure interaction study, Stroke 40(10), 3258–63 (2009)
17. Huang Y., Teng Z., Sadat U., He J., Graves M.J., Gillard J.H.: In vivo MRI-based simulation of fatigue process: a possible trigger for human carotid atherosclerotic plaque rupture, Biomed Eng Online 12, 36 (2013)
18. De Santis G., Trachet B., Conti M., De Beule M., Morbiducci U., Mortier P., Segers P., Verdonck P., Verhegghe B.: A computational study of the hemodynamic impact of open-versus closed-cell stent design in carotid artery stenting, Artif Organs 37(7), E96–106 (2013)
19. Kolachalama V., Bressloff N., Nair P.: Mining data from hemodynamic simulations via bayesian emulation. Biomed Eng OnLine, 6(1), 47 (2007)
20. Swillens A., Degroote J., Vierendeels J., Lovstakken L., Segers P.: A simulation environment for validating ultrasonic blood flow and vessel wall imaging based on fluid-structure interaction simulations: ultrasonic assessment of arterial distension and wall shear rate. Med. Phys. 37(8), 4318–4330 (2010)
21. Dong J., Inthavong K., Tu J.: Image-based computational hemodynamics evaluation of atherosclerotic carotid bifurcation models. Comput. Biol. Med. 43(10), 1353–1362 (2013)
22. Miller A.S., Blott B.H., Hames T.K.: Review of neural network applications in medical imaging and signal processing, Med. Biol. Eng. Comput. 30, 449–464 (1992)
23. Baldassarre D., Grossi E., Buscema M., et al.: Recognition of patients with cardiovascular disease by artificial neural networks. Ann Med 36, 630–640 (2004)
24. Grossi E.: The Framingham study and treatment guidelines for stroke prevention. Current Treatment Options in Cardiovascular Medicine 10, 207–215 (2008)
25. Hagan M.T., Menhaj M.B.: Training Feedforward Networks with the Marquardt Algorithm. IEEE Transactions on Neural Networks 5 (6), 989–993 (1994)
26. Conceição António C.A.: A Multilevel Genetic Algorithm for Optimization of Geometrically Non-Linear Stiffened Composite Structures. Structural and Multidisciplinary Optimization 24, 372–386 (2002)
27. Sousa L.C., Castro C.F., António C.C., Santos A., Santos R., Castro P., Azevedo E., Tavares J. M.R.S.: Haemodynamic conditions of patient-specific carotid bifurcation based on ultrasound imaging. Computer Methods in Biomechanics and Biomedical Engineering: Imaging & Visualization, Published online (2014)
28. Santos A.M.F., Santos R.M., Castro P.M.A.C., Azevedo E., Sousa L., Tavares J.M.R.S.: A novel automatic algorithm for the segmentation of the lumen of the carotid artery in ultrasound B-mode images. Expert Systems with Applications 40(16), 6570–6579 (2013)
29. Santos A., Sousa L., Tavares J., Santos R., Castro P., Azevedo E. Computer simulation of the carotid artery. Cerebrovasc. Dis. 33(Suppl 1):77 (2012)
30. Antiga L., Piccinelli M., Botti L., Ene-Iordache B., Remuzzi A., Steinman D.: An image-based modeling framework for patient-specific computational hemodynamics. Med Biol Eng Comput. 46, 1097–1112 (2008)
31. De Santis G., Mortier P., De Beule M., Segers P., Verdonck P., Verhegghe B.: Patient-specific computational fluid dynamics: structured mesh generation from coronary angiography. Med Biol Eng Comput. 48(4), 371–380 (2010)
32. Lee S.W., Antiga L., Spence J.D., Steinman D.A.: Geometry of the carotid bifurcation predicts its exposure to disturbed flow. Stroke 39(8), 2341–2347 (2008)

33. Long Q., Xu X.Y., Ramnarine K.V., Hoskins P.: Numerical investigation of physiologically realistic pulsatile flow through arterial stenosis. J. Biomech. **34**, 1229–1242 (2001)
34. Buratti P.: Analysis of Doppler blood flow velocity in carotid arteries for the detection of atherosclerotic plaques, Master Thesis, Politecnico di Milano (2011)
35. Kara S., Kemaloglu S., Güven A.: Detection of femoral artery occlusion from spectral density of Doppler signals using the artificial neural network. Expert Systems with Applications **29**, 945–952 (2005)
36. Sousa L.C., Castro C.F., António C.C., Tavares J.M.R.S., Santos A.M.F., Santos R.M., Castro P., Azevedo E.: Simulated hemodynamics in human carotid bifurcation based on Doppler ultrasound data. Int. J. of Clinical Neurosciences and Mental Health, accepted for publication (2014)

Computer Image Registration Techniques Applied to Nuclear Medicine Images

Raquel S. Alves and João Manuel R.S. Tavares

Abstract Modern medicine has been using imaging as a fundamental tool in a wide range of applications. Consequently, the interest in automated registration of images from either the same or different modalities has increased. In this chapter, computer techniques of image registration are reviewed, and cover both their classification and the main steps involved. Moreover, the more common geometrical transforms, optimization and interpolation algorithms are described and discussed. The clinical applications examined emphases nuclear medicine.

1 Introduction

Modern medicine has been using imaging as a fundamental tool to assist in diagnostic procedures, monitoring the evolution of pathologies and planning treatments and surgeries. However, in order to fully exploit digital medical images and their efficient analyses, suitable semi- or full-automated methods of image registration must be developed [1].

Computer techniques of image registration enable the fusion of different medical image modalities and the detection of changes between images acquired from different angles, at different acquisition times or even against an atlas that includes anatomical and functional knowledge. This task of image analysis can also point out changes in size, shape or image intensity over time and compare preoperative images and surgical planned outcomes with the physical world during interventions [2].

R.S. Alves
Faculdade de Engenharia, Universidade do Porto, Porto, Portugal

J.M.R.S. Tavares (✉)
Instituto de Engenharia Mecânica e Gestão Industrial,
Departamento de Engenharia Mecânica, Faculdade de Engenharia,
Universidade do Porto, Porto, Portugal
e-mail: tavares@fe.up.pt

© Springer International Publishing Switzerland 2015
J.M.R.S. Tavares and R.M. Natal Jorge (eds.), *Computational and Experimental Biomedical Sciences: Methods and Applications*, Lecture Notes in Computational Vision and Biomechanics 21, DOI 10.1007/978-3-319-15799-3_13

The aim of image registration techniques is to find the optimal transformation that best aligns the structures of interest in the input images. Accordingly, the techniques establish the spatial correspondence among features in the images or minimize an error measure or a cost function. To accomplish such goals, optimization algorithms are usually used to find the most suitable geometrical transformations, and interpolators are employed to resample the images into the registered discrete spaces.

The more usual applications of image registration techniques in nuclear medicine include correlative image interpretation, attenuation correction, scatter correction, correction for limited resolution and improvement of the reconstruction accuracy in emission tomography. These techniques have also been used in the co-registration of functional studies, for the transformation of images into standard spaces for their comparison against both normal cases and data from other modalities, and in conformal radiotherapy treatment. Also, these methods have been used to improve the interpretation of several functional studies based on static images, including brain, breast, chest, liver, kidneys and colon images, or to assist motion analyses as in cardiac and lung studies.

There have been previous reviews covering medical image registration in general [3–9], medical image classification [10], mutual-information-based registration methods [5], unsupervised registration methods [11], non-rigid image registration [12, 13], image registration of nuclear medicine images [14], image registration techniques for specific organs such as breast [15], brain [16, 17] and cardiac images [18]. In this chapter, the classifications of the registration methods suggested by several authors are reviewed. Then, techniques of image registration in general are introduced, including the geometric transforms, similarity measures, optimizers and interpolators. Finally, the main applications related to nuclear medicine imaging are examined.

2 Registration Methods: Classification

There are different classification criteria for image registration techniques depending on the authors. For example, image registration methods were classified into four categories: point methods, edge methods, moment methods and "similarity criterion optimization" methods [19]. Also, a classification based on: data dimensionality, origin of image properties, domain of the transformation, elasticity of the transformations, tightness of property coupling, parameter determination and type of interaction (interactive, semi-automatic or automatic) was proposed [10]. Moreover, registration techniques were also divided into: stereotactic frame systems, point methods, curve and surface methods, moment and principal axes methods, correlation methods, interactive methods, and atlas methods [19].

Registration methods can also be classified according to the subjects and the image modalities involved. Hence, intra-subject and intra-modality applications refer to the image registration of the same subject in images acquired using the same imaging modality. Intra-subject and inter-modality registration is the image registration between images of the same subject but acquired using different imaging modalities, which is a common case that involves Positron Emission Tomography (PET) and Single-Photon Emission Computed Tomography (SPECT) images [20]. Inter-subject and intra-modality registration consists of aligning images of different subjects but acquired by the same imaging modality. Finally, inter-subject and inter-modality is related to the alignment of images from different subjects and acquired by different imaging modalities.

Table 1 shows the classification of medical image registration methods that take into account the data dimensionality, nature of the registration basis, the nature and domain of the transformation, type of interaction, optimization procedure, imaging modalities, subject and object involved.

Registration methods based on pixel (or voxels in 3D) intensity are known as intensity based, while those based on the geometrical structures extracted from the images as feature or geometrical based; furthermore, frequency or Fourier based registration techniques use the image in the frequency domain and the Fourier transform properties. Feature space information, or techniques based on the amount of image information used, is another classification proposed in the literature [8].

3 Image Registration

Methods of image registration aim to find the optimal transformation that best aligns the structures of interest in the input images [21–23]. After the attribution of a common coordinate system, the images are transformed into this system. Usually, the registration methods are based on geometric approaches, known as feature-based or intensity-based methods. Feature-based methods start by establishing the correspondence between features in the input images and then compute the geometrical transformation that aligns these features. Intensity-based methods iteratively adjust the transformation that aligns the input images taking into account the intensity of the image pixels (or voxels in 3D), through the minimization of a cost function. Usually, the cost function consists of a similarity measure, i.e. the registration algorithms try to minimize an error measure [24]. In such approaches, optimization algorithms are needed to find the most suitable geometrical transformation, and interpolators are employed to resample the image data into the new common discrete space.

Landmark-based registration methods are based on the identification of the correspondence between landmarks in the two input images. These markers can be distinguished as extrinsic, anatomical and geometrical landmarks. External landmarks are well suited for validation studies; however, their routine application can be impracticable, since patient studies may be realized on different days and the location of the markers must not vary during a study. On the other hand, internal anatomical landmarks do not need marker preparation, but in common cases it is difficult to obtain a reliable and accurate localization; hence, they are not used in

Table 1 Classification of medical image registration methods (adapted from [8])

Classification criteria	Subdivision	
Dimensionality	Spatial dimension: 2D/2D, 2D/3D, 3D/3D	
	Temporal series	
Nature of the registration basis	Extrinsic	
	Invasive	Stereotactic frames
		Fiducials (screw markers)
	Non-invasive	Moulds, frames, dental adapters, etc.
		Fiducials (skin markers)
	Intrinsic	
	Landmark based	Anatomical
		Geometrical
	Segmentation based	Rigid models (points, curves, surfaces, volumes)
		Deformable models (snakes, nets)
	Voxel property based	Reduction to scalar/vectors (moments, principal axes)
		Using full image contents
	Non-image based (calibrated coordinate systems)	
Nature of transformation	Rigid (only rotation and translation)	
	Affine (translation, rotation, scaling and shearing)	
	Projective	
	Curved	
Domain of transformation	Local	
	Global	
Interaction	Interactive	Initialization supplied
		No initialization supplied
	Semi-automatic	User initializing
		User steering/correcting
		Both
	Automatic	
Optimization procedure	Parameters computed directly	
	Parameters searched (the transformation parameters are computed iteratively using optimization algorithms)	
Imaging modalities involved	Monomodal	
	Multimodal	
	Modality to model (register the coordinate system of the imaging equipment with a model coordinate system)	
	Patient to modality (register the patient with the coordinate system of the imaging equipment)	
Subject	Intra-subject	
	Inter-subject	
	Atlas	

(continued)

Table 1 (continued)

Classification criteria	Subdivision
Object	Head (brain, eye, dental, etc.)
	Thorax (entire, cardiac, breast, etc.)
	Abdomen (general, kidney, liver, etc.)
	Limbs
	Pelvis and perineum
	Spine and vertebrae

routine nuclear medicine, but just to access the efficiency of the registration methods. Geometrical landmarks consist of corners and other geometric features that can be identified automatically in the images, however, these features usually present low resolution and low signal-to-noise levels in nuclear medicine images [14]. These problems can be partially overcome using image registration algorithms based on different combinations of landmark-, surface-, attenuation- and intensity-based registration approaches [25, 26].

Boundaries or surfaces are more distinct in medical images than the usual simpler landmarks, and are therefore a valuable tool for registration methods based on surfaces. These methods require the establishment of correspondence between boundaries or surfaces that are defined in the input images, and they give good results in inter-modality registration, where both images can have very different pixel (or voxel) values [14]. There are four methods to carry out a surface registration, namely: feature, point, model and global similarity based methods. The criterion for selecting one of these is application-specific. The size of the transformation to be computed and its nature are also factors of choice [27].

Feature-based methods enable building explicit models of distinguishable anatomical elements in each image such as surfaces, curves and point landmarks, which can be aligned with their counterparts in the second image. The use of feature-based methods is recommended for images that contain enough distinctive and easily detectable features [15]. Figure 1 illustrates a typical feature-based registration algorithm.

Hybrid registration, using combined surface and volumetric-based registration methods, enables the extraction of relevant geometrical information from surface-based morphing and its following diffusion into the volume [28]. Surface alignment has been employed, for example, in image-guided surgery [29].

On the other hand, intensity based registration techniques align intensity patterns using mathematical or statistical criteria over the whole image without considering anatomical information. Combining geometric features and intensity features in registration should result in a more robust method. Therefore, hybrid algorithms involving intensity-based and model-based criteria allow the establishment of more accurate alignments, since these methods tend to average the error caused by noise or random fluctuations [12]. Figure 2 presents the general framework of the registration methods based on the minimization of a cost function. Image registration

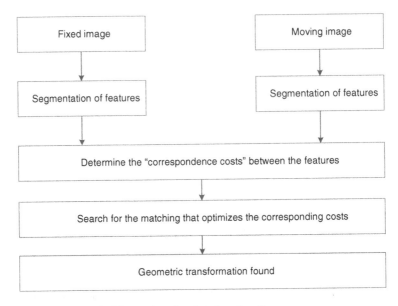

Fig. 1 Diagram of a typical feature-based registration algorithm

algorithms can also perform image correction by using the intensities of pixels (or voxels), locally or globally, in the two input images [30].

Image pre-processing is generally used before the registration to ensure that a suitable registration solution is successfully achieved, since it provides an enhanced definition of the object boundaries, and it enables intensity remapping in order to modify the range of the intensities that are used by the registration algorithms. However, it is fundamental that the pre-processing algorithms do not change the original images excessively and are not too time-consuming [14].

Rigid and affine registrations can be found in seconds; contrarily, non-rigid registrations can take minutes or hours [12]. Therefore, it is important to improve the speed of image registration techniques. Coarse-to-fine methods are commonly used, as they initially provide fast estimates and then gradually better-quality ones. Another solution to reduce the required registration time consists in sub-sampling the original images, involving spatial domain- or intensity-based procedures, and increase the image resolutions as the registration algorithm gets closer to the final solution [14].

3.1 Geometric Transformations

The goal of image registration algorithms is to find the transform involved between the two input images by means of geometrical transformations, whose number of parameters varies with the complexity of the transformation model used. The

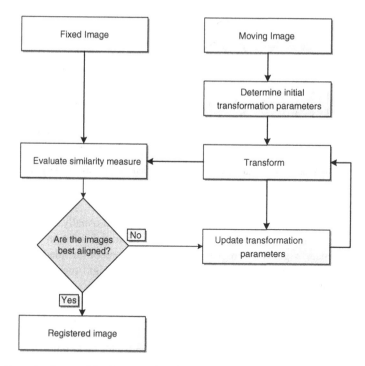

Fig. 2 General scheme of the image registration methods based on the optimization of a cost function (adapted from [14])

selection of the appropriate geometrical transformation model is crucial to the success of the registration process.

The geometrical transformation model can lead to rigid or non-rigid registrations. The simplest geometrical transformation model is based on a rigid transform that only considers rotations and translations, which is applied to all elements of one of the input images, usually known as moving images. Affine transform models include translations, rotations, scaling and shearing so that the straight lines of one image are kept as straight lines in a second image, and the parallel lines are preserved parallel [4]. An identity transformation maintains all the elements of the input image in their original configuration. Figure 3 illustrates these three types of transformation using squares. It should be noted that, a more complex transformation model implies a higher number of degrees of freedom leading to non-rigid transformations.

Image registration algorithms based on non-rigid transformations are required, for example, when the alignment between images of one individual and an atlas needs to be established [31], or when substantial anatomical variability among individuals needs to be accommodated [12, 13, 32, 33]. When compared with rigid transformations, non-rigid based registration algorithms have a higher number of degrees of freedom [34, 35]. They are frequently used in image registration when

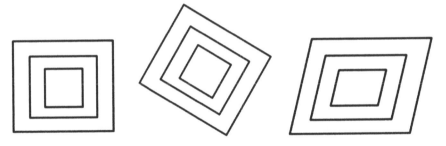

Fig. 3 Three types of geometrical transformations applied to squares: identity transformation (*left*), rigid transformation (*middle*) and affine transformation (*right*)

the image acquisition parameters are not known [36], and usually include an initial rigid body or affine transformation that provides an initial solution for the transformation. Hence, a good pre-registration method is recommended to obtain an initial position and orientation closer to the optima non-rigid registration solution. However, a higher number of parameters in the transformation model can introduce undesirable transformations and therefore, a regularization term must be taken into account [37–39]. Non-rigid image transformations can be achieved using basis functions such as a set of Fourier [40–43] or Wavelet basis functions [44].

Image registration using splines can be achieved with techniques based on the assumption that a set of control points are mapped into the target image from their corresponding counterparts in the source image [45], and a displacement field can be established and interpolated [46]. Therefore, spline-based geometrical transformations either interpolate or approximate the displacements at control points. Thin-plate splines (TPS) are based on radial basis functions and are used in surface interpolation of scattered data [32, 33]. Each basis function contributes to the transformation, and each control point has a global influence on the transformation. The modelling of local deformations can be more difficult with these functions, which requires the use of free-form transformations based on locally controlled functions [47, 48]. B-splines deform an object through the manipulation of an underlying mesh of control points generating a smooth continuous transformation. Thin-Plate Spline Robust Point Matching (TPS-RPM) algorithms have been used for non-rigid registration, showing robustness when aligning models with a large number of outliers [46].

Elastic, deformable or curved registration methods enable deforming and resampling similar to the stretching of an elastic material. Their limitations are because of the highly localized deformations that cannot be modelled due to stress deformation energy [45]. In the literature, there are reviews about the most promising non-linear registration strategies currently used in medical imaging, such as a novel curvature based registration technique that permits a faster image registration [51], the application of a deformable registration method in the automated hexahedral meshing of anatomical structures [52, 53], symmetric non-rigid registration [54] and Brownian Warps, which is a diffeomorphism registration algorithm

[55]. Also fluid registration and registration using optical flow are approaches that are equivalent to the equation of motion for incompressible flow [45].

3.2 Similarity Measures

The characteristics of the image modalities and the level of misregistration must be taken into account on choosing the similarity measure. Similarity measures can be classified into feature or intensity based metrics; however, some similarity metrics can be included in both classes. The similarity measure used in deformable image registration is commonly constituted by one term related to the pixel (or voxel in 3-D) intensity or to the matching between the structures in the images, and another one related to the deformation. Then, the cost function built is a trade-off between the pixel (or voxel) intensity or matching between the structures and the constraints imposed on the deformation field.

Concerning the feature based measures; the similarity measure commonly used represents the average distance between the corresponding features. Similarly, surfaces or edges based measures quantify an average distance between the corresponding surfaces, or between a surface extracted in one image and its corresponding set of points in the other image [9].

The simplest similarity measure compares the intensity values between the input images directly [14]. To register intra-subject and intra-modality images, the Correlation Coefficient (CC) has been an adequate similarity measure, since it involves the multiplication of the corresponding image intensities assuming a linear relationship between the intensity values. However, it is possible to subtract the corresponding image intensities instead of multiplying them, thus the search for the best alignment is based on the Smallest Sum of Squared Intensity Differences (SSD). However, due to the sensitiveness of SSD to a small number of voxels that have very large intensity differences between the input images [45], the Sum of Absolute Differences (SAD) is usually employed instead, as shown in Fig. 4 [56].

Ratio Image Uniformity (RIU), also known as Variance of Intensity Ratios (VIR), is an iterative technique similar to derived ratio images. The uniformity of the ratio image is quantified as the normalized standard deviation of the respective pixels [45]. This technique is used to find the transform that maximizes that uniformity. These similarity measures are used for intra-modality registration. Partitioned Intensity Uniformity (PIU) seeks to maximize the uniformity by minimizing the normalized standard deviation, and is usually used to register inter-modality images [4].

Image registration algorithms have also been developed based on information theory to solve both inter- and intra-modality registration problems. This image registration approach can be described as trying to maximize the amount of shared information between the two input images, which means that information can be used as a registration metric [57]. The joint entropy measures the amount of information existing in the combined images, and it has been used for rigid and non-rigid image registration [48, 49]. Mutual information can be given by the difference between the

Image #1	Image #2	SAD values between images #1 and #2

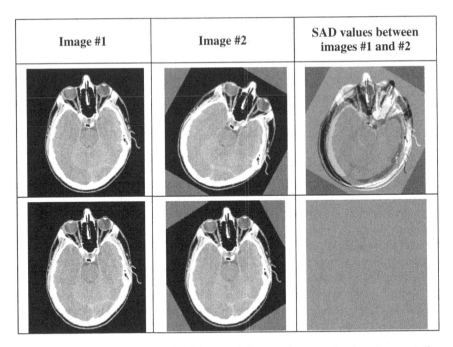

Fig. 4 Application of SAD to highlight the differences between the two images, before registration (*top*) and after registration (*bottom*). Before the registration, the original images present large absolute differences (*top-right image*), while after the registration, the aligned images present low or zero absolute differences (*bottom-right image*). Thus, the similarity measure indicates how well the images are aligned

sum of entropies of the individual images at the overlap regions and the joint entropy of the combined images [58]. Hence, it is the measure of how one image explains the other [45, 58, 60] and makes no assumptions about the functional form or relationship between the image intensities. Changes in very low intensity overlapped regions, such as those due to noise, can disproportionally contribute to artefacts [45] that affect the registration accuracy when based on mutual information, so this method is commonly used combined with the normalization of the joint entropy [45, 59].

3.3 Optimization

All the registration algorithms based on optimization require an iterative approach, whose initial estimate of the transformation is gradually refined by trial and error, by calculating the similarity measure, or cost function, at each iteration. So, the optimization process consists of both estimating the transformation and evaluating the similarity measure till the algorithm converges to a point when no new transformation can be found with a better similarity measure value [4]. Hence, the optimization algorithm evaluates the value of the similarity measure, searching for the subsequent alignment transformations that will end the registration process if an optimal value is reached. In other words, the registration is achieved by searching the transformation that increases or decreases the cost function until a maximum or minimum is found, depending on the type of the cost function used.

The optimization process is based on the fact that the quality of the matching of two images is balanced against some constraint. This constraint has the purpose of prohibiting implausible deformations and may be provided, for example, by some estimate of the energy required to physically induce the deformation [45].

One of the major difficulties of the registration methods is that the optimization algorithms can converge to an incorrect local optimum, because multiple optima can exist within the space of the transformation parameters [60–62]. The erroneous optima can be due to interpolation artefacts or good local matches between features or intensities; however it can be avoided by smoothing the original images. Also, the position and orientation associated to the two input images must be sufficiently close so the algorithm converges to the best solution within its functional range [45]. To choose the solution that has the best function cost value, a multi-start optimization can be used to get the global optimal solution [45, 60]. Additionally, the images can be initially registered at low resolution and then the transformation obtained is used as the starting transformation for registration at a higher resolution [63, 64].

3.4 Interpolation

A process of interpolation is commonly applied to transform an image space into the space of another image in order to register them; i.e. when it is necessary to estimate the values of the transformed image [14]. Thus, its goal is to estimate the intensity at the new position [8] and depends on the motivation for registering the images. The accuracy and speed of the registration process can be improved through the use of suitable interpolation solutions.

Nearest neighbour, linear interpolation or trilinear interpolation are the simplest interpolation methods, and consist of curve fitting, using linear polynomials. The interpolated image will be smoother than the original. When the interpolation complexity increases, the number of polynomial variables also increases and the smoothing effect can be more severe or even generate artefacts [14]. Recent interpolation methods between neighbouring image slices in grey-scale are based on B-splines [65], geometric multi-grid [66], using a modified control grid inter-polation algorithm [67] or adaptive 2D autoregressive modelling and soft-decision estimation [68].

The interpolation error can introduce modulations in the similarity measure used in the registration process, since the transformations involve pure translations of images with equal sampling spacing, and the period of the modulation is the same as the sampling spacing. Interpolation methods must be used with a practicable computational cost; for example, by using a low cost interpolation as trilinear or nearest neighbour first. Hence, it is a good practice to employ a more expensive interpolation approach just in the last iterations of the registration process or even take advantage of the spatial-frequency dependence of the interpolation error, by using, for example, cubic B-splines or windowed sinc interpolators. Finally, the use of a more robust interpolation solution in the optimization step may be imposed if the level of smoothness and robustness of the similarity measure is affected by interpolation imperfections [69].

4 Accuracy Assessment and Validation

The image registration methods must be validated, especially in medical applications. A verification process based on the comparison of the results obtained against a gold standard must be applied. Additionally, any process of accuracy assessment and validation should have a very low failure rate and be very accurate.

The visual assessment of registered images has been used as a standard method; however, this depends heavily on the clinical experience of the observers, besides being subject to inter- and intra-observer variability. To overcome this disadvantage, the software industry has already developed standards, protocols and quality assessment procedures [70]. The validation usually follows a sequence of measurements using computer-generated models, known as software generated phantoms [71], and the comparison of patients' images against the registration algorithms must be efficient. In order to extend the experimental validation of an image registration system to a clinical situation [72], the target registration error (TRE), which is a measure of error, is recommended to be used to monitor the clinical validation process [55], since it evaluates a target feature [73]. However, this can vary depending on the application, since there are different image modalities, anatomical structures and pathologies, and distinct positions within a view [74]. Several fiducial features can be used as registration cues, indicating the registration accuracy; this is a desirable method for rigid-body registration. Validation is accomplished by establishing statistical relationships between fiducial localization error (FLE) and TRE [75] to translate self-consistency into accuracy [74]. Furthermore, based on registration circuits, another self-consistency method [74] has also been considered, where a set of three or more images are registered in pairs.

The efforts to improve the registration validation methods have been focussed more on rigid registration than on non-rigid registration [74]. Improvement in these methods is fundamental for novel registration models to be accepted as a clinical tool, which is impossible without an optimal validation method.

5 Registration in Nuclear Medical Imaging

Nuclear image modalities have been widely used in healthcare diagnostics. They provide physiological diagnoses through the use of radiotracers to map the metabolism and fluid flow in tissues, organs or organ systems [76]. Nuclear medicine benefits from such integration and image registration plays a central role in this integration [18, 77–79].

In oncology, the completion of the medical Positron Emission Tomography (PET) examination, usually hybrid Positron Emission Tomography/Computed Tomography (PET/CT) [80, 81] enables the detection of tumours at early stages, As this exam is capable of detecting the development of a cancer it can help in the proper choice for the treatment and the later evaluation of the therapeutic response.

In cardiology, several studies have been developed, particularly in the study of chronic ischemia [20, 82–85], myocardial perfusion [18–20, 86–96], atherosclerosis rate [85, 97], post-transplantation [18] and cardiac nervous system. Registration of cardiac images is more complex than the registration of images of static organs, since it is a non-rigid moving organ inside a non-static body, and exhibits few easily distinguishable and accurate landmarks [18]. Non-rigid registration is, for example, a key requirement for the application of cardiac function biomechanical models, through the building of a generic cardiac model that is instantiated by linear elastic registration with cardiac images of a subject acquired using different modalities [12].

As regards the neurological and psychiatric disorders, molecular imaging registration has the ability to reveal non-detectable lesions by other imaging methods [98], and provides information on the physiological and biochemical properties and subsequent functional integrity of brain damaged adjacent regions [99]. The pre-surgical evaluation of epilepsy [14, 57] and guided biopsy in brain tumours [19], evaluation of primary brain tumours, dementia diagnosis and selection of stroke patients for surgical treatment [99] are usually based on the quantification of regions of interest in nuclear medicine images. Such quantification can be automated using techniques of image processing and analysis; such as image registration techniques for image correction. These techniques also allow the study of Parkinson's disease [85, 99], Alzheimer [100, 101], and movement disorders [102]. Monitoring changes in the individual by acquiring series of imaging scans and highlighting differences using image registration is a common practice and it is particularly useful in dementia where fluid registration is a cue to visualize patterns of regional atrophies [12].

Fully automatic multimodality image registration algorithms are also employed for aligning functional data with anatomic information, such as Magnetic Resonance/PET (MR/PET), Computerized Tomography/PET (CT/PET), and MR/SPECT inter-modality registrations.

6 Conclusions

Most current algorithms for medical image registration use rigid body transformations or affine transformations, and are restricted to parts of the body where the tissue deformations are small compared with the desired registration accuracy. Algorithms based on optimizing of a similarity measure and based on information theory can be applied automatically to a variety of imaging modality combinations, without the need of pre-segmenting the images, and can be extended to non-affine transformations. However, it is recommended to pre-register the input images with an image registration technique based on rigid transformation, and then finalize the process using another image registration technique based on deformable transformations.

Fully-automated inter-modality registration is still unusual in normal clinical practice, but this kind of image registration is being used in medical research, especially in neurosciences, where it is used in functional studies, in cohort studies and to quantify changes in structures during ageing and the development of diseases. However, its clinical use has logistical difficulties due to the need to acquire and register a large number of images in a reduced period, requiring advanced computational infrastructures as well as the storing of vast amounts of image data.

Due to the functional diagnosis that molecular imaging provides, computer techniques to register SPECT and PET images have been applied in clinical diagnosis, in order to assess the response to treatments and the delivery of targeted therapies. Image registration has proved its potential to aid the medical diagnosis, surgery and therapy. Examples include the combination of functional and high anatomical information to assist the localization and determination of abnormalities and the planning of their treatment. Besides, differences between two medical exams can be directly quantified, providing more objective evidences of the effects of intervention or responses to therapy in successive studies.

Acknowledgments This work was partially done in the scope of the project with reference PTDC/BBB-BMD/3088/2012, financially supported by Fundação para a Ciência e a Tecnologia (FCT), in Portugal.

References

1. Rao, A., Chandrashekara, R., Sanchez-Ortiz, G.I., Mohiaddin, R., Aljabar, P., Hajnal, J. V., Puri, B.K. & Rueckert, D. (2004). Spatial transformation of motion and deformation fields using nonrigid registration. Medical Imaging, IEEE Transactions on, 23(9), 1065-1076.
2. Fox, J.L., Rengan, R., O'Meara, W., Yorke, E., Erdi, Y., Nehmeh, S., Leibel, S. A. & Rosenzweig, K.E. (2005). Does registration of PET and planning CT images decrease interobserver and intraobserver variation in delineating tumor volumes for non–small-cell lung cancer?. International Journal of Radiation Oncology* Biology* Physics, 62(1), 70-75.
3. Maintz JBA, Viergever MA (1998) A survey of medical image registration methods. 2:1–36.
4. Hill, D. L., Batchelor, P. G., Holden, M., & Hawkes, D. J. (2001). Medical image registration. Physics in medicine and biology, 46(3), R1.
5. Pluim, J. P., & Fitzpatrick, J. M. (2003). Image registration. Medical Imaging, IEEE Transactions on, 22(11), 1341-1343.
6. Zitova, B., & Flusser, J. (2003). Image registration methods: a survey. Image and vision computing, 21(11), 977-1000.
7. Oliveira, F. P., Sousa, A., Santos, R., & Tavares, J. M. R. (2012). Towards an efficient and robust foot classification from pedobarographic images. Computer methods in biomechanics and biomedical engineering, 15(11), 1181-1188.
8. Oliveira, F. P., & Tavares, J. M. R. (2014). Medical image registration: a review. Computer methods in biomechanics and biomedical engineering, 17(2), 73-93.

9. Hutton, B. F., & Braun, M. (2003, July). Software for image registration: algorithms, accuracy, efficacy. In Seminars in nuclear medicine (Vol. 33, No. 3, pp. 180-192). WB Saunders.

10. Van den Elsen, P. A., Pol, E. J., & Viergever, M. A. (1993). Medical image matching-a review with classification. Engineering in Medicine and Biology Magazine, IEEE, 12(1), 26-39.

11. Zhang, H., Fritts, J. E., & Goldman, S. A. (2008). Image segmentation evaluation: A survey of unsupervised methods. computer vision and image understanding, 110(2), 260-280.

12. Crum WR (2004) Non-rigid image registration: theory and practice. British Journal of Radiology 77, S140–S153.

13. Holden, M. (2008). A review of geometric transformations for nonrigid body registration. Medical Imaging, IEEE Transactions on, 27(1), 111-128.

14. Hutton, B. F., Braun, M., Thurfjell, L., & Lau, D. Y. (2002). Image registration: an essential tool for nuclear medicine. European journal of nuclear medicine and molecular imaging, 29 (4), 559-577.

15. Guo, Y., Sivaramakrishna, R., Lu, C. C., Suri, J. S., & Laxminarayan, S. (2006). Breast image registration techniques: a survey. Medical and Biological Engineering and Computing, 44(1-2), 15-26.

16. Toga, A. W., & Thompson, P. M. (2001). The role of image registration in brain mapping. Image and vision computing, 19(1), 3-24.

17. Gholipour, A., Kehtarnavaz, N., Briggs, R., Devous, M., & Gopinath, K. (2007). Brain functional localization: a survey of image registration techniques. Medical Imaging, IEEE Transactions on, 26(4), 427-451.

18. Mariani, G., Bruselli, L., Kuwert, T., Kim, E.E., Flotats, A., Israel, O., Dondi, M. & Watanabe, N.(2010). A review on the clinical uses of SPECT/CT. European journal of nuclear medicine and molecular imaging, 37(10), 1959-1985.

19. Maurer, C. R., & Fitzpatrick, J. M. (1993). A review of medical image registration. Interactive image-guided neurosurgery, 17.

20. Declerck, J., Feldmar, J., Goris, M. L., & Betting, F. (1997). Automatic registration and alignment on a template of cardiac stress and rest reoriented SPECT images. Medical Imaging, IEEE Transactions on, 16(6), 727-737.

21. Lee, E., & Gunzburger, M. (2010). An optimal control formulation of an image registration problem. Journal of mathematical imaging and vision, 36(1), 69-80.

22. Shafique, K., & Shah, M. (2005). A noniterative greedy algorithm for multiframe point correspondence. Pattern Analysis and Machine Intelligence, IEEE Transactions on, 27(1), 51-65.

23. Shapiro, L. S., & Michael Brady, J. (1992). Feature-based correspondence: an eigenvector approach. Image and vision computing, 10(5), 283-288.

24. Leclerc, Y. G., Luong, Q. T., & Fua, P. (2003). Self-consistency and MDL: A paradigm for evaluating point-correspondence algorithms, and its application to detecting changes in surface elevation. International Journal of Computer Vision, 51(1), 63-83.

25. Johnson, H. J., & Christensen, G. E. (2002). Consistent landmark and intensity-based image registration. Medical Imaging, IEEE Transactions on, 21(5), 450-461.

26. Betke, M., Hong, H., Thomas, D., Prince, C., & Ko, J. P. (2003). Landmark detection in the chest and registration of lung surfaces with an application to nodule registration. Medical Image Analysis, 7(3), 265-281.

27. Audette, M. A., Ferrie, F. P., & Peters, T. M. (2000). An algorithmic overview of surface registration techniques for medical imaging. Medical Image Analysis, 4(3), 201-217.

28. Postelnicu, G., Zollei, L., & Fischl, B. (2009). Combined volumetric and surface registration. Medical Imaging, IEEE Transactions on, 28(4), 508-522.

29. Herline, A. J., Herring, J. L., Stefansic, J. D., Chapman, W. C., Galloway, R. L., & Dawant, B. M. (2000). Surface registration for use in interactive, image-guided liver surgery. Computer Aided Surgery, 5(1), 11-17.

30. Jia, J., & Tang, C. K. (2005). Tensor voting for image correction by global and local intensity alignment. Pattern Analysis and Machine Intelligence, IEEE Transactions on, 27(1), 36-50.
31. Hurvitz, A., & Joskowicz, L. (2008). Registration of a CT-like atlas to fluoroscopic X-ray images using intensity correspondences. International journal of computer assisted radiology and surgery, 3(6), 493-504.
32. Wu, C., Murtha, P. E., & Jaramaz, B. (2009). Femur statistical atlas construction based on two-level 3D non-rigid registration. Computer Aided Surgery, 14(4-6), 83-99.
33. Zagorchev, L., & Goshtasby, A. (2006). A comparative study of transformation functions for nonrigid image registration. Image Processing, IEEE Transactions on, 15(3), 529-538.
34. Bronstein, A. M., Bronstein, M. M., & Kimmel, R. (2009). Topology-invariant similarity of nonrigid shapes. International journal of computer vision, 81(3), 281-301.
35. Budd, C., Huang, P., Klaudiny, M., & Hilton, A. (2013). Global non-rigid alignment of surface sequences. International Journal of Computer Vision, 102(1-3), 256-270.
36. Kadyrov, A., & Petrou, M. (2006). Affine parameter estimation from the trace transform. Pattern Analysis and Machine Intelligence, IEEE Transactions on, 28(10), 1631-1645.
37. Ramsay, J. O., Hooker, G., Campbell, D., & Cao, J. (2007). Parameter estimation for differential equations: a generalized smoothing approach. Journal of the Royal Statistical Society: Series B (Statistical Methodology), 69(5), 741-796.
38. Stefanescu, R., Pennec, X., & Ayache, N. (2004). Grid powered nonlinear image registration with locally adaptive regularization. Medical image analysis, 8(3), 325-342.
39. Sorzano, C. O., Thevenaz, P., & Unser, M. (2005). Elastic registration of biological images using vector-spline regularization. Biomedical Engineering, IEEE Transactions on, 52(4), 652-663.
40. Andreetto, M., Cortelazzo, G. M., & Lucchese, L. (2004, September). Frequency domain registration of computer tomography data. In 3D Data Processing, Visualization and Transmission, 2004. 3DPVT 2004. Proceedings. 2nd International Symposium on (pp. 550-557). IEEE.
41. Larrey-Ruiz, J., Verdú-Monedero, R., & Morales-Sánchez, J. (2008). A fourier domain framework for variational image registration. Journal of Mathematical Imaging and Vision, 32(1), 57-72.
42. Oliveira, F. P., Pataky, T. C., & Tavares, J. M. R. (2010). Registration of pedobarographic image data in the frequency domain. Computer methods in biomechanics and biomedical engineering, 13(6), 731-740.
43. Pan, W., Qin, K., & Chen, Y. (2009). An adaptable-multilayer fractional Fourier transform approach for image registration. Pattern Analysis and Machine Intelligence, IEEE Transactions on, 31(3), 400-414.
44. Gefen, S., Tretiak, O., Bertrand, L., Rosen, G. D., & Nissanov, J. (2004). Surface alignment of an elastic body using a multiresolution wavelet representation. Biomedical Engineering, IEEE Transactions on, 51(7), 1230-1241.
45. Hajnal, J., Hill, D. L. G., & Hawkes, D. J. Medical image registration. (2001). Non rigid registration: concepts, algorithms and applications, 281-302.
46. Rueckert, D. (2001). Nonrigid registration: Concepts, algorithms, and applications. Medical Image Registration, 281-301.
47. Rogers, M., & Graham, J. (2007). Robust and accurate registration of 2-D electrophoresis gels using point-matching. Image Processing, IEEE Transactions on, 16(3), 624-635.
48. Šerifovic-Trbalic, A., Demirovic, D., Prljaca, N., Székely, G., & Cattin, P. C. (2009). Intensity-based elastic registration incorporating anisotropic landmark errors and rotational information. International journal of computer assisted radiology and surgery, 4(5), 463-468.
49. Bayro-Corrochano, E., & Rivera-Rovelo, J. (2009). The use of geometric algebra for 3D modeling and registration of medical data. Journal of Mathematical Imaging and Vision, 34 (1), 48-60.
50. Reyes-Lozano, L., Medioni, G., & Bayro-Carrochano, E. (2010). Registration of 2d points using geometric algebra and tensor voting. Journal of Mathematical Imaging and Vision, 37 (3), 249-266.

51. Fischer, B., & Modersitzki, J. (2004). A unified approach to fast image registration and a new curvature based registration technique. Linear Algebra and its applications, 380, 107-124.
52. Kybic, J., & Unser, M. (2003). Fast parametric elastic image registration. Image Processing, IEEE Transactions on, 12(11), 1427-1442.
53. Grosland, N. M., Bafna, R., & Magnotta, V. A. (2009). Automated hexahedral meshing of anatomic structures using deformable registration. Computer methods in biomechanics and biomedical engineering, 12(1), 35-43.
54. Tagare, H. D., Groisser, D., & Skrinjar, O. (2009). Symmetric non-rigid registration: A geometric theory and some numerical techniques. Journal of Mathematical Imaging and Vision, 34(1), 61-88.
55. Nielsen, M., Johansen, P., Jackson, A. D., Lautrup, B., & Hauberg, S. (2008). Brownian warps for non-rigid registration. Journal of Mathematical Imaging and Vision, 31(2-3), 221-231.
56. Sonka, M., & Fitzpatrick, J. M. (2000). Handbook of medical imaging (Volume 2, Medical image processing and analysis). SPIE- The international society for optical engineering.
57. Hoffer, P. B. (1995). Difference Images Calculated from Ictal and Interictal Technetium-. 99 m-HMPAO SPECIT Scans of Epilepsy.
58. Pluim, J. P., Maintz, J. A., & Viergever, M. A. (2003). Mutual-information-based registration of medical images: a survey. Medical Imaging, IEEE Transactions on, 22(8), 986-1004.
59. Seppa, M. (2008). Continuous sampling in mutual-information registration. Image Processing, IEEE Transactions on, 17(5), 823-826.
60. Collignon, A., Maes, F., Delaere, D., Vandermeulen, D., Suetens, P., & Marchal, G. (1995, June). Automated multi-modality image registration based on information theory. In Information processing in medical imaging (Vol. 3, No. 6, pp. 263-274).
61. Marques, J. S., & Abrantes, A. J. (1997). Shape alignment—optimal initial point and pose estimation. Pattern Recognition Letters, 18(1), 49-53.
62. Nguyen, M. H., & De la Torre, F. (2010). Metric learning for image alignment. International Journal of Computer Vision, 88(1), 69-84.
63. Marai, G. E., Laidlaw, D. H., & Crisco, J. J. (2006). Super-resolution registration using tissue-classified distance fields. Medical Imaging, IEEE Transactions on, 25(2), 177-187.
64. Telenczuk, B., Ledesma-Carbato, M. J., Velazquez-Muriel, J. A., Sorzano, C. O. S., Carazo, J. M., & Santos, A. (2006, April). Molecular image registration using mutual information and differential evolution optimization. In Biomedical Imaging: Nano to Macro, 2006. 3rd IEEE International Symposium on (pp. 844-847). IEEE.
65. Penney, G. P., Schnabel, J. A., Rueckert, D., Viergever, M. A., & Niessen, W. J. (2004). Registration-based interpolation. Medical Imaging, IEEE Transactions on, 23(7), 922-926.
66. Keeling, S. L. (2007). Generalized rigid and generalized affine image registration and interpolation by geometric multigrid. Journal of Mathematical Imaging and Vision, 29(2-3), 163-183.
67. Frakes, D. H., Dasi, L. P., Pekkan, K., Kitajima, H. D., Sundareswaran, K., Yoganathan, A. P., & Smith, M. J. (2008). A new method for registration-based medical image interpolation. Medical Imaging, IEEE Transactions on, 27(3), 370-377.
68. Zhang, X., & Wu, X. (2008). Image interpolation by adaptive 2-D autoregressive modeling and soft-decision estimation. Image Processing, IEEE Transactions on, 17(6), 887-896.
69. Oliveira, F. P., & Tavares, J. M. R. (2014). Medical image registration: a review. Computer methods in biomechanics and biomedical engineering, 17(2), 73-93.
70. Lee, J. S., Park, K. S., Lee, D. S., Lee, C. W., Chung, J. K., & Lee, M. C. (2005). Development and applications of a software for Functional Image Registration (FIRE). Computer methods and programs in biomedicine, 78(2), 157-164.
71. Dickson, J. C., Tossici-Bolt, L., Sera, T., Erlandsson, K., Varrone, A., Tatsch, K., & Hutton, B. F. (2010). The impact of reconstruction method on the quantification of DaTSCAN images. European journal of nuclear medicine and molecular imaging, 37(1), 23-35.
72. Mutic, S., Dempsey, J.F., Bosch, W.R., Low, D.A., Drzymala, R.E., Chao, K.S., Goddu, S. M., Cutler, P.D. & Purdy, J.A. (2001). Multimodality image registration quality assurance for

conformal three-dimensional treatment planning. International Journal of Radiation Oncology* Biology* Physics, 51(1), 255-260.

73. Wiles AD, Likholyot A, Frantz DD, Peters TM (2008). A statistical model for point-based target registration error with anisotropic fiducial localizer error. IEEE transactions on medical imaging 27:378–90.

74. Oliveira, F. P., & Tavares, J. M. R. (2011). Novel framework for registration of pedobarographic image data. Medical & biological engineering & computing,49(3), 313-323.

75. Nicolau, S., Pennec, X., Soler, L., & Ayache, N. (2003). Evaluation of a new 3D/2D registration criterion for liver radio-frequencies guided by augmented reality. In Surgery Simulation and Soft Tissue Modeling (pp. 270-283). Springer Berlin Heidelberg.

76. Wahl, R. L. (1999). To AC or not to AC: that is the question. Journal of Nuclear Medicine, 40(12), 2025-2028.

77. Stokking, R., Zuiderveld, K. J., Hulshoff Pol, H. E., Van Rijk, P. P., & Viergever, M. A. (1997). Normal fusion for three-dimensional integrated visualization of SPECT and magnetic resonance brain images. Journal of Nuclear Medicine, 38(4), 624-629.

78. Jacene, H. A., Goetze, S., Patel, H., Wahl, R. L., & Ziessman H. A. (2008). Advantages of Hybrid SPECT/CT vs SPECT alone. Open Med Imag J, 13(2), 67-79.

79. Bhargava, P., (2011). Overview of SPECT / CT Applications. 56th Annual Meeting of Southwestern chapter of the Society of Nuclear Medicine.

80. Townsend, D. W. (2008, May). Positron emission tomography/computed tomography. In Seminars in nuclear medicine (Vol. 38, No. 3, pp. 152-166). WB Saunders.

81. Gerasimou, G. P. (2006). Molecular imaging (SPECT and PET) in the evaluation of patients with movement disorders. Nuclear Medicine Review, 9(2), 147-153.

82. Slart, R. H., Tio, R. A., Zijlstra, F., & Dierckx, R. A. (2009). Diagnostic pathway of integrated SPECT/CT for coronary artery disease. European journal of nuclear medicine and molecular imaging, 36(11), 1829-1834.

83. Xue, Z., Shen, D., & Davatzikos, C. (2004). Determining correspondence in 3-D MR brain images using attribute vectors as morphological signatures of voxels. Medical Imaging, IEEE Transactions on, 23(10), 1276-1291.

84. Shekhar, R., Zagrodsky, V., Castro-Pareja, C. R., Walimbe, V., & Jagadeesh, J. M. (2003). High-Speed Registration of Three-and Four-dimensional Medical Images by Using Voxel Similarity 1. Radiographics, 23(6), 1673-1681.

85. Zaidi, H. (2006). Quantitative analysis in nuclear medicine imaging (pp. 141-165). New York: Springer.

86. Slomka, P. J., Radau, P., Hurwitz, G. A., & Dey, D. (2001). Automated three-dimensional quantification of myocardial perfusion and brain SPECT. Computerized medical imaging and graphics, 25(2), 153-164.

87. Hutton, B. F., Buvat, I., & Beekman, F. J. (2011). Review and current status of SPECT scatter correction. Physics in medicine and biology, 56(14), R85.

88. Garcia, E. V., Faber, T. L., Cooke, C. D., Folks, R. D., Chen, J., & Santana, C. (2007). The increasing role of quantification in clinical nuclear cardiology: the Emory approach. Journal of nuclear cardiology, 14(4), 420-432.

89. Cerqueira, M.D., Weissman, N.J., Dilsizian, V., Jacobs, A.K., Kaul, S., Laskey, W.K., Pennell, D.J., Rumberger, J.A., Ryan, T., Verani, M.S. (2002). Standardized myocardial segmentation and nomenclature for tomographic imaging of the heart a statement for healthcare professionals from the cardiac imaging committee of the Council on Clinical Cardiology of the American Heart Association. Circulation, 105(4), 539-542.

90. Hesse, B., Lindhardt, T.B., Acampa, W., Anagnostopoulos, C., Ballinger, J., Bax, J.J., Edenbrandt, L., Flotats, A., Germano, G., Stopar, T.G., Franken, P., Kelion, A., Kjaer, A., Le Guludec, D., Ljungberg, M., Maenhout, A.F., Marcassa, C., Marving, J., McKiddie, F., Schaefer, W.M., Stegger, L. & Underwood, R. (2008). EANM/ESC guidelines for radionuclide imaging of cardiac function. European journal of nuclear medicine and molecular imaging, 35(4), 851-885.

91. Slomka, P. J., & Baum, R. P. (2009). Multimodality image registration with software: state-of-the-art. European journal of nuclear medicine and molecular imaging, 36(1), 44-55.

92. Cherry, S. R. (2009, September). Multimodality imaging: Beyond pet/ct and spect/ct. In Seminars in nuclear medicine (Vol. 39, No. 5, pp. 348-353). WB Saunders.

93. Hosntalab, M., Babapour-Mofrad, F., Monshizadeh, N., & Amoui, M. (2012). Automatic left ventricle segmentation in volumetric SPECT data set by variational level set. International journal of computer assisted radiology and surgery, 7(6), 837-843.

94. Behloul, F., Lelieveldt, B. P. F., Boudraa, A., Janier, M. F., Revel, D., & Reiber, J. H. C. (2001). Neuro-fuzzy systems for computer-aided myocardial viability assessment. Medical Imaging, IEEE Transactions on, 20(12), 1302-1313.

95. Germano, G., Kavanagh, P.B., Waechter, P., Areeda, J., Van Kriekinge, S., Sharir, T., Lewin, H.C. & Berman, D.S. (2000) A new algorithm for the quantitation of myocardial perfusion SPECT. I: technical principles and reproducibility. Journal of nuclear medicine?: official publication, Society of Nuclear Medicine 41, 712–9.

96. Sharir, T., Germano, G., Waechter, P.B., Kavanagh, P.B., Areeda, J.S., Gerlach J, Kang, X., Lewin, H.C. & Berman, D.S. (2000). A new algorithm for the quantitation of myocardial perfusion SPECT. II: validation and diagnostic yield. Journal of Nuclear Medicine, 41(4), 720-727.

97. Rudd, J.H., Warburton, E.A., Fryer, T.D., Jones, H.A., Clark, J.C., Antoun, N., Johnström, P., Davenport, A.P., Kirkpatrick, P.J., Arch, B.N., Pickard, J.D., Weissberg, P.L. (2002). Imaging atherosclerotic plaque inflammation with [18F]-fluorodeoxyglucose positron emission tomography. Circulation, 105(23), 2708-2711.

98. Takalkar, A. M., El-Haddad, G., & Lilien, D. L. (2008). FDG-PET and PET/CT-Part II. The Indian journal of radiology & imaging, 18(1), 17.

99. Ci´žek, J., Herholz, K., Vollmar, S., Schrader, R., Klein, J., & Heiss, W. D. (2004). Fast and robust registration of PET and MR images of human brain. Neuroimage, 22(1), 434-442.

100. Fung, G., & Stoeckel, J. (2007). SVM feature selection for classification of SPECT images of Alzheimer's disease using spatial information. Knowledge and Information Systems, 11(2), 243-258.

101. Buckner, R.L., Snyder, A.Z., Shannon, B.J., LaRossa, G., Sachs, R., Fotenos, A.F., Sheline, Y.I., Klunk, W.E., Mathis, C.A., Morris, J.C. & Mintun MA (2005). Molecular, structural, and functional characterization of Alzheimer's disease: evidence for a relationship between default activity, amyloid, and memory. The Journal of Neuroscience, 25(34), 7709-7717.

102. Badiavas, K., Molyvda, E., Iakovou, I., Tsolaki, M., Psarrakos, K., & Karatzas, N. (2011). SPECT imaging evaluation in movement disorders: far beyond visual assessment. European journal of nuclear medicine and molecular imaging, 38(4), 764-773.

Segmentation and 3D Reconstruction of Animal Tissues in Histological Images

Liliana Azevedo, Augusto M.R. Faustino and João Manuel R.S. Tavares

Abstract Histology is considered the "gold standard" to access anatomical information at a cellular level. In histological studies, tissue samples are cut into very thin sections, stained, and observed under a microscope by a specialist. Such studies, mainly concerning tissue structures, cellular components and their interactions, can be useful to detect and diagnose certain pathologies. Thus, to find new techniques and computational solutions to assist this diagnosis, such as the 3D image based tissue reconstruction, is extremely interesting. In this chapter, a methodology to build 3D models from histological images is proposed, and the results obtained using this methodology in four experimental cases are presented and discussed based on quantitative and qualitative metrics.

Keywords Histology · Image analysis · Image segmentation · Image registration

1 Introduction

Nowadays, histology is an important topic in medical and biological sciences, since it stands at the intersections between biochemistry, molecular biology and physiology, and related disease processes [27].

The most commonly used procedure for tissue studies consists in the preparation of histological sections for microscopic observation. Because tissues are too thick to allow the passage of light, they must be sliced to obtain very thin sections. In order to make these very thin tissues slices, they need to undergo a series of prior treatments, such as Fixation (for preserving the tissue structure), Inclusion (the

L. Azevedo · J.M.R.S. Tavares (✉)
Instituto de Engenharia Mecânica e Engenharia Industrial,
Faculdade de Engenharia, Universidade do Porto, Porto, Portugal
e-mail: tavares@fe.up.pt

A.M.R. Faustino
Instituto de Ciências Biomédicas Abel Salazar, Universidade do Porto, Porto, Portugal

© Springer International Publishing Switzerland 2015
J.M.R.S. Tavares and R.M. Natal Jorge (eds.), *Computational and Experimental Biomedical Sciences: Methods and Applications*, Lecture Notes in Computational Vision and Biomechanics 21, DOI 10.1007/978-3-319-15799-3_14

technical process to impregnate the tissue with a rigid substance in order to be able to cut the sample into thin sections, such as paraffin) and Staining (to facilitate the distinction of tissue components) [3, 4].

The reconstruction of the three-dimensional (3D) structures of tissues from a series of 2D images, i.e. slices, is, at least in theory, a valuable tool to expand the 'hidden' microscopy dimension and thus be able to study the tissues and cells in depth. The possible approach to obtain such 3D models involves the digitalization of the histological slices, the preprocessing of the images obtained, the segmentation of the tissues in the pre-processed images, the registration, i.e. the aliment, of the segmented tissues and, finally, the 3D reconstruction of the tissues registered [5].

Whenever an original image is of poor quality due to, for example, the presence of severe noise, low contrast between relevant and irrelevant features, or intensity in homogeneity, image preprocessing techniques, such as image smoothing, denoising or intensity transformations, can be applied to enhance them [9].

On the other hand, algorithms of image segmentation try to extract the objects or regions of interest, here the tissues to be reconstructed into 3D, from images [9]. The algorithms for image segmentation can be classified into three main types: algorithms based on threshold [8, 22], algorithms based on clustering techniques and algorithms based on deformable models [28].

The goal of image registration is the geometrical alignment of two images—the reference image (also known as a fixed image) and the image to be aligned (also known as the moving image). Image registration is widely used, for example, in cartography, remote sensing and 3D reconstruction [29]. There are several methods to register images that can be divided according to: Dimensionality of the images, Nature of the transformation used, Domain of the transformation used, Degree of interaction, Optimization Procedures employed, Rules adopted, Subjects and Objects involved [13]. In general, the image registration methods can be divided into two major groups: feature-based methods (the alignment is made using distinct features from the images, like regions, lines or points) and intensity-based methods (the intensity values of the image are used directly) [29].

Registration accuracy of the algorithms can be evaluated using similarity measures, like the Sum of Square Differences (SSD) and Mean Square Error (MSE) [19, 20, 29], fiducial markers [6, 17, 23] and Dice Similarity Coefficient [1, 12].

In this work a methodology was developed to build 3D models from histological slices and then it was evaluated using experimental data.

2 Experimental Dataset

The histological images of the four dog tissues used in the experimental evaluation were produced at the Veterinary Pathology Laboratory of the Abel Salazar Institute of Biomedical Sciences, in Portugal.

After the selection of the tissue samples, the following steps were carried out: Fixation, Inclusion and Staining, according to standard procedures.

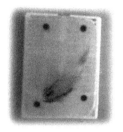 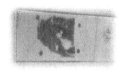

Fig. 1 Examples of a paraffin block (*left*) and of a tissue slide (*right*)

Table 1 Details about the tissue preparation procedures and images obtained

Case	Description	Number of original/final images	Tissue processing			Image digitalization
			Fixation	Inclusion	Staining	Scanner: olympus VS110, magnification: 20×
			Agent: formalin	Agent: paraffin	Protocol: hematoxylin and eosin (H&E Stain)	
#1	Testicular tumoral tissue	124/124	±2 days		±1 day	±7 days
#2	Normal lymph node	100/95	±1.5 day		±1 day	±5 days
#3	Lymph node tumor	100/100	±1.5 day		±1 day	±5 days
#4	Mammary gland tumor	96/95	±2 days		±1 day	±6 days

To slice the tissue paraffin blocks, a fully motorized Leica 2255 microtome, from Leica Microsystems (Germany), was used, Fig. 1. The slides obtained were then scanned, using an Olympus VS110 device from Olympus America Inc. (USA), in order to obtain the histological images.

After visual inspection, some of the images scanned were eliminated since several noisy artifacts were detected. Table 1 summarizes the procedures, time and tools adopted to obtain the images, i.e. the slices, for the four experimental cases.

3 Methodology

3.1 Image Preprocessing

Since the histological images are digital images, they are prone to various types of noise resulting from the acquisition. Image smoothing usually refers to spatial filtering in order to highlight the main image structures by removing image noise and fine details using for example a Gaussian filter [2, 10].

A Gaussian filter uses a 2D convolution operator in order to blur the input images and remove details and noise from them. The kernel used in the convolution represents the shape of a Gaussian hump [11]. A 2D Gaussian filter has the following form:

$$G(x, y) = \frac{1}{2\pi\sigma^2} e^{-\frac{x^2+y^2}{2\sigma^2}},$$

(1)

where (x, y) are the spatial coordinates and σ is the standard deviation of the distribution [11].

As reported in the literature [2], testing the images using different Gaussian filters showed that the higher the σ was the more apparent the blur was; however, this was not so dependent on the filter parameter in terms of the window size. Therefore, in order to obtain a good smoothing effect, but keeping the more relevant tissue details, a Gaussian filter with a window size of (3 3) and σ equal to 4 was applied to all experimental images.

3.2 Image Segmentation

Image Thresholding is commonly used in many applications of image segmentation because of its intuitive properties and simplicity of implementation; for example, one simple way to separate similar objects from the image background is by selecting a threshold T that separates the two classes involved, i.e. objects and background.

The Otsu method is a histogram based thresholding method where the gray-level histogram is treated as a probability distribution [8]. Supposing there is a dichotomization of the image pixels into two classes C_0 and C_1, then the Otsu method selects the threshold value k that maximizes the variance between classes, σ_B^2, which is defined as:

$$\sigma_B^2 = \omega_0(\mu_0 - \mu_T)^2 + \omega_1(\mu_1 - \mu_T)^2,$$

(2)

where ω_0 and ω_1 are the probability of occurrence, and μ_0 and μ_1 are the means of the two classes, respectively [8, 22].

In order to extract the tissues from the histological slices, the Otsu method was applied to the saturation component of the HSV (hue, saturation, value) colour space of the preprocessed images. Figure 2 shows that the smoothing step was essential to obtain suitable tissue segmentation masks.

In some of the tissue segmentation masks traces of loose tissue that were removed in order to reconstruct consistent tissue volumes were perceived, Fig. 3.

Afterwards, in order to obtain the final tissue segmentation, the preprocessed RGB images were transformed into grayscale images, and multiplication operations were performed between each tissue segmentation mask and the respective gray image, Fig. 4.

Fig. 2 Results of the Otsu
method on the saturation
channel of an original image
(**a**) and on the same channel
of the corresponding
smoothed image (**b**)

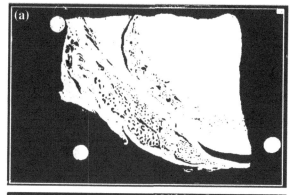

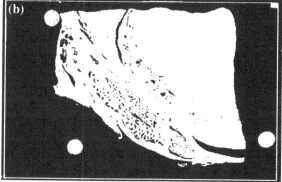

Fig. 3 Identification of the
regions (*in green*) to be
discarded from an
experimental image

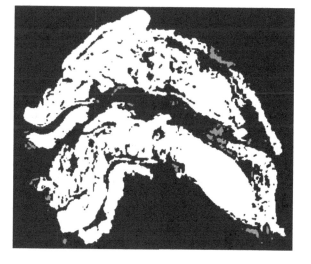

Fig. 4 An experimental
image in *grayscale* after been
multiplied with the
corresponding segmentation
tissue mask

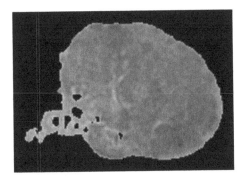

Since the image registration algorithm requires that the input images are the
same size, all experimental images were normalized to the same size.

3.3 Image Registration

Image registration is the process of overlapping two or more images of the same
scene acquired at different time points, from different views and/or by different
sensors. Usually, this process aligns geometrically two input images—the reference
image, also known as fixed image, and the moving image, by searching for
the optimal transformation that best aligns the structures of interest in the images
[21, 29].

In general, image registration methods can be divided into two major groups:
feature- and intensity-based methods. The first group is based on the detection and
matching of similar features, such as points, lines or regions, between the input
images [29]. This type of registration follows four steps: (1) Feature Detection; (2)
Feature Matching, i.e. the establishment of the correspondence between the
detected features; (3) Model Transformation Estimation, i.e. the estimation of the
parameters of the mapping function that register the features matched; and (4)
Interpolation and Transformation, i.e. the transformation of the moving image
according to the estimated parameters of the mapping function used. On the other
hand, the Intensity-based registration methods are preferably used when the input
images do not present prominent features that can be efficiently detected. To
overcome such difficulty, these methods use the intensity values of the pixels of the
input images in order to estimate the best mapping function by minimizing a cost
function, which is usually based on a similarity measure. The cost function is
computed using the overlapping regions of the input image and an optimizer tries to
obtain the best value possible. Additionally, an interpolator is used to map the
pixels (or voxels in 3D) into the new coordinate system according to the geometric
transformation found, Fig. 5.

Fig. 5 Diagram of a typical intensity-based registration algorithm (adapted from [21])

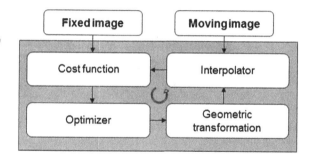

To register the histological images, the Intensity-based image registration algorithm in MATLAB (Mathworks, USA) was used [14, 15]. A monomodal registration was involved since the images were acquired using the same device and according to the same protocol. The geometric transformations compared were the rigid, affine and the similarity transformations. The projective transform was excluded because this transformation deals with the tilting transformation, and the slices used were obtained parallel to each other.

Additionally, the number of levels of the multiresolution pyramid used was specified to be equal to 3. For the cost function, the Root Mean Square Error (RMSE) was adopted since this metric is known to be appropriate for monomodal registration. This metric is computed by squaring the differences in terms of intensities of the corresponding pixels in each image and taking the mean of those squared differences. For the optimizer, the One Plus One Evolutionary also in MATLAB was used, which assumes a one-plus-one evolutionary optimization configuration, and an evolutionary algorithm is used to search for the set of parameters that produce the best possible registration result [18]. In this algorithm, the number of iterations equal to 1000 was adopted. The registration process started with the application of a rigid transformation to deal with the rigid misalignment involved between the images and simplify the posterior finer registration process and facilitate its convergence.

For the 3D reconstructing, the registration process started from an image in the middle of the image stack, since the slices closest to the center generally contain more information about the tissue [24]. Two approaches were tested: (1) Using a reference slice, the registration of each slice of the stack was done taking into account only its spatial information, i.e. all remainder slices were registered to the reference slice, Fig. 6a; (2) Using a pairwise strategy, the registration is made in cascade, starting from the center slice to the following neighbor slices in the stack, the next slice is registered with the previous one and so forth, Fig. 6b.

Three metrics were used to evaluate the registration accuracy:

1. RMSE—First the mean for the errors of the corresponding intensity pixels between each aligned image pair was calculated, and then the average error between all the images of the registered stack, given the Mean Square Error (MSE). Finally, the RMSE value was obtained by calculating the square root of

(a)   **(b)**

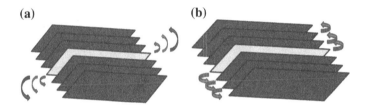

Fig. 6 Registration using the center slice as reference (**a**) and from the center slice to neighbor slices in the stack (**b**)

the correspondent MSE. The RMSE and its variations have been used in many image registration problems, including those with histological images [7, 25, 26].

2. The Dice Similarity coefficient (DSC or Dice)—The calculation of this metric is based on the overlap of two registered areas, and it has been a metric commonly used to evaluate the intersection of two areas. The DSC has values between 0 (zero) and 1 (one); the higher values represent registrations of better quality [1, 12]. This metric has been widely used to access the registration error of histological images [1, 12], and can be calculated as:

$$DSC = \frac{2A}{A + B},$$
(3)

where A and B are the registered areas.

3. Because the tissues may appear in the slices as a set of regions, in addition to the DSC, a DSC normalized by the total minor tissue area was defined:

$$Dice_n = \frac{R}{minor\ area},$$
(4)

where R is the area of intersection between total tissue area in slices A and B, and *minor area*, as the name suggests, is the total minor tissue area between these two.

3.4 3D Reconstruction

Finally, for the 3D reconstruction of the tissues presented in the experimental dataset, the surfaces were built using the isosurface algorithm included in MAT-LAB [16].

To enhance the visualization and facilitate the comparison among the four experimental cases under study, an adjustment on the reconstruction z scale was made, and different colors were chosen for the surfaces built.

4 Results and Discussion

The image preprocessing and the image segmentation were fundamental steps for preparing the images for the 3D registration. The intensity-based registration was carried out with success, but to find the best geometric transform, the registration accuracy needed to be evaluated, Table 2. Analyzing the data shown in Table 2, some conclusions can be pointed out:

The existence of a strong relationship between the metrics used to evaluate the registration accuracy (RMSE, Dice and $Dice_n$); the higher the quadratic registration error is, the lower the dice coefficient is; the registration improved the alignment of the tissue represented along the slices in each dataset.

In the preregistration step, a rigid transformation was used to place the tissue in the center of the image and then low error values and improved Dice values were achieved. The pairwise registration approach had better results than the reference slice based registration approach. Globally, and for the four cases used, the best registration results were obtained using the pairwise registration approach and the similarity transform. The worst results were obtained with the affine transformation: The RMSE values were high, and the dice values were low. The affine transformation copes with rotation, translation, scale and shear, which are too many degrees of freedom when histological images are involved. The registration based on the affine transform and pairwise registration approach was not successful for Case #1 and of bad quality in the other cases. On the other hand, the rigid registration only copes with rotation and translation (simple geometrical transformations), and the error and Dice values obtained indicated good registration results.

It was also possible to verify that the normalized dice ($Dice_n$) presented higher results than the normal dice (Dice). A plausible explanation for this is the fact that the $Dice_n$ is less affected by slices with different tissue areas, which is a common situation with histological images, since it is normal that the tissue appears with disconnected areas in each image slice.

Figures 7, 8, 9 and 10 show the 3D models built for the four experimental cases under study. These figures show that the best reconstructions built still had rough surfaces. This is due to the fact that the registration process is not totally perfect and also due to the procedure used to prepare the histological images, which is influenced by several features, such as dilation and retraction of the tissue.

Table 2 Assessment results for the four cases under study regarding the accuracy achieved using different geometrical transformations (rigid, similarity and affine) and a reference slice or pairwise based approach on the registration procedure

Case #1	Rigid			Similarity			Affine		
Without registration	RMSE = 9.3219	Dice = 0.8292	$Dice_n$ = 0.8458						
Pre-registration	RMSE = 8.6835	Dice = 0.9441	$Dice_n$ = 0.9635						
	RMSE	Dice	$Dice_n$	RMSE	Dice	$Dice_n$	RMSE	Dice	$Dice_n$
Reference slice	–	–	–	8.3307	0.9671	0.9753	8.8068	0.9377	0.9454
Pairwise	8.3255	0.9602	0.9798	8.1888	0.9676	0.9772	*	*	*

Case #2	Rigid			Similarity			Affine		
Without registration	RMSE = 9.5687	Dice = 0.8606	$Dice_n$ = 0.8734						
Pre-registration	RMSE = 7.9695	Dice = 0.9356	$Dice_n$ = 0.9517						
	RMSE	Dice	$Dice_n$	RMSE	Dice	$Dice_n$	RMSE	Dice	$Dice_n$
Reference slice	–	–	–	7.5954	0.9492	0.9598	8.6138	0.9066	0.9156
Pairwise	7.4857	0.9484	0.9651	7.3995	0.9515	0.9618	9.5232	0.7744	0.7820

(continued)

Table 2 (continued)

Case #3

	Rigid			Similarity			Affine		
	RMSE	Dice	Dice_n	RMSE	Dice	Dice_n	RMSE	Dice	Dice_n
Without registration							RMSE = 9.5544 Dice = 0.8222 Dice_n = 0.8423		
Pre-registration							RMSE = 7.7236 Dice = 0.8271 Dice_n = 0.8589		
Reference slice	-	-	-	7.2046	0.8679	0.8927	9.0429	0.6978	0.7211
Pairwise	6.8316	0.8774	0.9121	6.8222	0.8773	0.9052	9.4064	0.5922	0.6110

Case #4

	Rigid			Similarity			Affine		
	RMSE	Dice	Dice_n	RMSE	Dice	Dice_n	RMSE	Dice	Dice_n
Without registration							RMSE = 10.1506 Dice = 0.6705 Dice_n = 0.7135		
Pre-registration							RMSE = 9.9125 Dice = 0.7698 Dice_n = 0.8198		
Reference slice	-	-	-	9.7034	0.808	0.8471	10.0953	0.7273	0.7615
Pairwise	9.6133	0.8114	0.8613	9.5578	0.8191	0.8604	10.4697	0.5747	0.6061

–Not performed
*Erroneous registration

Fig. 7 3D reconstruction obtained for case #1

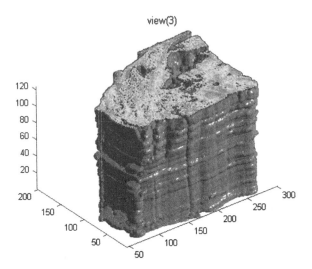

Fig. 8 3D reconstruction obtained for case #2

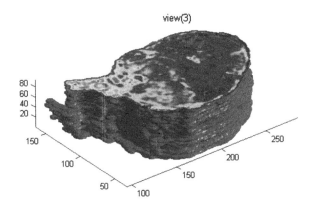

Fig. 9 3D reconstruction obtained for case #3

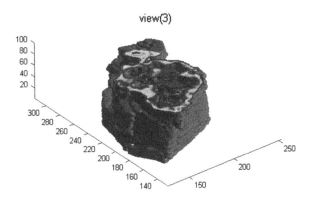

Fig. 10 3D reconstruction
obtained for case #4

view(3)

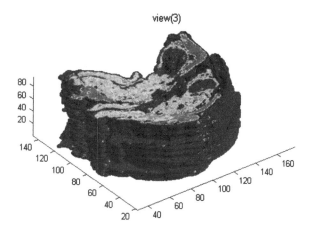

5 Conclusions

In this chapter, a straightforward and successful methodology to reconstruct the 3D
volumes of tissues from histological images was described. The methodology can
be resumed in three main steps: image preprocessing, segmentation and registration.

The image preprocessing step using a Gaussian filter proved to be efficient. The
Otsu thresholding method applied on the saturation component of the preprocessed
images also achieved good results.

The intensity-based registration algorithm used for the registration step proved to
be efficient. The similarity transform combined with the pairwise registration
approach proved to be useful for the 3D reconstructing of the four tissue types
addressed and led to a minimum of registration errors and more attractive
visualizations.

Acknowledgments This work was partially done in the scope of the project with reference
PTDC/BBB-BMD/3088/2012, financially supported by Fundação para a Ciência e a Tecnologia
(FCT), in Portugal.

References

1. Alterovitz, R., Goldberg, K., Pouliot, J., Hsu, I., Kim, Y., Noworolski, S., & Kurhanewicz,
J. (2006). Registration of MR prostate images with biomechanical modeling and nonlinear
parameter estimation. *Medical physics, 33*(2), 446–454.
2. Alves, A. (2013). Joint Bilateral Upsampling. Retrieved January 2, 2013, from http://lvelho.
impa.br/ip09/demos/jbu/filtros.html.
3. Bioaula. (2007). Histologia básica. Retrieved April 16, 2012, from http://www.bioaulas.com.
br/aulas/2006/histologia/apostilas/apostila_histologia_basica/apostila_histologia_basica_
demo.pdf.

4. Carneiro, J., & Junqueira, L. (2004). Histologia Básica. In G. K. S.A. (Ed.), *Histologia Básica* (10ª edição., pp. 1–22).
5. Cooper, L. A. D. (2009). *High Performance Image Analysis for Large Histological Datasets.* Ohio State University.
6. Danilchenko, A., & Fitzpatrick, J. (2011). General approach to firstorder error prediction in rigid point registration. *IEEE Transactions on Medical Imaging, 30*(3), 679–693.
7. Egger, R., Narayanan, R., Helmstaedter, M., De Kock, C., & M., O. (2012). 3D reconstruction and standardization of the rat vibrissal cortex for precise registration of single neuron morphology. *PLoS Computational Biology, 8*(12), 1–18.
8. Gonzalez, Rafael C.,Woods, Richard E. & Eddins, S. L. (2004). *Digital Image Processing Using MATLAB* (pp. 100,194,195,200,205, 378,404–406). PEARSON, Prentice Hall. doi:0-13-008519.
9. He, L., Long, LR., Antani, S. & Thoma, G. (2009). *Computer Assisted Diagnosis in Histopathology.* (Vol. 3, pp. 272–287).
10. He, L., Long, LR., Antani, S., Thoma, G. (2010) Computer Assisted Diagnosis in Histopathology. In: Zhao, Z., (Ed). *Sequence and Genome Analysis: Methods and Applications.* iConcept Press; pp. 271–287.
11. Ivanovska, T., Schenk, A., Dahmen, U., Hahn, H. & Linsen, L. (2010). A fast and robust hepatocyte quantification algorithm including vein processing. *BMC Bioinformatics., 11*(1), 1–18.
12. Klein, A., Andersson, J., Ardekani, BA., Ashburner J., Avants, B., Chiang, MC., Christensen, GE., Collins, DL., Gee, J., Hellier, P., Song, JH., Jenkinson, M., Lepage, C., Rueckert, D., Thompson, P., Vercauteren, T., Woods, RP., Mann, JJ. & Parsey, R. (2009). Evaluation of 14 nonlinear deformation algorithms applied to human brain MRI registration. *NeuroImage, 46* (3), 786–802.
13. Maintz, JBA. & Viergever, M. (1998). A survey of medical image registration. *Medical Image Analysis, 2*(1), 1–36.
14. Mathworks. (2013a). Estimate Geometric Transformation (R2013a). Retrieved March 4, 2013, from http://www.mathworks.com/help/vision/ref/estimategeometrictransformation.html.
15. Mathworks. (2013b). imregister (R2013a). Retrieved March 4, 2013, from http://www.mathworks.com/help/images/ref/imregister.html.
16. Mathworks. (2013c). Techniques for Visualizing Scalar Volume Data (R2013a). Retrieved April 6, 2013, from http://www.mathworks.com/help/matlab/visualize/techniques-for-visualizing-scalar-volume-data.html.
17. Mattes, D., Haynor, D., Vesselle, H., Lewellen, T., & Eubank, W. (2003). PET-CT image registration in the chest using free-form deformations. *IEEE Transactions on Medical Imaging, 22*(1), 120–128.
18. Mattes, D., Haynor, DR., Vesselle, H., Lewellyn, TK. & Eubank, W. (2001). Nonrigid multimodality image registration. *IEEE Transactions on Medical Imaging, 4322*, 1609–1620.
19. Oliveira, F. P. M. (2009). *Emparelhamento e alinhamento de estruturas em visão computacional: aplicações em imagens médicas.* Faculdade de Engenharia da Universidade do Porto.
20. Oliveira, F. P. M. & Tavares, J. M. R. S. (2011). Novel framework for registration of pedobarographic image data. *Medical and Biological Engineering and Computing, 49*(3), 312–324.
21. Oliveira, F. & Tavares, J. (2012). Medical image registration: a review. *Computer Methods in Biomechanics and Biomedical Engineering*, ISSN: 1025-5842 (print) - 1476-8259 (online), Taylor & Francis, 17(2), 73-93. doi: 10.1080/10255842.2012.670855.
22. Otsu, N. (1979). A Threshold Selection Method from Gray-Level Histograms. *IEEE Transactions on Systems, Man and Cybernetics., 9*(1), 62–66. doi:10.1109/TSMC.1979.4310076.
23. Pluim, J., Maintz, J. & MA., V. (2000). Image registration by maximization of combinedmutual information and gradient information. *IEEE Transactions on Medical Imaging, 19*(8), 809–814.

24. Robert, s N., Magee, D., Song, Y., Brabazon, K., Shires, M., Crellin, D., Orsi, NM., Quirke, R., Quirke, P. & Treanor, D. (2012). Toward Routine Use of 3D Histopathology as a Research Tool. *The American Journal of Pathology, 180*(5), 1835–1842.

25. Sharma, R. & Katz, J. (2011). Taxotere Chemosensitivity Evaluation in Rat Breast Tumor by Multimodal Imaging: Quantitative Measurement by Fusion of MRI, PET Imaging with MALDI and Histology. *IEEE Transactions on Medical Imaging, 1*(1), 1–14.

26. Sharma, Y., Moffitt, RA., Stokes, TH., Chaudry, Q. & Wang, M. (2011). Feasibility analysis of high resolution tissue image registration using 3-D synthetic data. *Journal of Pathology Informatics, 2*(6), 1–7.

27. Stevens, A. & Lowe, J. (1992). HISTOLOGY. In Mosby (Ed.), (pp. 1–6).

28. Zhen, M., Tavares, J. M. R. S., Natal, R. J., & Mascarenhas, T. (2010). Review of Algorithms for Medical Image Segmentation and their Applications to the Female Pelvic Cavity. *Computer Methods in Biomechanics and Biomedical Engineering, 13*(2), 235–246. doi:10. 1080/10255840903131878.

29. Zitová, B. & Flusser, J. (2003). Image registration methods: a survey. *Image and Vision Computing, 21*(11), 977–1000.

Ischemic Region Segmentation in Rat Heart Photos Using DRLSE Algorithm

Regina C. Coelho, Salety F. Baracho, Vinícius V. de Melo, José Gustavo P. Tavares and Carlos Marcelo G. de Godoy

Abstract Heart attack preceded by ischemia is responsible for many deaths worldwide. Thus, the detection of ischemic cardiac areas is very important not only to help the prevention of that mortal disease but also for teaching/learning purposes. This work presents the results of a new approach for ischemic region detection in rat heart photo. Such an approach is based on segmentation using "Distance Regularized Level Set Evolution" method (DRLSE). The DRLSE method is an improvement on "Level Set method". Evolving Interfaces in geometry, fluid mechanics, computer vision and materials sciences, 1999). The advantage of DRLSE is that the restart of level set function is not necessary. It was verified that the best identification of the ischemic region was obtained by using the yellow channel image in the processing, instead of the other color channels. Results show that the present approach is able to fairly segment ischemic regions in heart photos, being suitable for teaching/learning purposes.

1 Introduction

Cardiac ischemia that precedes infarction (heart attack) is an important cause of death worldwide [13]. Thus, many different techniques have been developed to help extraction (or segmentation) of ischemic regions of heart images [1, 3, 6, 11].

R.C. Coelho (✉) · S.F. Baracho · V.V. de Melo · J.G.P. Tavares · C.M.G. de Godoy
Universidade Federal de São Paulo—UNIFESP, São José dos Campos, SP, Brasil
e-mail: rccoelho@unifesp.br

S.F. Baracho
e-mail: saletybaracho@gmail.com

V.V. de Melo
e-mail: vinicius.melo@unifesp.br

J.G.P. Tavares
e-mail: padrao.tavares@hotmail.com

C.M.G. de Godoy
e-mail: gurjao.godoy@unifesp.br

© Springer International Publishing Switzerland 2015
J.M.R.S. Tavares and R.M. Natal Jorge (eds.), *Computational and Experimental Biomedical Sciences: Methods and Applications*, Lecture Notes in Computational Vision and Biomechanics 21, DOI 10.1007/978-3-319-15799-3_15

Although many authors use good resolution magnetic resonance images, such approach is, in most cases, not suitable for visual inspection of ischemia (or infarction) in a teaching/learning context. Therefore, the use of rat heart photos depicting well defined and experimentally controlled ischemia/infarction regions is appropriated for that purpose. However, the sharpness of those heart photos is not always enough for adequate visual diagnosis of ischemia/infarction regions [12].

The estimation of ischemic region is commonly performed by visual inspection after a cardiac reperfusion with a chemical marker [5]. However, that method can be inappropriate as the chemically marked ischemic region is frequently not evident enough for visual inspection. Thus, this work presents a semi-automatic method to extract the ischemic region in rat heart photos in order to help a suitable and didactical visual inspection of cardiac ischemia and/or infarction.

2 Materials and Methods

2.1 Obtaining Photos of the Rats Hearts

Photos were taken from hearts of rats anesthetized with urethane (1.25 g/kg IP) and fixed in the supine position. The animals were ventilated with room air (20 ml/kg body weight; 55 strokes/min). The chest was opened by a left thoracotomy and, after opening the pericardium, the heart was gently exteriorized. A silk ligature of descending left coronary was tied. After a 10 min period of coronary occlusion (ischemia), reperfusion was obtained by cutting the suture. Photos were taken from the rats hearts before, during, and after an ischemia. All procedures were approved by the Ethics Committee on Animal Experimentation of the Federal University of São Paulo-UNIFESP.

2.2 Segmentation Method

Distinct color channels (RGB and CMYK) were previously analyzed in order to improve performance of the calculations required for the segmentation process in the heart photos. The yellow channel presented the clearest ischemic region images (nine photos were evaluated), as can be seen in Fig. 1. Therefore, that color channel was adopted for the tests.

The segmentation method used to extract the pre-ischemic region was a variation of the Level Set method, so-called Distance Regularized Level Set Evolution [9]. This method is interesting because, in addition of being able to deal with topology changes (such as merging and splitting, as the conventional Level Set method), it can evolve from fixed Cartesian grid as initial seeds. It is distinct of other methods in which points have been chosen as input seeds of the algorithms.

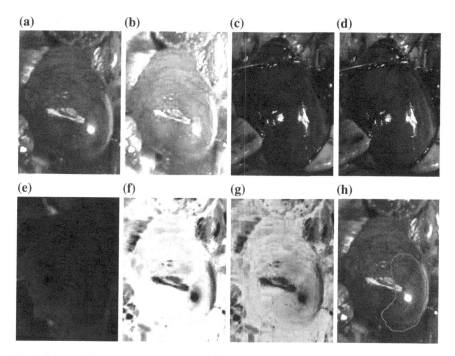

Fig. 1 Images of a rat heart with an ischemic region in different color channels. **a** Original photo; **b** red channel image; **c** green channel image; **d** blue channel image; **e** cyan channel image; **f** magenta channel image; **g** yellow channel image; **h** ischemic region manually marked by a specialist

Next section describes Level Set and next, Distance Regularized Level Set Evolution.

2.2.1 Level Set Method

The image segmentation consists of dividing an image in portions of interest. As for the present work, the goal is to separate the ischemic region image out of the heart photo. An interesting segmentation technique is the "Level Set Method" [14]. That method, widely used in the literature, defines a motion equation for a front propagation with curvature-dependent speed, based on the Hamilton-Jacobi equation [2, 4, 7–10]. In that segmentation method, the interface is considered to be the curve or surface that separates two environments interacting with each other. It can be quite difficult to follow the evolution of an interface, even if both motion speed and direction are known.

An interface is able to delimit the border between inside and outside of an object, thus allowing the differentiation of the ischemic region from the rest of the heart by propagating the interface. The propagated interface is the interface at time t after moving from a defined interface at $t = 0$. During this propagation the division, merging, or disappearance of the interface may occur depending on its geometry and the physical phenomena that influence it [15, 16].

The main idea of the Level Set method is to represent a particular interface as the initial interface (zero level set) of a higher level function (Level Set function). A Level Set function f is calculated based on the distance (d) from each point (x, y) with respect to level zero. The distance will be negative if the point is inside and positive if it is outside of the interface in evolution [16]. Thus, ϕ for $t = 0$ is calculated as:

$$\phi(x(t), y(t), t = 0) = \pm d. \tag{1}$$

The interface propagates according to the speed function F. This function determines how each point of the interface moves and gives the speed in the perpendicular direction to the curve. Thus, the evolution equation for ϕ is:

$$\phi_t + F|\nabla_\phi| = 0, \tag{2}$$

where ∇_ϕ is the gradient of ϕ.

To segment a region of an image it is necessary that the interface be moved to the edges of the object of interest but not beyond them. Therefore, the speed F is adjusted to detect the edge according to Sethian [16]:

- when the interface passes over places where the gradient of the image is small, it is assumed that the edge is not near and the curve should expand quickly;
- when the interface passes over places where the gradient of the image is large, it is assumed that the edge is near and the rate of expansion of the interface is decreased.

Therefore, F can be defined as:

$$F = g(x, y) \cdot (F_0 + F(K)) \tag{3}$$

where $K = \nabla \cdot \vec{n}$ and $\vec{n} = \frac{\vec{\nabla}\phi}{|\vec{\nabla}\phi|}$

Function $g(x, y)$ is calculated as:

$$g(x, y) = (1 + |\nabla G_\sigma * I(x, y)|)^{-p} \tag{4}$$

where

- $p \geq 1$ and
- $G_\sigma * I(x, y)$ is the convolution of image I with Gaussian kernel with standard deviation σ. The term $\nabla(G_\sigma * I(x, y))$ is zero, except near from edges, where the variation of σ is large [16].

An important advantage of that method is the fact that it is able to efficiently deal with topological changes and/or discontinuities that can appear during the propagation of the zero level contour.

2.2.2 Distance Regularized Level Set Evolution

In the Level Set method some irregularities can appear during the evolution of the ϕ function. Such irregularities can be represented by numerical errors and instabilities of the evolution. In order to avoid this, the level set function is periodically re-initialized as a signed distance function [7, 15, 16]. However, re-initialization can numerically affect the calculation accuracy. The Distance Regularized Level Set Evolution (DRLSE) method is an interesting as it eliminates re-initialization. It also allows the use of more general functions for the level set function initialization [8, 9] as, for instance, a binary step function [16]. Those functions define the regions for the initial seeds (Cartesian grid) selected. Thus, just a few iterations are sufficient to move the zero level set to the desired edge. DRLSE has two extra terms: one to regularize the distance function used in the level set function, and another term used to control the movement of the level zero contours so that it moves to the desired position. The distance regularization term allows eliminating the re-initialization. It is calculated using a potential function to force $|\nabla\phi|$ to one of its minimum points [8, 9]. In this method, p in Eq. 4 is equal to 2.

3 Results

Figure 2 presents results obtained by using the DRLSE segmentation method implemented with in MatLab (2012). The computing time (Intel Core I7-3770, 3.4 GHz, 16 GB RAM, Windows 7 Home Premium 64-bit) to process the images ranged from 5.02 s (220 × 300 image) to 81.24 s (454 × 590 image). As can be seen in Fig. 2 (row (a)), it is difficult to delimit the ischemic region only by visual inspection. On the other hand, the ischemic region in Fig. 2 (row (b)) seems easier to be delimited, as the region border contrast is more evident in the yellow channel photos.

The initial seeds are selected by the user, as well as the number of iterations. The rows (c), (d), (e) and (f) show, respectively, the selected seeds, an intermediate result, and final segmentation (only the segmentation contour). Table 1 presents the number of seeds used to segment the region in each photo and the number of iterations required to obtain both intermediate and final results.

In order to help verifying the suitability of using the yellow channel image in the method, Fig. 3 shows one photo and its corresponding yellow channel image. Coherently, in that example it is not possible to distinguish any ischemic region as, in fact, there is no ischemia in the represented heart.

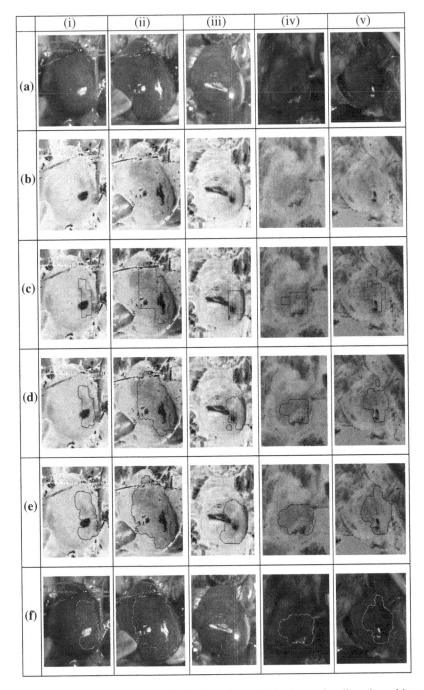

Fig. 2 Results of the segmentation of ischemic regions. **a** Color image; **b** yellow channel image; **c** initial seeds; **d** intermediate results; **e** and **f** final ischemia contour mark in yellow channel image and in color image, respectively

Table 1 Number of initial seeds and iterations to each figure shown in Fig. 2

	Number of initial seeds	Number of iterations of intermediate result	Number of iterations of final result
(i)	4	50	135
(ii)	4	100	270
(iii)	4	55	135
(iv)	3	85	185
(v)	4	60	160

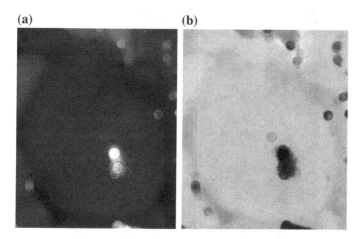

Fig. 3 Rat heart photos with no ischemic region. **a** Rat heart photo; **b** yellow channel image. Coherently, the segmentation method did not distinguish any ischemia

Columns (i) and (ii) of Fig. 2 represent the same heart in distinct moments in the ischemic-reperfusion experiment. Column (i) shows a photo of the heart in the beginning of the ischemia. Column (ii) shows the photo taken 5 min after the heart reperfusion. Thus, one may observe the ischemia evolution.

In order to qualitatively evaluate the method's capability of segmenting the ischemic region, the segmented regions found by the method were superimposed to photos with ischemic region contours manually marked by a specialist. Figure 4 shows that, in a qualitative evaluation, both contours are not depicting discrepant ischemic regions, indicating the method's suitability for visual inspection of ischemic regions in heart photos.

All segmented areas were validated by a physiologist and a cardiologist as being actual ischemic regions.

(a)   (b)   (c)

(d)   (e)

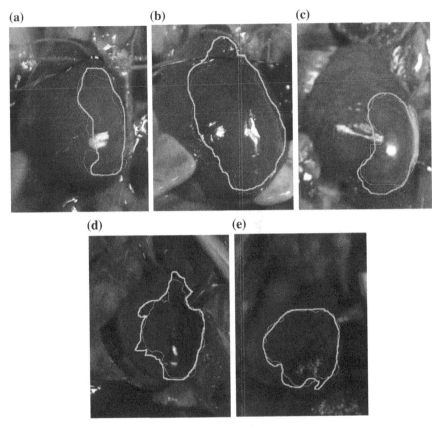

Fig. 4 Comparison between manual and DRLSE segmentation for each image of Fig. 2. The *green (thicker) lines* are manual ischemia contours drawn by the specialist. The *blue (thinner) lines* are the segmentation performed by DRLSE

4 Discussion and Conclusions

The DRLSE method was employed to segment the ischemic area in rat heart photos. The seeds and the number of the iterations are selected by the user. Those selections are necessary because heart photos normally do not exhibit enough contrasts for automatic segmentation of ischemic regions.

The presented approach was robust to detect the ischemic region in all tested rat ischemic heart photos. It was verified using of yellow channel images, instead of the original color images or other color channels, is more adequate to select the ischemic region in rat heart photos. The technique used in this work showed to be a suitable tool to help didactical teaching of an important cardiovascular disease: ischemia preceding heart attack. This semi-automatic segmentation is also suitable to evaluate the evolution of ischemic cardiac areas.

As a whole, the method may represent a relevant insight for the development of new tools for visual inspection or either ischemia or pre-ischemia in heart photos of other animals or humans.

Acknowledgments This work was supported by Fundação de Amparo à Pesquisa do Estado de São Paulo (FAPESP—Proc. No. 2012/01505-6).

References

1. Algohary A, Bialy AME, Kandil, AH, Osman, NF (2010) Improved Segmentation Technique to Detect Cardiac Infarction in MRI C-SENC Images. In: 5th International Biomedical Engineering Conference, Cairo, Egypt, 2010.
2. Balla-Arabé S, Gao X, Wang B (2013) A Fast an Robust Level Set Method for Image Segmentation Using Fuzzy Clustering and Lattice Boltzmann Method, IEE Transactions on Cybernetics, 43(3):910–920
3. Bervari RE, Block I, Redheuil A, Angelini E, Mousseaux E, Frouin F, Herment A (2007) An automated myocardial segmentation in cardiac MRI. In: 29th Annual International Conference of the IEEE, Lyon, France, 2007.
4. Brox T, Weickert J (2004) Level Set Based Image Segmentation with Multiple Regions, Pattern Recognition, Springer LNCC 3175:415–423.
5. Cagli K, Bagci C, Gulec M, Cengiz B, Akyol O, Sari I, Cavdar S, Pence S, Dinckan H (2005) In vivo effects of caffeic acid phenethyl ester on myocardial ischemia-reperfusion injury and apoptotic changes in rats, In: Annals of Clinical and Laboratory Science, 35(4):440–448, 2005.
6. Esteves T, Valente M, Nascimento D D, Pinto-do-'O P, Quelhas P (2012) Automatic Myocardial Infarction Size Extraction in an Experimental Murine Model Using an Anatomical Model. In: International Symposium on Biomedical Imaging, Porto, Portugal, 310–313, 2012.
7. Han X, Xu C, Prince J (2003) A topology preserving level set method for geometric deformable models, IEEE Trans. Patt. Anal. Mach. Intell. 25:755–768.
8. Li C, Xu C, Gui C, Fox MD (2005) Level Set Evolution Without Re-Initialization: A New Variational Formulation, IEEE Conference on Computer Vision and Pattern Recognition, Washington, DC. USA, 430–436.
9. Li C, Xu C, Gui C, Fox MD (2010) Distance Regularized Level Set Evolution and Its Application to Image Segmentation. IEEE Trans Image Process, 19(12):3243–3254.
10. Li C, Huang R, Ding Z, Gatenby J C, Metaxas, D N, Gore J C (2011) A Level Set Method for Image Segmentation in the Presence of Intensity Inhomogeneities with Application to MRI, IEEE Transactions on Image Processing, 20(7): 2007–2016.
11. Lu Y, Yang Y, Connelly K A (2012) Automated quantification of Myocardial Infarction Using Graph Cuts on Contrast Delayed Enhanced Magnetic Resonance Images. Quant Imaging Med Surg, 2(2):81–86.
12. McCoy CE, Menchine M, Anderson C, Kollen R, Langdorf M I, Lotfipour S (2011) Prospective randomized crossover study of simulation vs. didactics for teaching medical students the assessment and management of critically ill patients. Journal of Emergency Medicine, 40 (4), 448–455.
13. O'Gara P T, Kushner F G, et al. (2013) Guideline for the management of ST-elevation myocardial infarction, Circulation, 127(4), e362–e425.

14. Osher S, Sethian J (1988) Fronts propagating with curvature-dependent speed: Algorithms based on Hamilton-Jacobi formulations. Journal of Computational Physics, 79(1), 12–49.
15. Sethian, JA (1997) Level Set Methods: An Act of Violence. Evolving Interfaces in Geometry, Fluid Mechanics, Computer Vision and Materials Sciences.
16. Sethian JA (1999) Level Set Methods and Fast Marching Methods, Cambridge University Press, Cambridge, second edition.

Pectoral and Breast Segmentation Technique Based on Texture Information

Khamsa Djaroudib, Pascal Lorenz, Abdelmalik Taleb Ahmed and Abdelmadjid Zidani

Abstract Pectoral and breast segmentation is necessary and cumbersome step for the Computer Aided Diagnosis systems (CAD). This paper presents new pectoral and breast segmentation technique based on texture information from Gray Level Co-occurrence Matrix (GLCM). It showed good results to solve certain problems not yet resolved until presents, such as the presence of anomaly of mass or micro-calcification in the pectoral borders, omitted in breast segmentation step, and the confusion between the pectoral line and the pectoral border. First, we applied smoothing and enhancing techniques to enhance breast image. Second, we compute textural images representing statistics parameters from GLCM in any pixel of the breast image, to detect breast and pectoral borders. These techniques have been applied to the MIAS database, consisting of MLO mammograms. The results were evaluated by expert radiologists and are promising, compared to other related works.

Keywords Mammography · Segmentation · Breast · Pectoral muscle · Gray level co-occurrence matrices (GLCM)

1 Introduction

CAD systems must identify the breast region independently of the digitization system, the orientation of the breast in the image and the presence of noise, including imaging artifacts. Breast segmentation consists to extract breast and

K. Djaroudib (✉) · A. Zidani
Computer Science Department, University of Batna, UHL, Batna, Algeria
e-mail: k.djaroudib@yahoo.fr

P. Lorenz
University of Colmar, UHA, Alsace, France

A. Taleb Ahmed
LAMIH Laboratory, University of Valenciennes, Valenciennes, France

© Springer International Publishing Switzerland 2015
J.M.R.S. Tavares and R.M. Natal Jorge (eds.), *Computational and Experimental Biomedical Sciences: Methods and Applications*, Lecture Notes in Computational Vision and Biomechanics 21, DOI 10.1007/978-3-319-15799-3_16

pectoral borders, necessary and cumbersome step for typical CAD systems. Many studies focus on these problems. Raba et al. [1] review works on breast region segmentation with pectoral muscle suppression. At this date, no wok uses textural information for this purpose. Recently, a review of pectoral segmentation methods is summarized in [2]. It shows that breast tissue and pectoral muscle can have the same intensities and similar texture in mammogram [3–8]. So it embarrasses and disorientates the step of detection of cancerous anomalies. Peter and Sue [3] have used texture-based discrimination between fatty and dense breast types using granulometric techniques and texture masks. The main problem with the approach proposed by Ferrari et al. [4] is that the pectoral muscle is approximated by a line. These methods give poor results when the pectoral muscle contour is a curve. So authors focus on the segmentation of pectoral muscle as line and curve. Here we contribute and use texture parameters from GLCM to detect breast and pectoral borders, in order to get more efficient results to detect and segment pectoral muscle as a line or a curve shape, for CAD systems. The GLCM method not used before for this purpose, it used in order to give texture features in region approach. Here, we use these parameters in contour approach, to detect breast and pectoral borders, and then to extract breast region.

After this review of related works in pectoral muscle segmentation, we can say that three problems appear in previous methods. First, pectoral region can have the similar texture of breast region, which is the region of interest for the next stages in CAD systems, the stage of detection and/or segmentation of anomalies, and the classification stage. Second, the border of pectoral muscle must be considered as a curve and not a line. Third, researchers use a method for the pectoral muscle segmentation, and another method for the breast segmentation. For these three reasons we contribute and propose a semi-automatic approach using the GLCM to extract textural images, who allow detecting directly the pectoral muscle borders and the breast region, at the same time.

Four steps describe our approach and are detailed in the next paragraph: breast orientation step, the step of enhancing images and removing noise, the computation of textural images step, in order to detect the pectoral muscle borders and the breast region, step of computation mask with expert radiologist for segmentation and finally we present a evaluation of our segmentation approach.

2 Methods: GLCM for Breast and Pectoral Detection and Segmentation

The GLCM method is the statistic approach [9]. Theses matrices are widely used in the literature, but are generally used in order to extract textural features for segmentation or classification steps. Besides, in the literature, these matrices are known to give strong and complete information about the texture of an image. Here, we use these matrices to compute and extract textural images. Each point in these images represent one parameter of the Harralick parameters [10], computing in step 3.

Four steps are used for our approach:

2.1 Step 1: Breast Orientation

At first, we must flip the images where the breast is not well oriented as shown in Fig. 1.

2.2 Step 2: Enhancement Techniques

The performance of methods based on texture information is highly dependent on the pre-processing (enhancement) of the input image [11], so many researchers focus in this stage of CAD. For our approach, this stage is our key to have the best results for the pectoral segmentation stage. Most mammogram images have low intensity contrast, then we applied smoothing (denoising) and enhancing method to enhance breast image [12]. We suggested applying respectively, the anisotropic filter diffusion SRAD (Speckle Reducing Anisotropic Diffusion) [13] and Contrast-limited Adaptive Histogram Equalization (CLAHE) for enhancing image. Instead of most studies, in our approach and in the aim to perform texture information, denoising and enhancing steps are applied in whole breast image and then, we extract suspicious ROI image. So, our SRAD algorithm can take speckle for every image independently of another one which makes this approach is more efficiency for image speckle reducing.

We used the YU scripts for SRAD [13] and results of this step are shown in Fig. 4 (enhanced image). In this figure, the image of enhancement show clearly more regions in the breast image. The clear regions are even clearer and the dark regions are darker.

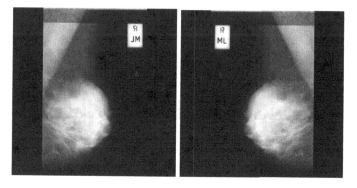

Fig. 1 Image MIAS: in *left*, bad orientation of the breast and in *right*, good orientation of the breast

2.3 Step 3: Edges Pectoral and Breast Detection by Computing Textural Images

We compute GLCM according to four important parameters: (1) direction (angle), (2) the distance, (3) a neighborhood size, (4) the texture descriptor of Harralick [10], and then we extract textural images.

2.3.1 Compute Direction

Compute one angle 0°, 45°, 90° or 135° do not give closed outlines, then we compute all directions and calculate their sum, see Fig. 2.

Figure 2 is an example of Brodatz image. We show images of texture which is contrast descriptor of Harralick [10], in direction 0°, 45°, 90°, 135° and image representing the sum of these four images. In the image sum, we see clearly more closed outlines.

2.3.2 Compute the Distance

The distance d = 1, it means that we consider the first pixel in the neighborhood.

2.3.3 Compute the Size of the Neighborhood

For synthetic 'Brodatz' images, we can see on Fig. 3 that in mask 3 × 3, edges are more smoothing than mask 7 × 7 and 9 × 9. The detected edges are more fuzzy if the neighborhood size is big. But in reality, the choice of the neighborhood size depends on textures of objects in image. For the mammographic images, neighborhood in mask size of 7 × 7 give better smooth edges than mask size of 3 × 3 and finer outlines than mask size of 9 × 9.

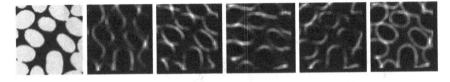

Fig. 2 From *left* to *right*, Brodatz D75 image, image contrast in 0°, image contrast in 45°, image contrast in 90°, image contrast in 135°, image contrast Sum (0° + 45° + 90° + 135°)

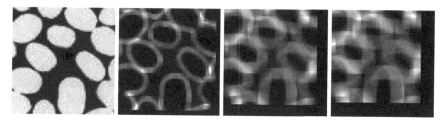

Fig. 3 From *left* to *right*, Brodatz D75 image, image contrast in mask 3 × 3, image contrast in mask 7 × 7 and image contrast in mask 9 × 9

2.3.4 Compute Texture Descriptor

Instead of taking the most known four descriptors extracted from GLCM, 'contrast', 'homogeneity', 'entropy' and 'correlation', we take only the 'contrast' descriptor, which measures the heterogeneity of an image and detect spatial variations of grey level intensity in image. Besides, it can summarize all the information of texture we needs.

2.3.5 Extract Texture Images

To extract texture images, and according to these previous parameters (direction, distance and the neighborhood size), we compute contrast descriptor of Harralick [10]. Each pixel of image is replaced by this descriptor.

In this work, we use "MatlabR2008b" formulation of contrast descriptor, Eq. (1):

$$contrast = \sum_{i,j} |i - j|^2 p(i,j) \tag{1}$$

But this equation returns only one measure of the intensity contrast between pixels $p(i, j)$ in the image. She represents only one value, while our algorithm computes this descriptor over the whole image, in every pixel. We obtain several measures which represent the number of pixels of the image.

2.4 Step 4: Extracting Mask

A mask is applied in texture images, according to the breast and the pectoral muscle borders, and the grounds truth of expert radiologist. The region of pectoral muscle is then deleted and breast region is extracted.

3 Results

3.1 Dataset

Our method was applied on the MIAS dataset. The images of the database originate from a film-screen mammographic imaging process in the United Kingdom National Breast Screening Program. The films were digitized and the corresponding images were annotated according to their breast density by expert radiologists.

We applied our methodology in the 'MIAS' database for MLO images, taking account breast orientation.

3.2 Results

Figures 4 and 6 represent different views of the breast image. Figures 5 and 7 show respectively the zoom of the Figs. 4 and 6, showing the region of the pectoral line and the pectoral border. Textural image in Fig. 4 shows the pectoral line (blue color) and the pectoral border (red color) detected by our algorithm, while the previous similar works detect only the pectoral line.

Textural image in the Fig. 6 shows also the pectoral line and the pectoral border detected by our algorithm.

Remark: Figure 4 shows that our algorithm detects the artifact border which is not visible in the MIAS breast image (input image), see the textural image. It shows the strength of the texture descriptor of the GLCM matrix. He is able to detect texture variations in the image.

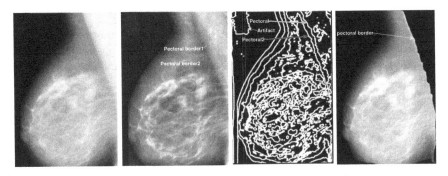

Fig. 4 From *left* to *right*, Input mdb019 image, Enhanced image, Textural image, The breast segmentation image with removal pectoral muscle

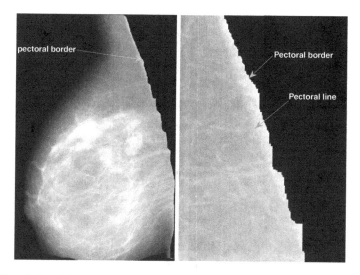

Fig. 5 From *left* to *right*, mdb019 segmentation image, zoom of pectoral muscle border

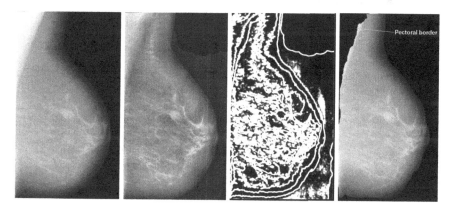

Fig. 6 From *left* to *right*, mdb012 image (input image), Enhanced image, Textural image, Breast segmentation image with removal pectoral muscle (output image)

3.3 Quantitative Evaluation of GLCM Methodology

We applied our methodology in the MIAS database for MLO images. To evaluate our pectoral segmentation approach, we have only used two categories (Acceptable, i.e., Good + Acceptable, and Unacceptable) since some papers do not consider other quality levels. And we compare with another similar methods in [14]: the method by Kwok et al. [15] that proposes an iterative thresholding together with a gradient-based searching, a statistical method based on AD measure [14], the work of Mustra

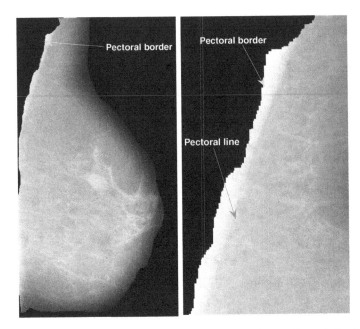

Fig. 7 From *left* to *right*, mdb012 segmentation image, zoom of pectoral muscle border

Table 1 Quantitative evaluation and comparison with other works

Methods	Images	% Acc.	% Unacc.
Kwok et al. [15]	322	83.6	16.4
Liu et al. [17]	100	81.0	19.0
Mustra et al. [16]	40	85.0	15.0
Raba et al. [1]	322	86.0	14.0
Molinara et al. [14]	55	89.1	10.9
Our method	55	90.1	12.0

et al. [16] proposing an hybrid with bit depth reduction and wavelet decomposition, an approach based on adaptive histogram proposed by Raba et al. [1] and the method of Molinara et al. [14]. The results in Table 1 show good performance on the considered images and our approach obtains better performance in terms of acceptable and unacceptable detection of the pectoral muscle, in 55 images.

4 Conclusions

In this study, we contributed to improve breast and pectoral muscle detection and segmentation, in order to extract breast region for CAD system, without forgetting the regions which can hide anomalies of cancer. Our approach based on texture information not used before for these problems. We used the texture descriptors extracted from these GLCM in a contour approach while mostly they are used in a region approach. Our techniques gives a method especially easier and fast in times of answer for the expert radiologist and outlines detected by this method are more precise compared with similar works.

References

1. D. Raba, A. Oliver, J. Mart´I and al. (2005), "Breast Segmentation with Pectoral Muscle Suppression on Digital Mammograms", Robotics and Computer Vision Group, http://vicorob. udg.es.
2. Karthikeyan Ganesana, U. Rajendra Acharyaa, Kuang Chua Chua and al. (2013), "Pectoral muscle segmentation: A review", Computer methods and proframs in biomedicine, 110, pp 48–57.
3. M. Peter, A. Sue (1992), "Classification of breast tissue by texture analysis", Image and Vision Computing 10 (June (5)) (1992) 277–282, 10.1016/0262-8856(92)90042-2, 0262-8856.
4. R. Ferrari, A. F. Frère, R. Rangayyan and al. (2004), "Identification of the breast boundary in mammograms using active contour models", Medical and Biological Engineering and Computing 42 (2) 201–208, doi:10.1007/BF02344632, ISSN: 0140-0118.
5. I. Domingues, J.S. Cardoso, I. Amaral and al. (2010), "Pectoral muscle detection in mammograms based on the shortest path with endpoints learnt by SVMs", Engineering in Medicine and Biology Society (EMBC), in: 2010 Annual International Conference of the IEEE, August 31–September 4, pp. 3158–3161, doi:10.1109/IEMBS.2010.5627168.
6. J. Grim, P. Somol, M. Haindl and al. (2009), "Computer-aided evaluation of screening mammograms based on local texture models", IEEE Transactions on Image Processing 18 (April (4)) 765–773, doi:10.1109/TIP.2008.2011168.
7. G. Qi, S. Jiaqing, F.R. Virginie (2006), "Characterization and classification of tumor lesions using computerized fractal-based texture analysis and support vector machines in digital mammograms", 4 (1) 11–25, doi:10.1007/s11548-008-0276-8.
8. C. Daniel, R. Mikael, D. Rachid, (1987), "A review of statistical approaches to level set segmentation: integrating color, texture, motion and shape", 72 (2) 195–215, doi:10.1007/ s11263-006-8711-1.
9. Sampat, M.P., Markey, M.K., Bovik, A.C. (2005), "Computer-Aided Detection and Diagnosis in Mammography", handbook.
10. Haralick, R. M., (1979), "Statistical and Structural Approaches to Texture," Proceedings of the IEEE, vol. 67, pp.786–804.
11. Richard Pfisterer and Farzin Aghdasi, (1999), "Comparison of Texture Based Algorithms for the Detection of Masses in Digitized Mammograms", 0-7803-5546-6/99/$10.00 0 IEEE.
12. Mencattini, A., Salmeri, M., Lojacono and al. (2008), "Mammographic Images Enhancement and Denoising for Breast Cancer Detection Using Dyadic Wavelet Processing", IEEE transactions on instrumentation and measurement, Vol. 57, No. 7.
13. Yongjian Yu and Scott T. Acton (2002), "Speckle Reducing Anisotropic Diffusion", IEEE Transaction on image processing", vol.11, no.11.
14. M. Molinara, C. Marrocco, F. Tortorella (2013), "Automatic Segmentation of the Pectoral Muscle in Mediolateral Oblique Mammograms", 978-1-4799-1053-3/13/, IEEE (CBMS 2013).
15. S.M. Kwok, R. Chandrasekhar, Y. Attikiouzel and al. (2004), "Automatic pectoral muscle segmentation on mediolateral oblique view mammograms", IEEE Transactions on Medical Imaging 23 (September (9)) 1129–1140, doi:10.1109/TMI.2004.830529.

16. M. Mustra, J. Bozek, M. Grgic, (2009), "Breast border extraction and pectoral muscle detection using wavelet decomposition", in: IEEE EUROCON 2009, EUROCON '09, 18–23 May 2009, 2009, pp. 1426–1433, doi:10.1109/EURCON.2009.5167827.
17. L. Liu, J. Wang, and T. Wang, (2011), "Breast and pectoral muscle contours detection based on goodness of fit measure", IEEE 5th International Conference on Bioinformatics and Biomedical Engineering, (ICBBE 2011).

Statistical and Physical Micro-feature-Based Segmentation of Cortical Bone Images Using Artificial Intelligence

Ilige S. Hage and Ramsey F. Hamade

Abstract At the micro scale, dense cortical bone is structurally comprised mainly of Osteon units that contain Haversian canals, lacunae, and concentric lamellae solid matrix. Osteons are separated from each other by cement lines. These micro-features of cortical bone are typically captured in digital histological images. In this work, we aim to automatically segment these features utilizing optimized pulse coupled neural networks (PCNN). These networks are artificially intelligent (AI) tools that can model neural activity and produce a series of binary pulses (images) representing the segmentations of an image. The methodology proposed combines three separately used methods for image segmentation which are: pulse coupled neural network (PCNN), particle swarm optimization (PSO) and adaptive threshold (AT). Two segmentation attributes were used: one statistical and another based on the physical attributes of the micro-features. The first, statistical-based segmentation method, where cost functions based on entropy (probability of gray values) considerations are calculated. For the physical-based segmentation method, cost functions based on geometrical attributes associated with micro-features such as relative size (i.e., elliptical) are used as targets for the fitness function of network optimization. Both of these methods were found to result in good quality segregation of the micro-features of micro-images of bovine cortical bone.

Keywords Bone image segmentation · Micro-structure · Neural networks · Optimization · Geometry · Statistics

I.S. Hage (✉) · R.F. Hamade
Department of Mechanical Engineering, American University of Beirut (AUB),
Beirut Riad El-Solh 1107 2020, Lebanon
e-mail: ish07@aub.edu.lb

R.F. Hamade
e-mail: rh13@aub.edu.lb

© Springer International Publishing Switzerland 2015
J.M.R.S. Tavares and R.M. Natal Jorge (eds.), *Computational and Experimental Biomedical Sciences: Methods and Applications*, Lecture Notes in Computational Vision and Biomechanics 21, DOI 10.1007/978-3-319-15799-3_17

229

1 Introduction

Bone image segmentation has been extensively utilized in many applications such as MR imaging to study necrotic lesions of the femoral head in [1, 2], in bone knee segmentation [3], in CT scan images for the wrist, foot, iliac and ankle [4, 5], in X-ray images [6] for fracture studies [7], and in age determination [8].

Segmentation of cortical bone images constitutes a challenge in medical image processing given the complexity of bone hierarchical structure at the heart of which lies the osteon unit. At the micro-scale, the cortical composite bone is made-up mostly of osteon units (concentric cylindrical system) at the center of each lies the Haversian canal. These canals are surrounded by concentric lamellae that are punctuated by small pores called lacunae which are in turn connected to each other via minute capillary channels called Canaliculi. Osteon units meet at what is known as 'cement lines'. Osteons constitute a repetitive structure throughout the cortical bone. This work aims to properly identify each micro-constituent of the osteon system via computer-based segmentation.

In this work, segmentation of cortical bone is accomplished by a hybrid methodology based mainly on PCNN. The PCNN algorithm is comprised of several parameters that need to be self-adapted. For this purpose, article swarm optimization (PSO) was used herein as a parameter optimizer for PCNN. A further enhancement is the use of the method of adaptive threshold (AT) where the PCNN algorithm is repeated until the best threshold T is found corresponding to the maximum variance between two segmented regions.

Two methods of preparing fitness functions for the purpose of segmentation: one is built based on statistical entropy and another on geometric attributes extracted from a training image. The PCNN-PSO-AT network was applied on training images of bone slices and high fidelity segmented images were obtained.

2 Materials and Image Acquisition

Cortical (mid femur) bones were extracted from bovine animal (cow both about 2 years old collected fresh from a butcher). The bone samples were immerged in formalin solution during a 3-day period for softening and fixation, than immerged in a decalcifying solution surgipath (hydrochloric acid <15 %wt., EDTA (ethylendiaminetetraacetic acid disodium salt) <5 %wt.) for 3 days. From the decalcified bone, a cortex of 2 mm thick was processed in a Leica machine model 300 where they were dehydrated and paraffin protected. This is followed by cutting the next day using a rotary microtome (model 340 E microm). Finally, bone slices were rehydrated using hot water. For better visualization, slices were exposed to Hematoxylin and Eosin (H&E) staining solutions. Finally, optical images of slices were acquired using a BX-41 M LED optical Olympus microscope at 20X magnification using Olympus SC30 digital microscope camera (based on 3.3 megapixel CCD chip with CMOS color sensor). One such resulting image is shown in Fig. 1.

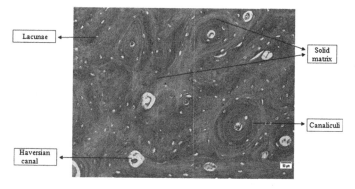

Fig. 1 Bone microstructures. Image captured with the SC 30 camera. The *arrows* point at examples of bone micro-constituents

3 PCNN-PSO-aT Framework

Pulse coupled neural networks [9–12] or particle swarm optimization [13] or adaptive threshold [12] are separately well known and used methods for image segmentation.

The ultimate aim of the hybrid methodology developed in this work is to obtain segmented images of high quality based on feature-specific (mainly geometrical) attributes and using only one training image. To that end, we had to automatically obtain an optimized set of 7 PCNN parameters that would be capable of extracting high fidelity segmented images from a number of testing microscope images. Specifically, the framework based on utilizing a combination of (3 separate methods previously used each separate for image segmentation) PCNN-PSO-AT is developed by the authors in [14, 15]. Two types of PSO fitness functions were developed: statistical and geometrical attributes (namely size).

3.1 Statistical-Based Segmentation

One bone image captured by the microscope was used as training in order to extract the feature to segment the images based on it. From the Statistical Pixel—Level (SPL) features the entropy was chosen since they reflect the information in an image. The training image was manually segmented into the 4 desirable bone micro-constituents mainly lacunae, Haversian canals, solid matrix and Canaliculi and the entropy of each image was calculated, Table 1 summarizes the target values of entropy.

Table 1 Features of entropy (H) values for the training image

Symbol	Lacunae	Haversian	Canaliculi	Solid matrix
Entropy, H	0.1255	0.1756	0.4856	0.5050

Table 2 PCNN parameters

	αl	αf	αθ	vl	vf	vθ	β
Lacunae	−0.2	−1.05	0.69	0.46	−0.48	−0.24	1.29
Haversian	−0.76	−0.06	−0.1	0.47	0.37	−0.34	−0.06
Canaliculi	−0.72	−0.09	−0.14	−0.85	−0.11	0.94	0.80
Solid matrix	0.57	0.22	−0.95	0.97	−0.51	−0.68	1.02

These 4 values constitute the targets building the fitness function. The algorithm constitutes of these steps as below:

1. Initialization of random population (random positions and velocities are initialized) for PSO and randomized parameters of PCNN.
2. The images were provided as input.
3. The iteration number of PCNN is set to be 5.
4. The evaluation begins were the entropy calculated are given as target for the fitness function and are evaluated by PSO using the fitness values for all the particles.
5. The position and the velocity of each particle update the population.
6. Evaluation using the fitness value of each particle.

Finally, if the terminal condition has not been satisfied, the algorithm is repeated; otherwise, the optimization process ends, and the output corresponds to the parameters of PCNN summarized in Table 2 for the lacunae, Haversian canals, canaliculi and for the matrix. The resultant segments for these 4 features are of high fidelity and are shown in Fig. 2.

3.2 Geometric (Size) Attributes

The resultant major-minor axis of the ellipse that has the same normalized second central moments as the region was used. The mean of these resultants were calculated for 3 manually segmented micro-features from the training image the lacunae, Haversian canals and the canaliculi.

$$resultant\, maj - \min axis = \sqrt{(maj\, axis\, length^2 + \min axis\, length^2)} \qquad (1)$$

Table 3 summarizes the mean major-minor axis length (in pixels) calculated by the resultant images.

The same method is used as above with a difference fitness function, here related to size attribute and with maj-min axis length targets. Table 4 shows the optimized PCNN parameters that yielded the shown segments.

Figure 3 displays the resultant pulses based on the geometrical (size of an ellipse) attribute. Since solid matrix does not have a predefined shape, it was obtained by

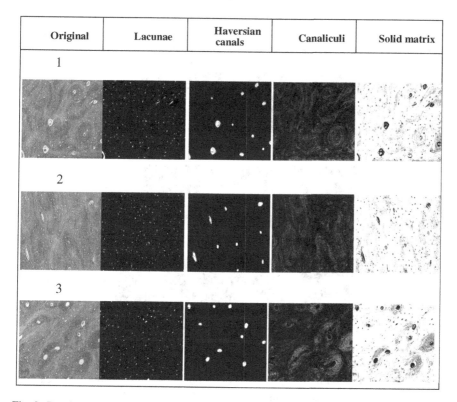

Original	Lacunae	Haversian canals	Canaliculi	Solid matrix
1				
2				
3				

Fig. 2 Resultant segments from the entropy attribute

Table 3 Mean resultant major-minor axis length (target values)

Target mean maj-min axis length (size) (pixels)	
Haversian	146.4943
Lacunae	22.7631
Canaliculi	13.1175

Table 4 PCNN parameters for the elliptical attribute

	αl	αf	αθ	vl	vf	vθ	β
Lacunae	−0.3393	−0.4150	−0.5467	−0.1914	−0.6591	0.5816	−0.4282
Haversian	0.7763	0.6059	0.7585	−0.5500	0.1511	−0.0961	0.2296
Canaliculi	−0.156	0.3114	0.5844	0.3574	0.6982	0.4862	0.3109

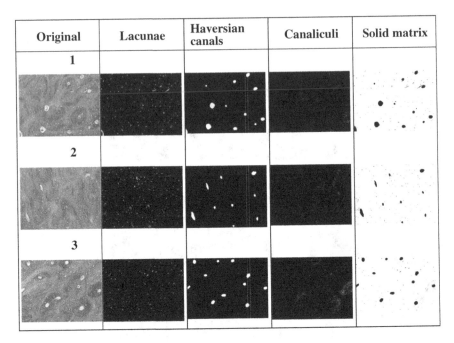

Original	Lacunae	Haversian canals	Canaliculi	Solid matrix
1				
2				
3				

Fig. 3 Resultant pulses from Elliptical attribute algorithm

subtracting the original image from the 3 other obtained segments of micro-features namely: lacunae, Haversian canals, and canaliculi. the fitness function based on the physical attributes yielded high fidelity segments.

4 Summary

In this work, a methodology was developed based on 3 main methods previously used separately for image segmentation: pulse coupled neural networks (PCNN), particle swarm optimization (PSO) and adaptive threshold (AT). Two different fitness functions were used based on either (1) statistical entropy or (2) geometrical (mainly elliptical size) attribute. The functions were extracted from one manually segmented training image and then used on other test images as targets. Both fitness functions yielded high fidelity segments. As seen in the figures below the lacunae which are small features (pores) where osteoblasts reside were detected in both methods successfully as well as the Haversian canals. For the canaliculi, tiny delicate features, they were auspiciously segmented which is a testament to the effectiveness and robustness of the developed methodology which was shown to be based on either of two fitness functions: statistical-based or geometrical-based. This segmentation may be used in future applications such as in the determination of bone porosity, an critical measure of osteoporosis.

References

1. Zoroofi R A, Nishii T, Sato Y, Sugano N, Yoshikawa H, Tamura S (2001) Segmentation of avascular necrosis of the femoral head using 3-D MR images. Comput Med Imaging Graph 25: 511

2. Zoroofi R A, Sato Y, Nishii T, Sugano N, Yoshikawa H, Tamura S (2004) Automated segmentation of necrotic femoral head from 3D MR data. Comput Med Imaging Graph 28: 267–278

3. Bourgeat P, Fripp J, Stanwell P, Ramadan S, Ourselin S (2007) MR image segmentation of the knee bone using phase information. Med Image Anal 11: 325–335

4. Calder J, Tahmasebi A M, Mansouri A (2011) A variational approach to bone segmentation in CT images. SPIE Medical Imaging 79620B-79620B-15

5. Zhang J, Yan C, Chui C, Ong S, Fast segmentation of bone in CT images using 3D adaptive thresholding. Comput Biol Med, 40: 231–236

6. Cernazanu-glavan C, Holban S (2013) Segmentation of Bone Structure in X-ray Images using Convolutional Neural Network. Advances in Electrical and Computer Engineering 13: 87–94

7. Jiang Y, Babyn P (2004) X-ray bone fracture segmentation by incorporating global shape model priors into geodesic active contours. Int Congr Ser 1268: 219–224

8. Morris D T, Walshaw C F (1994) Segmentation of the finger bones as a prerequisite for the determination of bone age. Image Vision Comput 12: 239–245

9. Xiao Z, Shi J, Chang Q (2009) Automatic image segmentation algorithm based on PCNN and fuzzy mutual information. Computer and Information Technology 241–245

10. Cai H, Zhang X Y, Dai H T and Zhou D M (2012) An Image Segmentation Method Using Image Enhancement and PCNN with Adaptive Parameters. Advanced Materials Research 490: 1251–1255

11. Wei S, Hong Q, Hou M (2011) Automatic image segmentation based on PCNN with adaptive threshold time constant. Neurocomputing 74: 1485–1491.

12. Gao K, Dong M, Jia F, Gao M (2012) OTSU image segmentation algorithm with immune computation optimized PCNN parameters. Engineering and Technology (S-CET) 1–4

13. Du F (2005) Infrared image segmentation with 2-D maximum entropy method based on particle swarm optimization (PSO).Pattern Recognition Letters 26: 597–603.

14. Hage I, Hamade R (2013) Smart segmentation of Bone histology slides using Pulse coupled neural networks (PCNN) optimized by particle-swarm optimization (PSO). In: 6th ECCOMAS Conference on Smart Structures and Materials, SMART2013, Politecnico di Torino, 24–26 June 2013

15. Hage I, Hamade R (2013) Structural Feature-attribute-based Segmentation of Optical Images of Bone Slices Using Optimized Pulse Coupled Neural Networks (PCNN). In: Proceedings of the ASME 2013 International Mechanical Engineering Congress & Exposition IMECE 2013, San Diego, California, USA, 12–15 November 2013

Human Motion Segmentation Using Active Shape Models

Maria João M. Vasconcelos and João Manuel R.S. Tavares

Abstract Human motion analysis from images is meticulously related to the development of computational techniques capable of automatically identifying, tracking and analyzing relevant structures of the body. This work explores the identification of such structures in images, which is the first step of any computational system designed to analyze human motion. A widely used database (CASIA Gait Database) was used to build a Point Distribution Model (PDM) of the structure of the human body. The training dataset was composed of 14 subjects walking in four directions, and each shape was represented by a set of 113 labelled landmark points. These points were composed of 100 contour points automatically extracted from the silhouette combined with an additional 13 anatomical points from elbows, knees and feet manually annotated. The PDM was later used in the construction of an Active Shape Model, which combines the shape model with gray level profiles, in order to segment the modelled human body in new images. The experiments with this segmentation technique revealed very encouraging results as it was able to gather the necessary data of subjects walking in different directions using just one segmentation model.

1 Introduction

Human motion analysis from images is strictly related to the development of computational techniques capable of automatically identifying, tracking and analyzing relevant structures of the human body. Many systems designed for this purpose begin with the feature extraction task, which is to identify the structures to

M.J.M. Vasconcelos (✉) · J.M.R.S. Tavares
Instituto de Engenharia Mecânica e Gestão Industrial, Faculdade de Engenharia,
Universidade do Porto, Rua Dr. Roberto Frias s/n, 4200-465 Porto, Portugal
e-mail: maria.vasconcelos@fe.up.pt

J.M.R.S. Tavares
e-mail: tavares@fe.up.pt

© Springer International Publishing Switzerland 2015
J.M.R.S. Tavares and R.M. Natal Jorge (eds.), *Computational and Experimental Biomedical Sciences: Methods and Applications*, Lecture Notes in Computational Vision and Biomechanics 21, DOI 10.1007/978-3-319-15799-3_18

be analyzed in the image sequences, and then followed by the establishment of feature correspondences, which is to address the problem of matching features from two consecutive frames, and, finalizing with high level analysis of human movements and poses.

Most of the methods proposed for human motion analysis until now have used models to fit body parts to the input images. The human body structure can therefore be represented by means of stick figures, 2D contours or volumetric models. While stick figures are mainly built to learn the 3D variability of the human posture and perform gait detection, as in [1, 2]; 2D contours, instead, are often extracted to perform human detection and tracking [3, 4]; on the other hand, volumetric models have many potential applications, including advanced Human Computer Interaction, 3D animation and robot control [5]. Therefore, in this work, we intended to build a model combining information from the stick figures and from the 2D silhouette contours in order to obtain the advantages of both modelling methodologies.

Active Shape Models (ASMs) [6] have commonly been used in different domains of Computational Vision for image segmentation purposes, in areas such as medicine, industry and security. The aim here was to build a Point Distribution Model (PDM) [7] that combines the human silhouette contour and the specific anatomical joints from the stick figure and then to construct an ASM in order to segment the modelled body further into new images.

In [8] the authors proposed a model-based on a pose of the human body using ASMs with stick figures for frontal poses and they obtained good results. However, their research did not take into account the influence of illumination and was restricted to one view of the human pose. Recently, [9] introduced Active Shape Feedback Segmentation, which is based on the Grab-cut segmentation framework and ASMs, but the authors claim that there were still some problems to be solved to be able to use the system in real situations. Also, a small dataset was used, and the time required was a drawback.

A rich collection of gait datasets have been collected, which the research community has been using for comparative performance evaluations. Examples of those databases include CMU Mobo, HID-UMD datasets, SOTON databases, HumanID Gait Challenge, CASIA databases and TUM GAID [10]. A description of the existing gait databases through to 2010 can be found in [11].

There are various applications for human motion analysis. Clinical studies, for instance, require accurate motion knowledge for the diagnosis of locomotion difficulties or abnormalities in patients. Another application is in sports, where it is commonly used to find potential improvements in an athlete's performance.

This chapter is organized as follows: in the next section, the methodology adopted is presented, starting by describing the image database used and also explaining the construction of Point Distribution Models and Active Shape Models. Afterwards, the model built and their application in the segmentation of the human body in new images are presented, and the results are shown and discussed. Finally, the conclusions are made and some considerations for future work are pointed out.

2 Materials and Methods

2.1 Database

The CASIA Gait Database [12], which is a large multiview gait database created in January 2005 and widely adopted by the Computational Vision community, was used here in order to test the efficiency of the models built. In addition to the original video files, the referred database also contains the human silhouettes extracted from them. All video sequences were stored as video files encoded with MJPEG, a frame rate of 25 fps and a frame size of 320 × 240 pixels. The database also has information about the 124 subjects involved, which were mostly young Asians aged between 20 and 30.

In this work information from 14 subjects walking in four different directions (0°, 36°, 54° and 90°) in relation to the camera was used (Fig. 1). Table 1 depicts the number of images used in the construction of the models built, as well as the number of images used to test their segmentation accuracy.

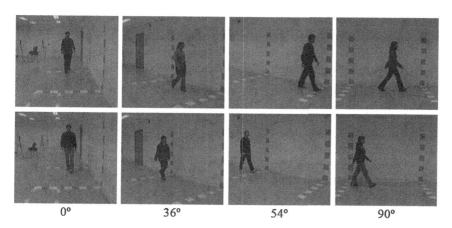

| 0° | 36° | 54° | 90° |

Fig. 1 Examples of subjects walking in different directions (images used for training in the first row, and testing in the second row)

Table 1 Summary of the data used to construct (training) and test the segmentation models built

Direction	# Training images	# Testing images
00	746	73
36	696	52
54	695	65
90	597	25
Total	2734	215

2.2 Point Distribution Models and Active Shape Models

A Point Distribution Model expresses the mean shape of the modelled object in addition to the admissible variations in relation to the same mean shape [7]. In this work, the silhouette contour and the anatomical landmark points of the human body structure were modelled by a PDM from a set of 2,734 images. Those images include various configurations of the human body acquired while different persons were walking (Fig. 1).

In order to obtain a robust PDM, the images used in the training process needed to adequately represent the variability of the human shape during walking. Moreover, each human silhouette presented in the training set had to be described by a group of labelled landmark points conveying important aspects of the body contour. Hence, 100 contour points were chosen to be extracted from the silhouettes available on the dataset and a further 13 extra points indicating the anatomical points from the human stick figure were manually selected, leading to a total of 113 landmark points to represent the structure of the human body. In more detail, the landmark points used were the following:

- From the silhouette contour:

  - 45 points from the left side (equally spaced);
  - 45 points from the right side (equally spaced);
  - 10 points between the feet of the subject (equally spaced);

- From the stick figure:

  - 1 point in the centre of the head (1);
  - 1 point on each shoulder (2);
  - 1 point on each elbow (2);
  - 1 point on each hand (2);
  - 1 point on left and right of the hip (2);
  - 1 point on each knee (2);
  - 1 point on the backside of each foot (2).

In all the images here, the landmark points corresponding to the silhouette contour appear connected by fictitious line segments to enhance their visualization, while the anatomical landmark points are represented with an "x". Figure 2 shows examples of some images used with the corresponding extracted landmark points.

In order to learn the variability of the coordinates of the landmark points in the training shapes, the points need to be aligned using, for example, dynamic programming. Only afterwards, it is possible to calculate the mean shape and apply the Principal Component Analysis (PCA) to the deviations from the mean shape and obtain the modes of variation, which characterize the manner in which the landmarks of the modelled object tend to move together. Once the PDM of the object under study is built, it can be further used to generate new shapes of the object as well as to segment it in new images through an Active Shape Model developed for the same object as will be explained next.

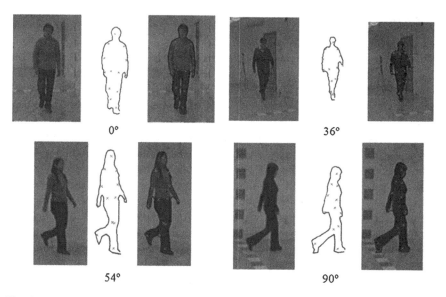

0°   36°

54°   90°

Fig. 2 The landmark points used to build the models in an example image of each direction studied

Similarly to the coordinates of the landmark points, the local gray level surroundings of each landmark can be considered in the statistical modelling of objects from images. Thus, statistical information about the mean and covariance of the gray level values of the pixels around each landmark can be used in the object modelling.

The PDM and the gray level profiles of each landmark point used in the construction of the PDM may be used to segment the object modelled into new images through an Active Shape Model [6]. ASMs use an interactive technique that fits flexible models to objects represented in images based on an optimization scheme, which is combined with PDMs to refine the initial estimated shapes of the objects to be segmented. The refining process adopted can be summarized into following steps: (1) The displacement required to move the model to a more suitable position, that is, closer to the final shape, is calculated at each landmark point; (2) The calculation of the changes in the overall shape position, orientation and scale that most effectively satisfy the local displacements found in (1); (3) Make the required adjustments in the parameters of the model, by analyzing the residual differences between the current shape of the model and the final shape sought.

The image segmentation process with the support of ASMs was improved in [13] by adopting a multiresolution approach. In this approach, a multiresolution pyramid of the input images is built by applying a Gaussian mask; then, the gray level profiles at the various levels of the pyramid built are studied. As such, the former process enables the ASMs to segment the input images more quickly and in a reliable manner.

3 Results

To extract the landmark points from the silhouettes on CASIA Gait Database, an algorithm in MATLAB was developed to automatically identify and extract the coordinates of the 100 contour points according to the rule described in the previous section. Afterwards, the 13 anatomical landmark points corresponding to the stick figure of the human body were manually extracted from each frame, and the associated coordinates were concatenated with the contour related landmarks.

The Active Shape Model software [14] was used for the ASM building process. In this process 95 % of all object shape variance in the geometrical modelling (i.e. in PDM) was adopted and a 7 pixels width profile was used for the gray level modelling. As a stopping criterion for the segmentation process, a maximum of 6 iterations for each resolution level was applied. As 3 resolution levels were defined based on the dimensions of the images under study, only 18 iterations were performed. Finally, for the segmentation quality assessment, the mean and standard deviation values of the Euclidean distances between the landmark points of the final shape and the groundtruth reference points were calculated.

The adequacy of the modelling process to characterizing the human shape is shown by the more significant modes of variation of the PDM built in Fig. 3. For instance, it is clear that the first mode of variation gathers the information on the walking stance of the subjects, whilst the second and third modes of variation gather the direction in which the subject is walking. In contrast, smaller and more specific variations can be seen in the fourth mode.

Figure 4 depicts several steps of the active search performed in order to segment an image from the test set; not included in the training set used, and the adaptation of the ASM built along the iteration process to reach an optimal result can be seen. Other examples, in this case, just showing the final position for the 4 directions studied are represented in Fig. 5. These images show that the landmarks corresponding to contour points have a much more reliable behaviour than those corresponding to the anatomical points. In fact, this behaviour was expected since the

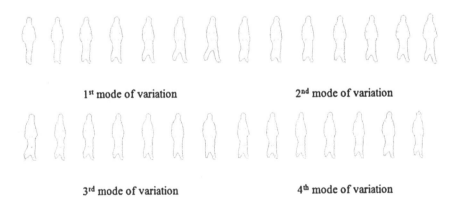

1st mode of variation   2nd mode of variation

3rd mode of variation   4th mode of variation

Fig. 3 First four modes of variation of the PDM built (mean shape ±1 standard deviation)

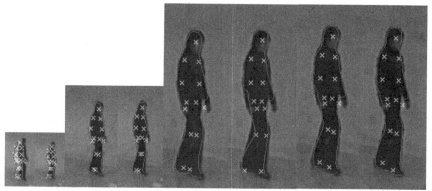

Iteration process of ASM

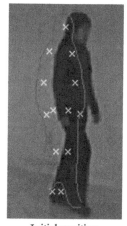

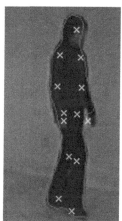

Initial position   Final position

Fig. 4 Example of the iteration process using an active shape model in a new image in the first row, and, in the second row, the initial and final (i.e. the segmentation result) positions of the model

ASM searches for the gray level information around the point positions, and the anatomical landmark points are more likely to have similar neighbours around them, making it more difficult to choose the right position in comparison to the landmark contour points.

In order to conclude on the variation errors of the model, besides the mean Euclidean error distribution calculation for all 113 points, one also decided to study the mean Euclidean error distribution for each subgroup of points: the contour landmarks and the anatomical landmarks (i.e. from the stick figure), separately. In other words, the error distribution was calculated using 113, 100 and 13 points, corresponding to the all the points, the contour points and the stick model.

As expected, from the observation of data distribution obtained, see Fig. 6, one can confirm that the mean error distribution is slightly worse for the subgroup of the stick points. If we take into account that the images under study have 320×240

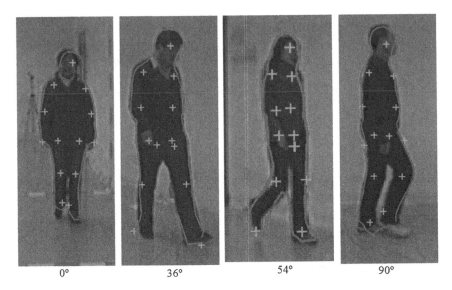

Fig. 5 Examples of segmentation results obtained in images for the 4 directions studied

Fig. 6 Mean error distribution according to the landmark point set used

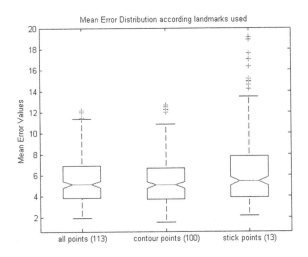

pixels in size, it is worth noting that the results achieved with the suggested segmentation model are extremely satisfactory, within the 25th–75th percentile interval ranging from 4 to 7 pixels, which translates into very accurate segmentation results. Even the mean error distribution considering only the stick points achieves good results, with the 25th–75th percentile ranging from 4 to 8 pixels.

We also studied the segmentation quality in terms of the direction in which the subjects were walking, Fig. 7. Analyzing this figure, an interesting conclusion can be reached: considering all directions against each direction separately, equivalent

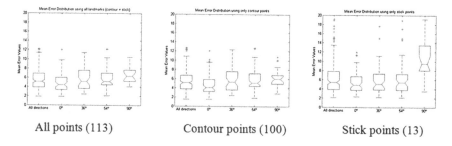

Fig. 7 Mean error distributions according to the direction of the subjects and using all the 113 landmark points; only the landmark points from the contour; or just the anatomical landmark points

error ranges were achieved. This behaviour is repeated independently of the landmark points. In summary, the ASM built could successfully segment the human body structure in images independently of the direction the subjects were walking, which is an important goal in studies concerning human motion analysis from images.

4 Conclusions

In this work, a widely used database, CASIA Gait Database, was used to build the Point Distribution Model of the structure of the human body. The training image dataset used was composed of 14 subjects walking in four directions, and each shape of the training set was represented by a set of 113 labelled landmark points, which combines information of the contour of the silhouette and the anatomical stick points.

In order to obtain the mean shape of the human silhouette as well as its admissible shape variations a PDM was built. This model was then used to construct an Active Shape Model, which combines the shape model (i.e. PDM) with gray level profiles, with the purpose of segmenting the modelled silhouettes into new images.

The good results obtained through the use of the ASM built to perform human body segmentation in new images strongly suggest that this type of deformable model can be used in this task. In addition, just one segmentation model gathers the necessary information to segment the structure of the human body independently of the direction the subjects were walking.

A future work would be to develop methodologies that can combine, more accurately, the human silhouette with important anatomical joint positions, mainly for use in biomechanical studies related to human motion. As soon as the use of simple image cameras allows the robust and detailed analysis of real movements performed by subjects in their daily life, it will be possible to obtained new levels of information of the subjects from the input images. Up until now, this has been only achieved from images acquired under well controlled conditions and in significantly restricted environments, which consequently demands more robust techniques of image segmentation, motion tracking and analysis.

Acknowledgments The first author would like to thank the support of the Ph.D. grant with references SFRH/BD/28817/2006 from *Fundação para a Ciência e Tecnologia* (FCT), in Portugal. This work was partially developed under the scope of the project with reference PTDC/BBB-BMD/3088/2012 financially supported by FCT. The research described in this chapter use CASIA Gait Database collected by Institute of Automation, Chinese Academy of Sciences.

References

1. Ogawara K, Li X, Ikeuchi K. Marker-less Human Motion Estimation using Articulated Deformable Model. IEEE International Conference on Robotics and Automation, 2007. p. 46–51.
2. Wei XK, Chai J. Intuitive Interactive Human-Character Posing with Millions of Example Poses. IEEE Computer Graphics Applications, 2011. 31(4): p. 78–88.
3. Al-Huseiny M, Mahmoodi S, Nixon M. Gait Sequence Synthesis and Reconstruction. IEEE Transactions on PAMI 2008. 30.8: p. 1385–1399.
4. Das Choudhury S, Tjahjadi T. Gait recognition based on shape and motion analysis of silhouette contours. Computer Vision and Image Understanding, 2013. 117(12): 1770–85.
5. Tran C, Trivedi MM. Human body modelling and tracking using volumetric representation: Selected recent studies and possibilities for extensions. Second ACM/IEEE International Conference on Distributed Smart Cameras, 2008. p. 1–9.
6. Cootes TF, Taylor CJ, Cooper DH, Graham J. Active Shape Models-Their Training and Application. Computer Vision and Image Understanding, 1995. 61(1): p. 38–59.
7. Cootes TF, Taylor CJ, Cooper DH, Graham J. Training Models of Shape from Sets of Examples. BMVC92. Springer London, 1992. p. 9–18.
8. Jang C, Jung K. Human pose estimation using Active Shape Models. Proceedings of World Academy of Science: Engineering & Technology 46 (2008).
9. Pourjam E, Ide I, Deguchi D, Murase H. Segmentation of Human Instances Using Grab-cut and Active Shape Model Feedback. Proceedings of IAPR Conference on Machine Vision Applications (MVA) 2013. p. 77–80.
10. Hofmann M, Geiger J, Bachmann S, Schuller B, Rigoll G. The TUM Gait from Audio, Image and Depth (GAID) database: Multimodal recognition of subjects and traits. Journal of Visual Communication and Image Representation 2014. 25(1): p. 195–206.
11. Nixon MS, Tan T, Chellappa R. Human Identification Based on Gait. Vol 4, Springer; 2010.
12. Yu S, Tan D, Tan T. A Framework for Evaluating the Effect of View Angle, Clothing and Carrying Condition on Gait Recognition. 18th International Conference on Pattern Recognition, 2006. p. 441–444.
13. Cootes TF, Taylor CJ, Lanitis A. Multi-resolution search with active shape models. Proceedings of the 12th IAPR International Conference on Pattern Recognition, 1994. Vol.1 p. 610–612.
14. Hamarneh G. Active Shape Model Software [Internet]. 1999. Available from: http://www.cs.sfu.ca/~hamarned/software/code/asm.zip Last accessed June 2012.

3D Vocal Tract Reconstruction Using Magnetic Resonance Imaging Data to Study Fricative Consonant Production

Sandra M. Rua Ventura, Diamantino Rui S. Freitas, Isabel Maria A.P. Ramos and João Manuel R.S. Tavares

Abstract The development of Magnetic Resonance Imaging (MRI) has grown rapidly in clinical practice. Currently, the use of MRI in speech research provides useful and accurate qualitative and quantitative data of speech articulation. The aim of this work was to describe an effective method to extract vocal tract and compute their volumes during speech production from MRI images. Using a 3.0 Tesla MRI system, 2D and 3D images of the vocal tract were collected and used to analyze the vocal tract during the production of fricative consonants. These images were also used to build the associated 3D models and compute their volumes. This approach showed that, in general, the volumes measured for the voiceless consonants are smaller than the counterpart voiced consonants.

Keywords Magnetic resonance imaging (MRI) · Fricative consonants · Vocal tract imaging · 3D models · Volumetric measurements

S.M. Rua Ventura
Área Técnico-Científica da Radiologia, Centro de Estudos do Movimento e Actividade Humana (CEMAH), Escola Superior de Tecnologia da Saúde, Instituto Politécnico do Porto, Porto, Portugal

D.R.S. Freitas
Departamento de Engenharia Electrotécnica e de Computadores, Faculdade de Engenharia, Universidade do Porto, Porto, Portugal

I.M.A.P. Ramos
Serviço de Radiologia do Centro Hospitalar de S. João, EPE, Faculdade de Medicina, Universidade do Porto, Porto, Portugal

J.M.R.S. Tavares (✉)
Instituto de Engenharia Mecânica e Gestão Industrial, Departamento de Engenharia Mecânica, Faculdade de Engenharia, Universidade do Porto, Porto, Portugal
e-mail: tavares@fe.up.pt

© Springer International Publishing Switzerland 2015
J.M.R.S. Tavares and R.M. Natal Jorge (eds.), *Computational and Experimental Biomedical Sciences: Methods and Applications*, Lecture Notes in Computational Vision and Biomechanics 21, DOI 10.1007/978-3-319-15799-3_19

1 Introduction

This chapter has a particular interest for professionals related to speech study and rehabilitation, medical imaging and bioengineering. It is organized as follows: the Introduction section starts with a review from the literature about the use and feasibility of MRI to study the vocal tract, in particular, during speech production of fricative consonants. In addition, some articulatory phonetic concepts of Portuguese sounds are introduced. In the second section, the methodology adopted for the MRI acquisition and image data assessment is described. In the Results and Discussion sections the key aspects of the 2D and 3D visualization of the vocal tract during the production of sustained consonants are illustrated and discussed. In the final section, the conclusions are presented and some suggestions for future works are indicated.

1.1 Magnetic Resonance Imaging of the Vocal Tract

The first Magnetic Resonance Imaging (MRI) scan of the entire human body was carried out by Raymond Damadian, in 1977, to diagnose cancer. Since then the use of this imaging modality has grown rapidly in clinical practice. Its use is of interest in various medical areas and at the same time has opened up new fields of research.

Magnetic Resonance Imaging is a recognized and powerful non-ionizing diagnostic tool, employed for the diagnosis of various disorders, such as cancer, soft tissue damage, cardiology and neurology. The technique uses a magnetic field and radiofrequency waves to create detailed images of the organs and tissues, and relies on the nuclear magnetic resonance of the hydrogen nucleus. Compared with images from other techniques, MRI provides excellent anatomical details [19] and is superior to computed tomography (CT) in distinguishing various tissue characteristics [13].

The images produced have good signal-to-noise ratio and contrast; however, the temporal resolution of MRI is very low when compared with radiographic techniques. In addition, some safety and contraindication issues must be taken into consideration, namely metallic fragments, clips or patients with magnetically activated implants and devices.

The vocal tract consists of a set of open air-cavities surrounded by soft-tissue, where sounds are produced. This region is similar to a long tube with a non-linear shape that extends from the vocal folds to the lips, with a side branch leading to the nasal cavity. Vocal tract organs (also called articulators) include the tongue, lips, teeth and alveolar ridge, hard palate, velum (soft palate), and the pharynx. All these organs (except the teeth) are well defined on MR images due to their good signal-to-noise ratio.

The main resonance cavities of the vocal tract include: nasal cavity (and nasopharynx), oral cavity, oropharynx and hypopharynx as shown in Fig. 1.

Fig. 1 Sagittal MR image of the vocal tract and its main resonance cavities

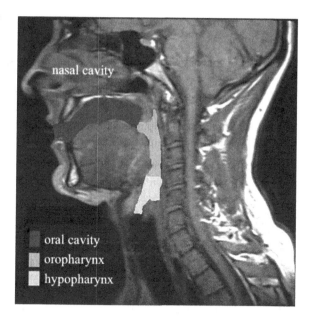

nasal cavity

oral cavity
oropharynx
hypopharynx

As can be seen in Fig. 1, air has a low signal in MR images compared with the high signals of the fat and surrounding soft tissues of the vocal tract. This air conducting tube that extends along the lips and the glottis presents an irregular shape, controlled by the movement of the articulators during speech production.

The tongue is the most important articulator, mainly because it is the largest one, and performs a wide range of movements during speech production.

1.2 Measuring and Modelling Speech: A Review

The task of modelling the vocal tract for articulatory synthesis systems aims to obtain the complete geometrical information concerning the vocal tract measured by different techniques, especially MRI [11, 14]. Currently, the use of MRI in speech research provides useful and accurate qualitative and quantitative data of speech articulation [21–24].

Modelling of the vocal tract has traditionally been limited to two-dimensional (2D) images [2, 17] although, with the improvement of MRI acquisition techniques, three-dimensional (3D) modelling has become available [3, 5, 16]. Between 1986 and 1996, most of the vocal tract models to study speech production and articulatory synthesis relied on the extraction of midsagittal distances and cross-sectional area functions. These previous MRI studies were based on 2D multi-slice acquisitions requiring artificially sustained sounds or multiple repetitions of the same sound during long scan acquisition times. With this data, it was theoretically possible to try to reconstruct the vocal tract shape, but some important problems still remained, such as:

1. Air-tissue boundaries were hard to segment, i.e. to identify, and were time consuming;
2. Several image artefacts due to the long scan acquisition time;
3. Low signal from the teeth;
4. Hardware constraints: supine position imposed on the subjects and MRI system noise that inhibits high-quality audio recording.

To obtain more detailed information about the relation between vocal tract shape and speech sounds, 3D data are required [15, 18, 25]. For this purpose, only the MRI technique provides excellent structural differentiation of all the vocal tract organs and without harmful effects. At present, MRI is the most reliable and powerful imaging tool to acquire the full geometry of the vocal tract and to provide quantitative volumetric data.

Although multiplanar scanning may have been performed, only one MR image stack in one orientation (transversal, sagittal or coronal) is usually used in vocal tract reconstruction. Several researchers also used this approach, due to the common MRI-related constraints: acquisition times, costs and fatigue of the subjects under study. In order to improve vocal tract modelling, some techniques have been proposed that combine manually [1, 4, 14] or even automatically [26] orthogonal image stacks. On the other hand, the first application of compressed sensing to high-resolution 3D upper airways was provided in [9]. The authors demonstrated that it is possible to acquire 3D imaging data of the vocal during a single sustained sound production stack (without sound repetitions). In line with this work, other studies have been performed, particularly for European Portuguese sounds [12, 24].

1.3 Articulatory Phonetics: Sounds of Portuguese Speech

The standard European Portuguese speech system consists of nine oral and five nasal vowels, three diphthongs and nineteen consonants (six plosives, six fricatives, three nasals and four liquids). There are two main classes of consonants: plosives and fricatives. Plosives are sounds in which the air streams from the lungs are interrupted by a complete closure in some part of the vocal tract. In fricative sounds, the air passes usually through a narrow constriction that causes the air to flow turbulently and thus create a loud sound [7]. The other classes of consonants that are found in the majority of languages (nasals, "liquids" and vowel-like approximants) are voiced in the overwhelming majority of cases.

Consonants can be classified according to three major features:

- Place of articulation—specifies where the constriction in the vocal tract is;
- Manner of articulation—how narrow the constriction is, whether air is flowing through the nose, and whether the tongue is dropped down on one side;

- Voicing—specifies whether the vocal folds are vibrating.

One of the major ways that consonants differ from each other is in the accompanying action of the larynx; most larynx settings allow air to flow freely between the vocal folds versus others when the vocal folds vibrate to produce regular voicing.

For the European Portuguese language, the distribution of the sounds between voiced and voiceless counterparts in the fricative consonants is /v, z, ʒ/, and /f, s, ʃ/, respectively. The main configuration of the vocal tract during the production of fricative consonants is illustrated in Table 1.

2 Methodology

2.1 Magnetic Resonance Imaging: Protocol and Procedures

The MRI data used in this study were acquired at the Radiology Department of the Centro Hospitalar de S. João, Porto, in Portugal, using a MAGNETOM Trio 3.0 Tesla MRI system (Siemens AG, Germany) and two integrated coils: a 32-channel head coil and a 4-channel neck matrix coil, with the subjects in the supine position.

The experiments were performed with two young native European Portuguese (EP) subjects, one male and one female and according to the MRI safety procedures. In addition, a questionnaire was carried out before any procedure to screen any contraindications. The subjects were previously informed and instructed about the study, and their informed consents were collected. Verbal communication was maintained with the subjects through an intercom.

The speech corpus included the sustained sounds of the EP language: three pairs of fricative consonants /f v/, /s z/ and /ʃ ʒ/ according to the International Phonetic Alphabet (IPA).

The first MRI dataset was collected using a turbo spin echo 2D sequence, to be used as the sound articulation references, and consisted of one T1-weighted 4 mm thick midsagittal slice for each sound. The following imaging acquisition parameters were adopted: a repetition time of 400 ms, an echo time of 10 ms, an echo train length of 5, a square field of view of 240 mm, a matrix size of 512 × 512 pixels, and a pixel size of 0.469 × 0.469 mm^2. The acquisition time lasted around 8.07 s for each sound. Afterwards, a 3D volumetric MR acquisition of the vocal tract resonance cavities was carried out using a flash gradient echo sequence. A 120 mm thick transversal slab was acquired according to the following parameters: repetition time of 5.8 ms, echo time of 2.17 ms, flip angle = 10°, a square field of view of 270 mm, a matrix size of 256 × 256 pixels and a pixel spacing of 1.055 × 1.055 mm^2. The imaging acquisition lasted around 16.12 s for each sound. From this slab, 60 2-mm-thick slices were reconstructed automatically.

Table 1 Vocal tract configuration associated to the European Portuguese fricative consonants

Fricative consonant	Description	Vocal tract configuration
[f]	Voiceless labiodental Reference word: /fé/(faith)	
[v]	Voiced labiodental Reference word: /vê/(see)	
[s]	Voiceless alveolar Reference word: /sol/(sun)	
[z]	Voiced alveolar Reference word: /casa/(home)	
[ʃ]	Voiceless post-aveolar Reference word: /já/(already)	
[ʒ]	Voiced post-aveolar Reference word: /chave/(key)	

2.2 Image Processing and Analysis: Tasks and Techniques

The segmentation of the vocal tract, for the image processing and analytical tasks, was automatically performed in each slice followed by image-based reconstruction of the vocal tract shape using the ITK-SNAP software (version 2.1.4-rc1), which was developed at the Penn Image Computing and Science Laboratory (PICSL) in USA. Similar to other imaging software packages for 3D analysis, this software provides reliable and accurate volume segmentation of the oropharynx for upper airway assessment [20].

The three-dimensional models were built from the subset of sagittal images defining the whole vocal tract, the oral cavity and the pharynx. The original set of 60 2-mm-thick slices, and without any gap between them, was segmented using the active contour method, usually known as snakes, proposed by Kass et al. [8], which has revealed robustness against image noise and efficiency in images with low signal-to-noise ratio as is the case of MR images. Active contours are curves that are moved and deformed by internal and external forces until they reach the object's boundary in the image to be segmented.

In order to segment the vocal tract, a pre-processing of the original images was performed in order to adjust the range of the airway voxel intensities (threshold interval selection). After the segmentation, a 3D model of the airway of each resonance cavity was automatically built from the contours segmented in each slice. As a result of the automated segmentation and labelling of each resonance cavity, the software could compute the volume of the vocal tract.

3 Results

The complete 2D MR image dataset is depicted in Fig. 2. The images have good signal-to-noise ratio and resolution, which allows a clear visualization of the different vocal tract shapes produced for each EP sound. These reference images were then used to define the slices acquired and also to confirm the proper production of the intended sound.

For the segmentation of each consonant imaged, first the vocal tract was segmented as a whole, and then the oral cavity and pharynx were segmented individually.

The analysis of the whole vocal tract by means of the 3D models built confirms the occurrence of important articulatory changes, as shown in Fig. 3. The 3D models show that the main difference found is the increase of the overall volume of the vocal tract, especially in the pharynx cavity.

In order to get measurable data concerning the articulatory changes found in the morphology of the vocal tract and the major resonance cavities, the volumes were calculated and then compared. The results obtained are shown in Table 2 according to each speaker.

4 Discussion

In this chapter, a morphological assessment of the vocal tract during sustained production of EP by MRI is presented. From the approach adopted, morphologic information can be extracted in both 2D and 3D MRI sequences concerning the

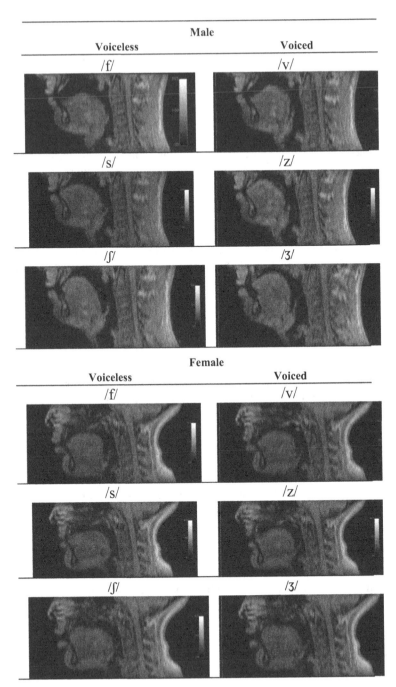

Fig. 2 Midsagittal MR slices of the vocal tract of a male and a female during EP speech production

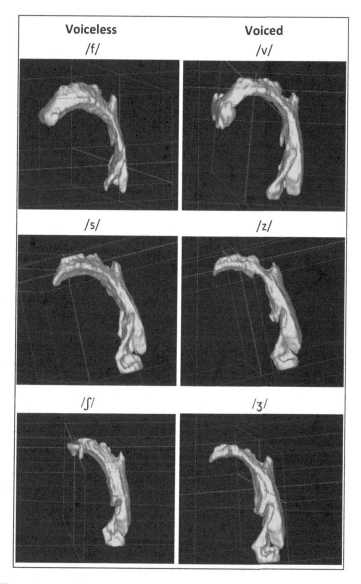

Voiceless	Voiced
/f/	/v/
/s/	/z/
/ʃ/	/ʒ/

Fig. 3 3D vocal tract models built for the voiceless fricative consonants from the image dataset of the male subject

shape and dimensions, respectively, of the vocal tract and the two major resonance cavities during the production of EP fricative consonants.

On the 2D sagittal images acquired, only subtle differences can be observed among each pair of fricative consonants, especially for the male subject. The vocal tract shapes associated to the female subject were more difficult to establish in the MR images acquired due to the smaller anatomy.

Table 2 Volumetric measurements of the major resonance cavities computed for each pair of fricative consonants (voiceless versus voiced) for each subject under study

	Volumes (mm³)	/f/	/v/	/s/	/z/	/ʃ/	/ʒ/
Male	Total vocal tract	52,007	64,717	62,014	75,075	86,704	107,420
	Oral cavity	28,432	22,614	19,711	24,287	26,383	48,770
	Pharynx	23,575	42,103	42,303	50,788	60,321	58,650
Female	Total vocal tract	47,777	50,207	52,142	54,830	37,361	44,055
	Oral cavity	12,240	13,192	17,159	17,488	12,062	12,718
	Pharynx	35,537	37,015	34,983	37,342	25,299	31,337

The results obtained using the 3D models built and the quantitative measurements made, confirmed the important articulatory changes among the fricative consonants and for each subject. The main difference found between the subjects was that the volumes measured for the voiceless consonants were smaller than their counterpart voiced consonants. Excluding the male subject for the consonant /f/, all pharynx volumes measured were superior to the oral cavity volumes. The study in [14] also found larger pharyngeal volumes in voiced fricatives by means of vocal tract lengths and area function measurements. Equivalent results were also reported in [16] where the authors observed some supraglottal volume changes of pharyngeal articulation during the production of voiced and voiceless fricative consonants.

The volumes of the resonance cavities of the male subject are larger for the alveolar and post-alveolar sounds; additionally, the highest volumetric value was attained during the production of the consonant /ʒ/.

Comparing the volumes obtained for the female subject, larger dimensions were observed associated to labiodental and alveolar sounds, and the largest volume measured was during the production of the consonant /z/.

One issue that should be taken into account in this study is the artificiality of the speech task. MRI requires a supine posture and unnaturally long times to sustain sounds for 3D imaging sequences. Several authors have discussed these problems but without finding a solution [6, 10]; however, they should not affect the fundamental findings of this work. The larger pharyngeal volume, found in this study, in voiced fricatives is consistent with the study in [16]. In addition, the MRI acquisition times in this work were considerably lower (around 16 s) than the sustain times used in that study (around 36 s).

This study has addressed only the morphological aspects of the vocal tract and major resonance cavities during the production of EP fricative consonants; however, there are many aspects of fricative production and voicing, which remain to be investigated.

5 Conclusion

The approach used to visualize the vocal tract during the production of fricative consonants in MR images, and posterior building of the associated 3D models proved to be very effective. Quantitative measurements of volumes for each pair of fricative consonants (voiceless versus voiced) for each subject were also successfully attained.

The 3D models built for the vocal tract showed that the volumes measured for the voiceless consonants are smaller than the counterpart voiced consonants.

Applying the present technology, volumetric MRI can be successfully applied to obtain 3D models, as well as measurable data concerning the vocal tract resonance cavities and all the articulators involved. More phonetic data are required to endorse the differences in the volume measures of each fricative consonant, and to reduce some inconsistencies observed between subjects and at different places of articulation.

Due to the developments that have recently taken place in MRI systems, namely the use of 3.0 Tesla magnetic fields, new applications and image refinements are expected, and consequently, significant improvements in the quality of the data acquired for articulatory events during speech production. This 3D enhanced knowledge about the speech organs could be very important, especially for clinical purposes (for example, for the assessment of articulatory impairments followed by tongue surgery in speech rehabilitation), and also for a better understanding of the acoustic theory in speech production.

Until today, the automatic and robust interpretation of biomedical images is still a major goal. Thus, a future development concerning medical image processing and analysis will be the increased integration of such algorithms and their applications in clinical practice.

Acknowledgments The images were acquired at the Radiology Department of the Hospital S. João, Porto, in Portugal, with the collaboration of the technical staff, to whom we are most grateful. The first author would like to thank the support and contribution of the PhD grant from Escola Superior de Tecnologia da Saúde (ESTSP) and Instituto Politécnico do Porto (IPP), in Portugal. This work was partially done in the scope of the project with reference PTDC/BBB-BMD/3088/2012, financially supported by Fundação para a Ciência e a Tecnologia (FCT), in Portugal.

References

1. Baer T, Gore JC, Gracco LC, Nye PW (1991) Analysis of vocal tract shape and dimensions using magnetic resonance imaging: vowels. Journal of Acoustical Soc. Am. 90(2): 799–828
2. Badin P, Bailly G, Raybaudi M, Segebarth C (1998) A three-dimensional linear articulatory model based on MRI data. In: Proceedings of the 5th International Conference on Spoken Language Processing (ICSLP 98), pp 417–420

3. Badin P, Serrurier A (2006) Three-dimensional modeling of speech organs: Articulatory data and models. IEIC Technical Report of the Institute of Electronics, Information and Communication Engineers 106(177): 29–34

4. Demolin D, Metens T, Soquet A (1996) Three-dimensional Measurement of the Vocal Tract by MRI. In: Proceedings of the 4th International Conference on Spoken Language Processing (ICSLP 96), pp 272–275

5. Doel KVD, Vogt F, English R, Fels S (2006) Towards Articulatory Speech Synthesis with a Dynamic 3D Finite Element Tongue Model. In: Proceedings of the International Seminar on Speech Production, pp 59–66

6. Engwall O and Badin P (2000) An MRI study of Swedish fricatives: coarticulatory effects. In: Proceedings of the 5th Seminar on Speech Production: Models and Data, pp 297–300

7. Jackson P and Shadle C (2000) Aero-acoustic modelling of voiced and unvoiced fricatives based on MRI data. In: Proceedings of 5th Speech Production Seminar, pp 2–5

8. Kass M, Witkin A, Terzopoulos D /1987) Snakes: active contour models. International Journal of Computer Vision 1(4): 321-331

9. Kim Y-C, Narayanan SS, Nayak KS (2009) Accelerated three-dimensional upper airway MRI using compressed sensing. Magnetic Resonance in Medicine 61(6): 1434–1440

10. Kitamura T, Takemoto H, Honda K, Shimada Y, Fujimoto I, Syakudo Y, Masaki S, Kuroda K, Oku-uchi N, Senda M (2005) Difference in vocal tract shape between upright and supine postures: Observations by an open-type MRI scanner. Acoustical Science and Technology 26 (5): 465–468

11. Kröger B and Birkholz P (2009) Articulatory synthesis of speech and singing: State of the art and suggestions for future research. Esposito A, Hussain A, Marinaro M, Martone R (Eds.). Multimodal Signals: Cognitive and Algorithmic Issues, Lectures Notes in Computer Science 5398 pp 306–319

12. Martins ALD, Mascarenhas NDA, Suazo CAT (2010) Temporal Resolution Enhancement of Vocal Tract MRI Sequences Based on Image Registration. In: 17th International Conference on Systems, Signals and Image Processing (IWSSIP 2010), pp 190–193

13. Muller NL (2002) Computed tomography and magnetic resonance imaging: past, present and future. European Respiratory Journal 19(35): 3s–12s

14. Narayanan SS, Alwan AA, Haker K (1995) An articulatory study of fricative consonants using magnetic resonance imaging. The Journal of the Acoustical Society of America 98(3): 1325–1347

15. Niikawa T, Matsumura M, Tachimura T, Wada T (2000) Modeling of a speech production system based on MRI measurement of three-dimensional vocal tract shapes during fricative consonant phonation. In: Interspeech, pp 174–177

16. Proctor MI, Shadle CH, Iskarous K (2010) Pharyngeal articulation in the production of voiced and voiceless fricatives. The Journal of the Acoustical Society of America 127(3): 1507–1518

17. Serrurier A and Badin P (2005) Towards a 3D articulatory model of velum based on MRI and CT images. Papers in Linguistics 40(1): 195–211

18. Shadle C, Proctor M, Iskarous K (2008) An MRI study of the effect of vowel context on English fricatives. In: European Conference on Noise Control, pp 5101–5106

19. Symms M, Jäger HR, Schmierer K, Yousry TA (2004) A review of structural magnetic resonance neuroimaging. Journal of Neurology, Neurosurgery, and Psychiatry 75(9): 1235–1244

20. Weissheimer A, Macedo de Menezes L, Sameshima GT, Enciso R, Pham J, Grauerf D (2012) Imaging software accuracy for 3-dimensional analysis of the upper airway. American Journal of Orthodontics and Dentofacial Orthopedics 142(6): 801-813

21. Vasconcelos MJ, Ventura SR, Freitas DR, Tavares JMRS (2011). Inter-speaker speech variability assessment using statistical deformable models from 3.0 Tesla magnetic resonance images. Proceedings of the Institution of Mechanical Engineers, Part H: Journal of Engineering in Medicine 226(3): 185–196

22. Ventura SR, Freitas DR, Ramos IM, Tavares JMRS (2011) Requisitos e condicionantes da imagem por ressonância magnética no estudo da fala humana. In: Congresso de Métodos Numéricos em Engenharia (CMNE), pp 1–12

23. Ventura SR, Freitas DR, Tavares JMRS (2011) Toward dynamic magnetic resonance imaging of the vocal tract during speech production. Journal of Voice 25(4): 511–518

24. Ventura SR, Freitas DR, Ramos IM, Tavares JMRS (2013) Morphological Differences in the Vocal Tract Resonance Cavities of Voice Professionals: An MRI- based Study. Journal of Voice 27(2): 132–140

25. Ventura SR, Freitas DR, Tavares JMRS (2009) Application of MRI and biomedical engineering in speech production study. Computer Methods in Biomechanics and Biomedical Engineering 12(6): 671–81

26. Zhou X, Woo J, Stone M, Prince JL, Espy-Wilson CY (2013) Improved vocal tract reconstruction and modeling using an image super-resolution technique. The Journal of the Acoustical Society of America 133(6): 439–445

Printed in the United States
By Bookmasters